Long Night's Journey into Day

Prisoners of War in Hong Kong and Japan, 1941-1945

Long Night's Journey into Day

Prisoners of War in Hong Kong and Japan, 1941-1945

Charles G. Roland

Wilfrid Laurier University Press

WLU

This book has been published with the help of a grant from Associated Medical Services Inc., through the Hannah Institute for the History of Medicine Program. We acknowledge the support of the Canada Council for the Arts for our publishing program. We acknowledge the financial support of the Government of Canada through the Book Publishing Industry Development Program for our publishing activities.

National Library of Canada Cataloguing in Publication Data

Roland, Charles G., 1933–

    Long night's journey into day: prisoners of war in Hong Kong and Japan, 1941–1945

Includes bibliographical references and index.
ISBN 0-88920-362-8

1. World War, 1939–1945—Prisoners and prisons, Japanese.   2. World War, 1939–1945—Medical care—Japan.   3. Prisoners of war—Health and hygiene—Japan.   4. Prisoners of war—China—Hong Kong.   5. Prisoners of war—Japan.   I. Title.

D805.H85R64 2001   940.54'7252   C2001-930465-X

© 2001 Wilfrid Laurier University Press
Waterloo, Ontario, Canada   N2L 3C5

Cover design by Leslie Macredie. Front cover photograph of HMCS *Prince Robert* returning to Canada with ex-prisoners of war, October 1945. Back cover photographs, top to bottom: Salesian Mission near Shau Kei Wan, Hong Kong; aerial view of Camp 5B, Niigata; interior of barracks at Sham Shui Po POW Camp, 1944; Lye Mun Passage separating mainland and Hong Kong Island.

Printed in Canada

Dedication

This book is dedicated to the medical officers, nurses, and medical orderlies who endured captivity in the Far East and who laboured under the most appalling difficulties to care for their patients,

and

to Connie Rankin Roland, who participated actively in the research and who helped and inspired in many other ways.

"We live not as we would but as we can."
—Menander

Contents

Illustrations and Tables xi

Preface xiii

Acknowledgments xvii

Abbreviations xxi

Hong Kong Chronology xxv

1. Hong Kong before 8 December 1941 1

2. The Eighteen-Day War: 8-25 December 1941 13

3. The Prisoner-of-War Camps and Hospitals 45

4. Prisoner-of-War Life in Hong Kong 91

5. Trying to Cope with Too Little Food 127

6. In Sickness, Rarely in Health: Life and Death
   in the Camps and Hospitals 155

7. The Overseas Drafts 207

8. POW Camps in the Japanese Home Islands 225

9. Less than Perfect Soldiers 303

10. The Journey Ends—But It Never Does 321

Notes 329

Bibliography 375

Index 403

Illustrations and Tables

Illustrations

Figure 1.1   Lt.-Gen. Tanaka Ryosaburo signing surrender
papers at Hong Kong, September 1945 1

Figure 1.2   Bowen Road Military Hospital, Hong Kong
Island, 1930s 6

Figure 1.3   Loading of Canadian military equipment
aboard HMT *Awatea*, in Vancouver, en route
to Hong Kong, 27 October 1941 10

Figure 2.1   Map showing outline of Hong Kong
and New Territories 14

Figure 2.2   Map showing Hong Kong Island and
Kowloon with sites of military hospitals 16

Figure 2.3   LaSalle College, Kowloon, used as temporary
hospital briefly in December 1941 21

Figure 2.4   Lye Mun Passage separating mainland
(background) and Hong Kong Island 22

Figure 2.5   Salesian Mission near Shau Kei Wan,
Hong Kong, September 1945; scene of Japanese
atrocities, 19–20 December 1941 31

Figure 2.6   Dr. S. Martin Banfill, 1946 or 1947 32

Figure 2.7   Drawing of Salesian Mission and area, based
on a sketch made by Norman Leath 33

Figure 2.8   St. Stephen's College, Hong Kong,
September 1945 36

Figure 3.1   Ward in British Military Hospital, Bowen
Road, Hong Kong Island, 1930s 50

Figure 3.2   Plan of North Point POW Camp in 1942,
based on exhibit from war crimes trial 57

Figure 3.3   Plan of North Point POW Camp, 1942 60

Figure 3.4   Aerial view of Sham Shui Po Camp,
Jubilee Buildings in the background 63

Figure 3.5   The Jubilee Buildings, Sham Shui Po, taken
in 1941 just before war began 64

Figure 3.6   Plan of the layout of Sham Shui Po
POW Camp, Hong Kong 66

Figure 3.7   Interior of barracks at Sham Shui Po
POW Camp, 1944 69

Figure 3.8   Capt. Saito Shunkishi, IJA, formerly senior
                medical officer at POW headquarters,
                Hong Kong, ca. 1946 70

Figure 3.9   Cartoon-style drawing of Maj. Cecil Boon,
                RASC 76

Figure 3.10   The former Argyle Street POW Camp,
                Kowloon, Hong Kong 80

Figure 3.11   Maj. (Acting) Leopold W. Ashton-Rose,
                IMS (1896-1957) 87

Figure 4.1   Sham Shui Po, theatre scene 98

Figure 4.2   Colour drawing of "Sonny" Castro, HKVDC,
                wearing his famous "Carmen Miranda"
                costume and makeup 99

Figure 4.3   Col. Tokunaga Isao (far left) being interrogated
                by Lt.-Col. S.E.H. White, Royal Scots 121

Figure 6.1   Former IJA interpreter, the Reverend
                Watanabe Kiyoshi, "Uncle Jon" 162

Figure 6.2   Lt.-Col J.N.B. Crawford, RCAMC (1906-1997),
                testifying during war crimes trials in Tokyo, 1946 169

Figure 6.3   Photograph of Dr. Tokuda Hisakichi, commandant
                and senior Japanese medical officer at Shinagawa
                Hospital, Tokyo, 1943-1945 188

Figure 6.4   Surgeon, dentist, and anesthesiologist with a mock
                patient, using POW-made operating table,
                Sham Shui Po POW Camp, 1945 189

Figure 7.1   Flowchart of movements of Canadian servicemen
                captured by the IJA at Hong Kong,
                December 1941 212

Figure 8.1   Plan of Oeyama POW Camp, Japan 226

Figure 8.2   Graph of weight changes of POWs held in
                Oeyama Camp 231

Figure 8.3   Graph of deaths at Niigata POW Camp 235

Figure 8.4   Aerial view of Camp 5B, Niigata 239

Figure 8.5   Plan of Omori POW Camp, Tokyo Bay, Japan 280

Figure 9.1   Sign at Stewart, BC, July 1929 316

Figure 10.1   HMCS *Prince Robert* entering harbour at Esquimalt,
                BC, carrying Canadian ex-prisoners of war
                home to Canada, October 1945 322

Tables

Table 5.1   Report on Rations, December 1943 134

Table 5.2   Weight Loss among POWs at Oeyama
                Camp, Japan 135

Table 6.1   Monthly Returns, 1942 156

Table 6.2   Sources of Funds to Purchase Supplies for
                POWs (in Swiss francs) 198

Table 7.1   Work Performed by POWs, by Industry,
                May 1944-August 1945 209

Preface

World War Two prisoners of war (POWs) had an unenviable existence. No matter where one is captured or by whom, at the time of capture there is always the frightening possibility that one will be killed on the spot. Then, once men have surrendered and survived, they have to cope with the psychological crisis of believing that they have failed in their military duty. For western POWs, this worry could be temporarily depressing; for POWs from Japan's military services, the failure had cultural connotations that often led them to commit suicide.

Moreover, as soon as men cease to be military "effectives" they also cease to be of day-to-day interest to their parent military establishment. This can have long-term connotations to permanent-service soldiers, who, after the war and their captivity ends, usually and not unnaturally find that they are permanently retarded in terms of promotion. Often, they return home to dislocated families and have to struggle to cope with a world significantly changed from the one they knew before captivity.

Nevertheless, twentieth-century POWs in general have had an infinitely better prospect than was the case in previous centuries. Until the eighteenth century, prisoners routinely could expect to be mutilated, killed, or enslaved by their captors.

Beginning in the 1700s, ad hoc arrangements began to be made in the field, between opposing generals, that permitted the repatriation of the prisoners they might take in ensuing battles. In the 1800s, more generalized arrangements began to be made. The United States codified a humane set of rules for managing the existence of POWs during the Civil War, a groundbreaking formulation known as the Lieber Code after Francis Lieber, its author. These rules were promulgated by the Union in May 1863 as General Orders No. 100, "Instructions for the

---

Notes to Preface are on p. 329.

xiii

Government of Armies of the United States in the Field."[1] But the appalling fate of so many Union and Confederate POWs makes it clear that a Code, by itself, can do little to prevent suffering and death.

The next significant advance came through the efforts of Henri Dunant, a Swiss. He was on the battlefield after the battle of Solferino in 1859, and had been so horrified by the desperate plight of the wounded and sick, both prisoners and non-prisoners, that he began what became the Red Cross movement. The first step in that direction, in 1862, was the publication of Dunant's *A Memory of Solferino*.[2] One crucially important consequence of the movement was that a series of multnational conferences were convened to devise regulations assuring proper treatment of wounded and imprisoned soldiers. Over several decades, conferences were held in Geneva, Switzerland, and in The Hague, The Netherlands; the resulting multnational agreements were identified both by the name of the host city and by the year the particular compact was signed. The first so-called Geneva Convention was signed by 12 nations in 1864; the 1929 version was the one that provided restraint and guidance to the actions of most of the nations involved in World War Two. Those countries that did not sign or ratify the 1929 Geneva Convention had, in some important instances such as Japan, fully ratified the 1908 Hague Convention, to the terms of which they were bound theoretically in international law.

There are two stages in the process of accepting an international agreement of this type and formally committing a nation to adhere to it. The first consists in having one or more officials sign the Convention—at Geneva or The Hague—on behalf of their country. The second stage requires the government to ratify the agreement after appropriate discussions in its own parliament. Only then does that government formally undertake to abide by the Convention.

The 1929 International Convention Relative to the Treatment of Prisoners of War was signed in Geneva on 27 July 1929; among the signatories were Yoshida Isaburo,[3] Shimomura Sadamu,[4] and Miura Seizo, the official representatives of the Emperor of Japan. Yoshida was Envoy Extraordinary and Minister Plenipotentiary of Japan at Berne, the other two were military officers.[5] A second Convention, signed at the same time, dealt with the treatment of the sick and wounded in the field. Japan signed this document also.

In the Diet, the country's parliamentary body, Japan ratified the Convention on treatment of the sick and wounded in the field, but did not ratify the Convention on POWs. In discussions within the Japanese government in 1934, the army decided to "refrain from petitioning the Emperor for his ratification."[6] No specific reasons seem to have been identified. Naval leaders itemized four reasons why they believed that ratification would work to Japan's detriment. Since Japanese fighting men "do not expect any possibility of becoming war prisoners" the obligations of the treaty would be unilateral on Japan; the expectation of lenient treatment by the Japanese might encourage such acts as bombing raids from distances so great that enemy fliers could not return to their base; permitting unobserved interviews between prisoners and representatives of the Protecting Powers would harm the war effort; and treaty provisions on punishment of POWs were more advantageous to Allied POWs than corresponding Japanese law would be to Japanese soldiers, thus necessitating a change in Japanese codes and laws.[7] The Convention was not ratified.[8]

Thus Japan had no legal obligation in international law to follow the precepts of that particular Convention. Naturally, this was a source of great anxiety to the governments of those nations whose troops faced the Japanese in their rapid advances dating from 7-8 December 1941. On 3 January 1942, in a communication that may have been a direct result of the capitulation of Hong Kong on Christmas Day 1941, the Argentine Ambassador in Tokyo, Erasto M. Villa, wrote to Togo Shigenori, Minister for Foreign Affairs. He conveyed to Minister Togo the information that the governments of Great Britain, Canada, Australia, and New Zealand "will observe towards Japan the terms of the International Convention on the treatment of prisoners of war" and enquired on behalf of these governments whether Japan was prepared to make a similar declaration.[9] On 29 January 1942, Togo responded, giving the views of the Imperial Japanese Government. In translation, the pertinent item read as follows:

> The Imperial Government has not yet ratified the Convention relating to treatment of prisoners of war of 27 July 1929. It is therefore not bound by the said Convention. Nevertheless it will apply *mutatis mutandis* the provisions of that Convention to...prisoners of war in its power.[10]

In a later communication, Togo further stated that his government intended to take into consideration the national and racial customs of POWs and civilian internees when distributing provisions and clothing.[11] In considering these commitments, which should have assured reasonably good conditions for the prisoners of the Japanese, one must wonder what decisions or external circumstances led to their abandonment or to their being ignored. For most certainly the 1929 Geneva Convention on Prisoners of War was not adhered to with regularity by Japan, as will become evident in the following pages.

The experiences of Allied servicemen who became prisoners of war at Hong Kong in December 1941 are examined in this book. These experiences agreed, in fundamental generality, with those of POWs all over Japan's Greater East Asia Co-Prosperity Sphere, as the Japanese called their wartime expanded empire. Because of this essential similarity, the Hong Kong captive years can be seen as a sort of case study of POW life in the Far East.

The purpose of this book is to tell what happened to the men captured in the Crown Colony of Hong Kong. The primary emphasis will be on the 1,900 Canadians who arrived there on 16 November 1941. But the account will by no means be limited to them. About the same number of both British soldiers and Indian troops were there also, as well as Royal Air Force aviators and ground crew, Royal Navy personnel, and of course, the citizens of Hong Kong, thousands of whom took part in the battle and shared the grim years of defeat and imprisonment. Moreover, in the camps in Japan where many of the Hong Kong prisoners ended the war, American, British, Dutch, and Australian POWs laboured, and sickened, and often died as well.

I am a medical historian. My thesis is that the story of the Allied forces at Hong Kong—three weeks of fighting and 191 weeks of captivity—is explicitly a medical story and therefore may be told particularly effectively and appropriately from the viewpoint of a medical ßhistorian. Every POW was a patient at some time during those 191 weeks, many of them spending substantial portions of that time starving or seriously ill, with limited medical assistance. A high percentage were ill enough that they did not last the 191 weeks.

I have depended upon three kinds of evidence in documenting the events to be described: archives, books, and interviews. Archival collections in many countries have provided information from sources ranging from official reports and military war diaries to tattered clandestine diaries, maintained at great risk and eventually taken home. Hundreds of men and a few women have written personal memoirs about their experiences, and scores of historians have recorded and analyzed various aspects of the war; a complete listing appears at the end of the book. But perhaps the most significant source has been the interviews conducted with many dozens of survivors of the camps in the Far East. Their first-hand knowledge has been invaluable, and I can only hope that the picture I shall draw will reflect their generous contributions of time and, often, deep emotion at the re-telling of mostly painful experiences.

Their experiences cannot be fully understood when told exclusively in traditional political and military historical terms. The reality of constant disease pervaded and influenced every other aspect of life in the camps. In this book, the reasons for the existence of so much disease, and the responses to it, take centre stage. In Chapter one, that stage is set as the months of 1941 recede into history.

Acknowledgments

*T*his project has had an existence of more than 20 years and, therefore, there are many persons and institutions to be recognized. I have been helped by so many selfless people in so many ways that it is humbling to look back and contemplate such cooperation.

First, I must recognize all the men and women who agreed with my requests to interview them about their experiences during World War Two. For many, these recollections were complicated by intensely emotional moments as painful memories rose to the surface. Without these individuals this book would not exist. Their names all are cited in the bibliography and I offer them here a collective vote of gratitude.

Numerous individuals assisted by reading portions of the manuscript, responding to specific questions about various historical matters, and providing encouragement. The following alphabetical list is an inadequate recognition of this assistance; I am nonetheless deeply appreciative: Steve Anderson (Hamilton), Miss Judy Au (Hong Kong), Dr. S.R. Bakshi (New Delhi), Dr. Solomon Bard (Hong Kong and Australia), Monte Brown (Ocean City, NJ), Philip Bruce (Hong Kong), Dr. Chen (Hong Kong), Sanjeev Chawla (New Delhi), David Clinton (Hong Kong), Dr. Amand Date (Muscat, Oman), Dr. Gavan Daws (Hawaii), Prof. Jacalyn Duffin (Kingston, Ontario), Alan Fraser (Isaacs, Australia), Dr. Marianne Gideon (Ocean City, NJ), Arthur Gomes (Hong Kong), Dr. Arthur Gryfe (Toronto), Miss Helen Ho, OBE (Hong Kong), Hoshi Kenichi (Tokyo), Fred W. Hunter (Chicago), Dr. Robert J.T. Joy (Bethesda, MD), Dominique Junod (Comité International de la Croix-Rouge, Geneva), Kondo Junichi (Niigata), Prof. Philip Leon (Charleston, SC), Dr. Douglas W. MacPherson (Hamilton), Brian McDouall (Hong Kong), Ms. Trudy McLaren (Edmonton), Dr. Darlene Miltenberg (Toronto), Dr. David Parsons (St. John's, Newfoundland), Robert Perrins (Hamilton), Ms. Flora Ricciuti

(Hamilton), Dr. T.R. Sareen (New Delhi), Dr. Sasagawa Tsutomu, (Niigata, Japan), Dr. Harry Shannon (Hamilton), Suresh Sharma (New Delhi), Ms. Lori Smith (Hamilton), Dr. Ian Stewart (Hamilton), Sumitani Yuko (Tokyo), Tajima Tatsuya (Niigata), Ms. Utsumi Aiko (Tokyo), Stuart Winn (Bath, Ontario), and Mrs. D.M. Woodward (Ivanhoe, Victoria, Australia).

The interviews were transcribed meticulously by Sue Glover, Cora Miszuk, Jeanne Pengelly, and Maureen Potter.

Historians are constantly in debt to libraries and archives, to librarians and archivists. I am no exception, and wish to mention with gratitude the following institutions and individuals: at McMaster University, reference librarians Linda Baker, Rabia Bond, and Tom Fleming; Ms. Angela Grigg (Australian War Memorial, Canberra); the National Archives of Canada (Ottawa); Canadian War Museum (Ottawa); Public Record Office (Kew, England); Armed Forces Institute of Pathology (Washington); Oral History Department, National Archives of Singapore; Mrs. Kwek-Chew Kim Gek, archivist, National Archives of Singapore; Institute of Southeast Asian Studies, National University of Singapore; Urban Council Public Libraries Office, City Hall (Hong Kong); Hung On-To Memorial Library, Hong Kong Collection, University of Hong Kong Libraries; Government Records Service, Public Records Office (Hong Kong); National Archives and Records Administration, Washington, DC (Suitland and College Park, Maryland); Richard Boylan, archivist, NARA; Operational Archives, US Naval Historical Center (Washington, DC); Armed Forces Institute of Pathology (Washington, DC); Royal Army Medical Corps Archives (Aldershot, England); Philip Reed, Stephen Walton, Roderick Suddaby, and Anthony Richards, Department of Documents, Imperial War Museum (London); North Texas State University, Oral History Collection (Denton, Texas); Ms. Susan Hart, Provincial Archives of British Columbia (Victoria, BC); Wellcome Library for the History of Medicine, Contemporary Medical Archives Centre (London); Australian War Memorial, Research Department (Canberra); Australian National Archives (Mitchell, ACT); National Archives of India, Government of India (New Delhi); National Archives Research Library, National Archives of India, Government of India (New Delhi); Delhi Public Library, Reference Department (Old Delhi, India); Kate O'Brien, Liddell Hart Centre for Military Archives, King's College London, University of London (London); D. Lawrence and Ian Baxter, India Office Library and Records, The British Library (London); Timothy Dubé, NAC Manuscript Division (Ottawa); Dr. Thomas Lau, Mr. Kelvin Chow, and Mr. Osman Chen, Hong Kong Museum of History (Hong Kong); Mr. Y.C. Wan, Special Collections Librarian, University Library, University of Hong Kong; Reference Library, City Hall, Urban Council Public Libraries (Hong Kong); Rhodes House Library, Bodleian Library, University of Oxford (Oxford); and Dr. Linda Washington, National Army Museum, Chelsea, London, England.

Translations of various documents have been made by the following persons, all courteous volunteers: Beatrix and Richard Robinow (Toronto: translations from Dutch and German); Dr. Terashima Yasushi (Tokyo: translations from Japanese); Dr. Jans Muller (Indianapolis: translations from Dutch); Dr. Frederick W. Klutzow (Wichita, Kansas and Florida: translations from Dutch); Saito Takeshi (Tokyo: translations from Japanese); Roy Ito (Hamilton: translations from Japanese); Dr. Hiraga Minako (Tokyo: translations from Japanese).

The financial contributions of several agencies have made the research possible. Chief among these has been the ongoing generosity of the John P. McGovern Foundation, Houston, Texas. Funding has also been provided by Associated Medical Services and The Hannah Institute for the History of Medicine (Toronto) and by the Social Sciences and Humanities Research Council of Canada (Ottawa).

Finally, I recognize the special contributions made to this book, and to the research upon which it depends, by Connie Roland. She has laboured in archives in several parts of the world, organized and catalogued photographs, and, most importantly, has throughout the long and sometimes discouraging process, encouraged my work enthusiastically.

Though much aided by all the individuals and institutions named, I alone am responsible for any errors, omissions, or misinterpretations.

Permission to reprint from Charles G. Roland, "Massacre and Rape in Hong Kong: Two Case Studies Involving Medical Personnel and Patients," *Journal of Contemporary History* 32 (1997): 43-61 is kindly provided by Sage Publications.

Abbreviations

AAMS	Australian Army Medical Corps
ABS	Able-Bodied Seaman
A/C	Aircraftsman
ADMS	Assistant Director Medical Services
AWM	Australian War Memorial, Canberra
BAAG	British Army Aid Group
BBC	British Broadcasting Corporation
BGH	British General Hospital
BMH	British Military Hospital
BOR	British Other Ranks
CADC	Canadian Army Dental Corps
CCS	Casualty Clearing Station
CDC	Canadian Dental Corps
CMAJ	Canadian Medical Association Journal
CPC	Canadian Postal Corps
CWM	Canadian War Museum
DDMS	Deputy Director of Medical Services
DJAG	Deputy Judge Advocate General
FANY	First Aid Nursing Yeomanry
F/Lt	Flight Lieutenant
F/O	Flying Officer
GOC	General Officer Commanding
HKPRO	Hong Kong Public Record Office
HKVDC	Hong Kong Volunteer Defence Corps
ICO	Indian Commissioned Officer (see VCO)
ICRC	International Committee of the Red Cross
IGH	Indian General Hospital
IJA	Imperial Japanese Army
IJN	Imperial Japanese Navy
IMS	Indian Medical Service

Note to Abbreviations is on p. 329.

IMTFE	International Military Tribunal for the Far East
IWM	Imperial War Museum
KIA	Killed in Action
KCO	King's Commissioned Officer (see VCO)
KNIL	Koninklijk Nederlands-Indisch Leger (Royal Netherlands Indies Army)
MBE	Member of the (Most Excellent Order of the) British Empire
MSR	Middlesex Regiment
NAAFI	Navy, Army, and Air Force Institutes
NAC	National Archives of Canada
NARA	National Archives and Records Administration, USA
NCO	Non-Commissioned Officer
NEI	Netherlands East Indies (Indonesia)
OBE	Officer of the (Most Excellent Order of the) British Empire
OC	Officer Commanding
OR	Other Rank, i.e., the privates, able-bodied seamen, etc.
P/O	Pilot Officer
POW	Prisoner of War
PRO	Public Records Office, UK
QAIMNS	Queen Alexandra's Imperial Military Nursing Service
RA	Royal Artillery
RAAF	Royal Australian Air Force
RAF	Royal Air Force
RAFVR	Royal Air Force Volunteer Reserve
RAMC	Royal Army Medical Corps
RAN	Royal Australian Navy
RAOC	Royal Army Ordnance Corps
RAP	Regimental Aid Post
RCAF	Royal Canadian Air Force
RCAMC	Royal Canadian Army Medical Corps
RCASC	Royal Canadian Army Service Corps
RCCS	Royal Canadian Corps of Signals
RCN	Royal Canadian Navy
RE	Corps of Royal Engineers
REME	Royal Electrical and Mechanical Engineers
RN	Royal Navy
RNEIA	Royal Netherlands East Indian Army
RNVR	Royal Navy Volunteer Reserve ("Wavy Navy")
RRC	Royal Rifles of Canada
RSM	Regimental Sergeant–Major
SBA	Sick Berth Attendant
SBMO	Senior British Medical Officer
SBO	Senior British Officer
SEAC	South-East Asia Command

Sig.T.O.	Signalman Trained Operator [naval]
S/L	Squadron Leader
SMO	Senior Medical Officer
USAAF	United States Army Air Force
USAMC	United States Army Medical Corps
USMC	United States Marine Corps
USN	United States Navy
VAD	Volunteer Aid Detachment
VCO	Viceroy's Commissioned Officer[1]
W/C	Wing Commander
WG	Winnipeg Grenadiers
YMCA	Young Men's Christian Association

Hong Kong

Chronology

1941

November 16: Canadians arrive in Hong Kong
December 8: Japanese attack
13: Japanese demand for Hong Kong surrender rejected by Governor
18-19: Japanese invade Hong Kong Island
Massacre at Shau Kei Wan
20: first use of North Point to house POWs
25: British forces capitulate
Massacre and rape at St. Stephen's College
30: Sham Shui Po set up as POW Camp

1942

January 5: Japanese fix the rate of exchange at 2 HK$ to 1 Military Yen; in July 1942 this became 4 HK$ to 1 MY.
6: performance by IJA band, Sham Shui Po
21: Indians at North Point move to Argyle Street Camp
23: Canadians at Sham Shui Po move to North Point Camp
24: British and HKVDC at North Point to Sham Shui Po Camp
February 5: regular "muster" parades begin at Sham Shui Po
15: electricity restored in Sham Shui Po
27: 4 MOs, 20 RAMC orderlies, and ca. 30 nurses (QARNS & VADs) sent to St. Teresa's (80 beds) to set up a POW hospital for Sham Shui Po and Argyle Street camps
28: first issue of meat at Sham Shui Po

March 10: illuminations seen in Kowloon; surrender of Dutch East Indies

19: buffalo meat issued in Sham Shui Po

April 1: first issue of pay to officers

7: first whale-meat issue in Sham Shui Po

10: escape from Sham Shui Po of Pearce, Clague, White, and Bosanquet

15: first yeast issue in Sham Shui Po

18: senior officers above rank of captain move to Argyle Street Camp

May 22: non-escape oath demanded by IJA

June n.d.: first ICRC visit to Bowen Road Hospital

4: canteen opens, Argyle Street Camp

6: allowed to write first mail home

27: first diphtheria death among British at Sham Shui Po

July 3: first visit of ICRC representative, Rudolf Zindel, to Sham Shui Po

August 7 : first case of diphtheria diagnosed among Canadians at North Point Camp

7: transfer of Col. Shackleton, RAMC, from Bowen Road; Maj. Donald Bowie takes over

12: St. Teresa closed; patients to Bowen Road Military Hospital or Sham Shui Po

19-20: escape of Payne, Berzenski, Adams, and Ellis, Winnipeg Grenadiers, from North Point Camp

September 4: first draft leaves for Japan

8: Chinese in Sham Shui Po released (105, 97 of these from HKVDC)

16: first Kai Tak work party from Sham Shui Po

25: 2nd draft boards *Lisbon Maru*

26: 1,404 Canadians and 27 Dutch move from North Point to Sham Shui Po; North Point Camp closes

27: 2nd draft of British POWs (1,816) leaves on *Lisbon Maru*

October 8: *Lisbon Maru* sunk

17: Japanese beat Maj. Crawford and berate medical orderlies because so many POWs are dying

25: first Allied air raid on Hong Kong

28: 70 "bad cases" [Edwards, IWM] sent from Sham Shui Po to Bowen Road Hospital

November 1: first issue of ghee in Sham Shui Po

21: first issue of Red Cross stores (bully beef and raisins)

28: first Red Cross parcels issued

December 21: first visit of ICRC delegate from Japan, C.A. Kengelbacher and Pestalozzi, to Hong Kong camps

1943

January 19: 663 Canadians to Japan on *Tato Maru* or *Tatsuta Maru*, including Capt. John Reid, RCAMC, plus 451 regulars (British), and 83 HKVDC. Edwards (IWM) identifies the ship as the *Asama Maru*.

22: Lt. Tanaka O/C Argyle Street Camp succeeds Lt. Sanemore

March 30: first mail received, Sham Shui Po

April 9: bath house opens at Sham Shui Po

May 3: Dr. Selwyn Selwyn-Clarke arrested by Kempeitai

August 4: 14 senior officers to Formosa

15: 4th draft: 376 Canadians, 83 British, 23 Dutch, 17 RAF, and 2 HKVDC to Japan on *Manryu Maru*

19: all Canadian senior officers to Argyle Street

27: Gnr. Mathiew killed on wire at Sham Shui Po

September 5: typhoon begins

14: complete search of Sham Shui Po, 8:30 a.m. till 5:45 p.m., during which time no food or drink

December 15: 5th draft, 204 HKVDC, 200 British, and 98 Canadians to Japan on *Toyama Maru*

1944

January 1: hut collapses at Niigata Camp 5B, Japan, killing eight men

April 20: 11 MOs to Sham Shui Po en route to Japan (no Canadians)

29: 47 Canadians to Japan on *Naura Maru*

May 4: first group of officers move from Argyle Street Camp to Sham Shui Po Camp "N"

11: second group of officers move from Argyle Street Camp to Sham Shui Po Camp "N"

22: third group of officers move from Argyle Street Camp to Sham Shui Po Camp "N"

June, n.d.: Indian POWs move from Ma Tau Chung Camp to the now-vacant Argyle Street Camp

July 17: Lt. Goodwin escapes from Sham Shui Po

August 10: ICRC inspection: Barnett incident

October 16: heavy air raid; camp hit

26: partridge and pheasant in Sham Shui Po Camp "N"

27: Canadian Red Cross parcels issued

December 8: massive US air raid, Kai Tak bombed heavily

19-24: daily heavy air raids

1945

January 16: heaviest air raid on Hong Kong, 8:30 a.m. to 7 p.m.

March 3: British Red Cross parcels (1942 vintage) at Sham Shui Po

24: patients and staff at Bowen Road Military Hospital move to Sham Shui Po

April 9: patients and reduced staff from Bowen Road move to Central British School

August 6: atom bomb dropped on Hiroshima

9: atom bomb dropped on Nagasaki

15: Emperor Hirohito broadcasts to his subjects

19: Crawford MO in charge of Camp "N"; Ashton-Rose MO in charge of Ma Tau Chung

30: British fleet arrives in Hong Kong harbour

September 5: POWs leave Niigata Camp 5B for Tokyo

16: Maj.Gen. Okada and Vice-Adm. Fujita formally surrender all Japanese forces in the Hong Kong area to Adm. Sir Cecil Harcourt, RN

1948

March 31: last judgment rendered in Hong Kong war crimes trials; 48 cases involving 129 Japanese had been tried

Chapter 1

Hong Kong before
8 December 1941

*W*ars end in different ways for different participants. World War Two ended at Hong Kong formally and officially on 16 September 1945. On that day, in the afternoon, in Government House, Maj.-Gen. Okada Umekichi and Vice-Admiral Fujita Ruitaro surrendered formally to Rear-Admiral Cecil Halliday Jepson Harcourt, CB, CBE.

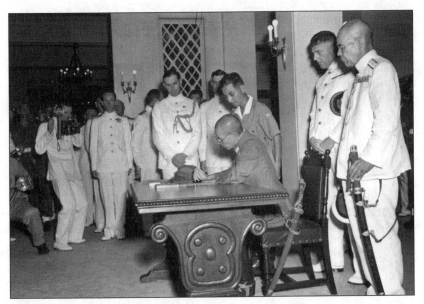

Figure 1.1. Lt.-Gen. Tanaka Ryosaburo signing surrender papers at Hong Kong, September 1945. Vice-Admiral Fujita (r) waits his turn. (National Archives of Canada, National Photographic Collection, PA 147118.)

Notes to Chapter 1 are on pp. 330-31.

For Canadian Rifleman Gabriel Guitard, the war ended on 22 February 1944, in Japan. He had been ill for some time, in and out of makeshift hospitals; he was admitted for the final time to the hospital at Niigata Camp 5B, northern Japan, on 1 February 1944: "Moved in hospital have diarrhoea cramps and passing blood. Off eats." Somehow, he had kept a terse but eloquent pencilled diary while he was at Niigata.

Guitard also recorded the contents of his final message home by postcard, a poignant effort to downplay his condition so as not to worry his wife: 6 February 1944: "Dearest Eugenie and Terry: Just a word to say hello to you all at home. I am well enough. Hope this word finds you all the same. Give my love to Mother and family. How are the boys and Dad. Well Sweet I will close with love and kisses. From husband. Gabriel." On 15 February he wrote what turned out to be his final diary entry: "Weather cloudy and snowing cold meals fair. on small diet. in hospital. diarrhoea is bad few cramps side is sore frequent." That same day, looking ahead still, he pencilled in the next few dates, leaving himself a line or two blank so that he could make his painful notations. But nothing appears alongside these dates. He died of dysentery on 22 February: emaciated, dehydrated, dirty, verminous, finally too weak to move and soiling his own bed space with the bloody discharges over which he had no longer any control.[1]

For Arthur Thomas, Winnipeg Grenadiers, the war didn't end until 29 March 1953. He had been seriously ill as a prisoner, hospitalized continuously from April 1942 till war's end. He returned to Canada nearly blind, with both legs weak and with troublesome abnormal sensations. The state of his legs worsened over the next year, his blindness did not improve, and he received a 100 percent pension. He died of a myocardial infarction at age 43. His post-mortem examination showed that there were permanent defects in his spinal cord and in the nerves governing vision, changes that certainly began in Japanese captivity.[2]

One man, Rifleman David M. Schrage, didn't get as far as Hong Kong in 1941. He died aboard the transport ship *Awatea*, somewhere on the Pacific Ocean, on 31 October 1941. Schrage was a victim of patriotism and bravado and lethally bad luck. And improperly self-treated diabetes.

What was this place these men travelled so far to defend and, too often, to die for?

The Colony of Hong Kong

The Crown Colony of Hong Kong consisted, until 1 July 1997, of Hong Kong Island and, across a narrow channel, a portion of the mainland bordering China. The Island of Hong Kong was ceded to Great Britain in 1841; 19 years later, the peninsula of Kowloon with the surrounding islands were also ceded to Britain. In 1898, an agreement with the Chinese government was signed for an extension of the lease to the area adjoining Kowloon. This area of about 400 square miles, known as the New Territories, was leased to Britain for 99 years. That lease ended in 1997.

The Island covers an area of 32 square miles, with a chain of mountainous ridges extending throughout its length of 11 miles. The low mountains are broken by deep valleys, and their precipitous slopes are covered by dense vegetation. The island's highest point is Victoria Peak. On the northwest corner of the island, below Victoria Peak, lies the capital of Victoria, which occupies a narrow strip extending along the northern shore for about four miles, a large section of which is dominated by massive skyscrapers constructed since 1945—Hong Kong's famous skyline.

Kowloon is sited immediately across the straits from Victoria and connected to it by the famous Star Ferry (and, long after the war, by tunnels). In 1941, the mainland to the north of Kowloon consisted of sparsely populated villages hidden amidst mountainous, inaccessible ground, much of it covered by forest. Most of the largely Chinese population lived in Kowloon. Forty miles from Kowloon and Victoria lies the city of Canton, now named Guangzhou. In 1941, only two good roads connected Canton and the Chinese frontier with Kowloon: the Castle Peak road to the west and the Tai Po road to the east. Hong Kong's only aerodrome was at Kai Tak on the eastern edge of Kowloon, used for both commercial and military purposes.

The colony's population in 1941 was about 1,750,000, the vast majority Chinese. As many as 750,000 were refugees from the Japanese aggression that had wracked the mainland in Manchuria since 1931 and particularly severely in China after 1937.

Hong Kong was the headquarters and base of the Royal Navy's China Station, and for a century had been a "defended port" of some strength.[3] When Great Britain was still great and controlled the high seas, Hong Kong was a significant node in an effective military chain that included Singapore, Australia, Ceylon (Sri Lanka), Burma (Myanmar), and India, in the East. But in 1941, with much of the Royal Navy heavily engaged in the Atlantic, Mediterranean, and North Sea campaigns, the situation at Hong Kong had altered. The Royal Navy was unable to mass fighting ships in the area, and Hong Kong suddenly became largely indefensible, a fact Prime Minister Winston Churchill and his professional strategists recognized early in the war.

In 1938, the Imperial Japanese Army had landed about 35,000 men at Bias Bay, 35 miles from Hong Kong. They occupied Canton and effectively cut off communications between Hong Kong and mainland China. The Imperial Japanese Navy made shipping hazardous even before fighting began in December 1941. Hong Kong was almost entirely cut off, particularly after the Japanese occupied Hainan Island early in 1939, thus threatening the sea link with Singapore.

There were four regiments in Hong Kong in the summer of 1941. As war loomed, the British had several options, not all of them realistic. They could abandon Hong Kong completely: impossible because of the impact on prestige and the blow to honour. They could cut losses by removing one or two regiments, but this would have destroyed morale. They could leave status quo. Or they could strengthen the defences. They chose the last course, and two inadequately trained and equipped Canadian battalions became part of the ill-fated garrison.

Before the Canadians arrived, Maj.-Gen. C.M. Maltby, an Indian Army officer who was General Officer Commanding the Hong Kong Garrison, had under his command the 2nd Battalion, Royal Scots (who had been in Hong Kong since January 1938), 1st Battalion, Middlesex Regiment (arrived August 1937), plus 5th Battalion, 7th Rajput Regiment, and 2nd Battalion, 14th Punjab Regiment, both of the Indian Army (arrived June 1937 and November 1940, respectively).

Naval strength included three destroyers, but two of these sailed for Singapore on the day the Japanese attacked, leaving only HMS *Thracian*. There were four gunboats, HMS *Cicala*, *Tern*, *Robin*, and *Moth*, a modest flotilla of eight motor torpedo-boats, and miscellaneous smaller vessels.

There were four regiments of artillery—a Coastal Regiment of the Royal Artillery and a Medium Defence Battery manning the coastal guns, one AA Regiment, and the 1st Hong Kong Regiment of the Hong Kong and Singapore Royal Artillery. The last was responsible mainly for the mobile artillery and comprised two mountain batteries equipped with 3.7 howitzers using pack mules and with 4.5 howitzers on wheels. The coastal defences comprised 29 guns. The total complement of RAF planes were three obsolete Vildebeeste torpedo-bombers and two Walrus amphibians.[4] As well, there were the almost 3,000 members of the Hong Kong Volunteer Defence Corps and the Hong Kong Naval Volunteer Reserve. Canada's "C" Force arrived 16 November 1941. Thus the garrison on 8 December 1941 amounted to 8,919 British, Canadian, and Hong Kong personnel, 4,402 Indians, and 660 Chinese.[5]

Medical Planning

When war began in Europe in 1939, military medical officials at Hong Kong worked to bring medical defence up-to-date. The report for 1939 indicated that their efforts included the planning of first-aid posts, casualty clearing stations, and relief hospitals; recruiting and training personnel; and collecting ambulances, stretchers, instruments, dressings, and medications.[6] Auxiliary hospitals were to be sited at various places (described in the next chapter). An Auxiliary Nursing Service (ANS), created in March 1939, was made a part of the Hong Kong Volunteer Defence Corps.

The medical personnel came from three sources. Those members of the Royal Army Medical Corps (RAMC) who were not attached to specific regiments were consolidated into 27 Company RAMC just prior to the beginning of the war in Europe in 1939.[7] There were the regimental medical officers and other personnel. And there were the members of the medical section of the Hong Kong Volunteer Defence Corps; some of these men had had previous military service but they were in civilian practice in Hong Kong until mobilized in 1941. A few individuals from the first group, a Canadian medical officer from the second group, and the bulk of the third were formed into the Hong Kong Field Ambulance late in 1941.

The established military medical institutions were segregated, as was routine practice at the time, with separate facilities being maintained for Indian soldiers. This segregation vanished during the fighting in December 1941. The two main hospitals were the British Military Hospital on Bowen Road, on Hong Kong Island (168 beds), and the Indian Hospital in Whitfield Barracks, Kowloon (120 beds). The latter hospital was to be replaced by the facilities on the island at Tung Wah Eastern Hospital, Causeway Bay, in the event of the mainland having to be evacuated.[8] Once hostilities began, St. Albert's Convent, on the Island, would provide another 400 beds. In addition, a potential 400 beds could be provided in an emergency hospital to be set up at St. Stephen's College, near the town of Stanley on the southeastern side of the island, and 200 beds in the Hong Kong Hotel, Victoria.

The Army Medical Store was located on the mainland until August 1941. It was then moved to St. Albert's Convent on the island. The staff was accommodated at the nearby Bowen Road Military Hospital. However, the war plan called for St. Albert's to become a hospital. Accordingly, early in October the Stores moved to a "permanent" home at the Salesian Mission at Shau Kei Wan (or Shaukiwan). "One would have thought this to be a most unlikely site in which to place all the Colonies [sic] reserves of medical supplies,"[9] because of the distance between Shau Kei Wan, near North Point on the eastern part of the island, and the main military hospital, British Military Hospital, Bowen Road, in the west above Victoria City. All too soon, the unhappy placement of this depot would become grimly clear, though for reasons unrelated to the location of Bowen Road Military Hospital.

That institution opened 1 July 1907. It was a conspicuous red-brick building of three storeys commanding a magnificent view of

Victoria, Hong Kong Harbour, and Kowloon from a hillside high above the city. In peacetime the location was ideal. The hospital consisted of two wings of wards plus a central administrative block that also housed the operating rooms and the x-ray department.

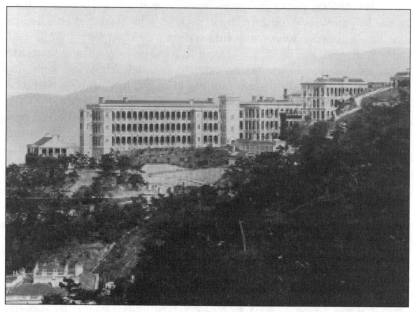

Figure 1.2. Bowen Road Military Hospital, Hong Kong Island, 1930s. (Reproduced by permission of the Urban Council of Hong Kong, collection of the Hong Kong Museum of History, P69.143.)

For reasons unrecorded, the roadway to the hospital had been so built that an ordinary army ambulance could not reach Bowen Road Hospital directly. The last three-quarters of a mile was only a narrow path over which a specially constructed, narrow, one-stretcher ambulance transferred patients from the end of the nearest roadway. Fortunately, this bizarre and anomalous situation was resolved in 1938 when a proper road was extended into the courtyard of the hospital. Had this not been done, the use of the hospital during December 1941 would have been severely restricted.

Another important pre-war project was the creation of an underground operating suite and x-ray department in renovated basement space. An emergency generator was installed and the Royal Engineers constructed a water reservoir in the hospital grounds, both measures proving to be of great value during and after hostilities. In addition, in autumn 1941 the accommodation at Bowen Road was increased from 168 to 250 beds to handle a severe outbreak of malaria that particularly affected the Royal Scots, already undermanned because of rampant venereal disease.[10] A Nursing Sister voiced what was widely known:

"The second Battalion of the Royal Scots had been abroad for seven years and was riddled with VD and malaria and was unfit to fight."[11] Malaria reached epidemic proportions after manoeuvres in October, so that, as one surgeon put it, "there must have been many of those manning the mainland defenses whose legs felt weak and shaky following the fever and anaemias of the disease as they covered the hilly and terribly uneven country they were called on to defend."[12] When hostilities began the total bed capacity at Bowen Road was increased to 400.[13]

On the civilian side, many efforts were carried forward in preparation for the medical needs of war. For example, volunteers were asked to have their blood typed.[14] Air raid drills were routine, reflecting the grim realities of life in Great Britain at the time. A young woman wrote in her diary that on 29 November 1941: "We took Mum to pictures—good one 'Sun Valley Serenade.' The Exercise was on so there was a blackout and we had to walk most of the way there and back, because syrens [sic] blew at inconvenient times. It looked like a good blackout—saw a plane drop a pretend parachute."[15]

There was a considerable and unfortunate alteration in key Allied personnel in 1941. The changes may have been necessary for strategic or political reasons, but in retrospect it is obvious that the changes occurred too soon before the outbreak of fighting. For example, it was only on 11 September 1941 that Sir Geoffrey Northcote turned over the governorship of the colony to Sir Mark Young. That same month the replacement for the former Commander of the Garrison (a Canadian, Maj.-Gen. A. Edward Grasett) arrived to take up his heavy task; this was Maj.-Gen. Christopher M. Maltby, MC.[16] Thus these key figures had less than three months to acquire the detailed knowledge of plans, terrain, and men necessary to permit efficient leadership.

Canada's Military Involvement

Britain asked Canada for two battalions and a brigade headquarters to aid in the defence of Hong Kong on 19 September 1941, in a telegram dispatched from the Dominions Office, London. The War Committee of the Canadian Cabinet considered the telegram on 23 September but deferred its decision pending examination by the General Staff, headed by Lt.-Gen. H.D.G. Crerar,[17] and consultation with the Minister of National Defence, Col. James Layton Ralston, who was then out of the country. Inevitably, one event swayed General Crerar (and, probably, others in authority) towards acceding to the request: the consultation he had held with Maj.-Gen. Grasett the previous month. Grasett, a Canadian but a member of the British regular army, was en route to the United Kingdom at the conclusion of a two-year assignment as Commander-in-Chief, China Command (Hong Kong). As Crerar said later: "Major-General Grasett informed me during our conversation that the addition of two or more battalions to the forces then at Hong Kong would render the garrison strong enough to withstand for an extensive period of siege an attack by such forces as the Japanese could bring to bear against it."[18] Grasett proved to be tragically wrong, but his opinion, as the outgoing Commander at Hong Kong and as a fellow Canadian, must have weighed heavily in Ottawa.

On 27 September a message arrived from Col. Ralston conveying his approval and specifying that the units should be sent from troops then in Canada, not from those previously transported to England. On the 29th Prime Minister William Lyon Mackenzie King cabled to the Dominions Office that his government had agreed in principle to send two battalions to strengthen the Hong Kong garrison.[19]

The Royal Rifles of Canada (from Quebec) and the Winnipeg Grenadiers were chosen for Hong Kong because they represented both eastern and western Canada, and French- and English-speaking Canadians. Actually, the Royal Rifles was technically an English-speaking unit, though a substantial proportion of its men had French as their first language. Some, it turned out, had little English at all. Both battalions had been on garrison duties, the Royal Rifles in Newfoundland, and the Grenadiers in Jamaica. It was assumed that there would be ample time for them to receive necessary additional training after arriving in Hong Kong.[20]

The Royal Rifles of Canada was founded in 1862 when six independent companies were combined at Quebec. Some units fought in the North-West Rebellion of 1885 and during the South African war, and others in France and Flanders in the First World War as reinforcements to the Canadian Corps. In spite of the Regiment's long history, the Hong Kong campaign proved to be its first active service fighting as a formed body. After mobilization in July 1940, the Royal Rifles, including many soldiers from the Gaspé (a substantial proportion of the men came to the regiment through the 7th-11th Hussars[21]) were posted to Newfoundland.

The Winnipeg Grenadiers, formed in Manitoba in 1908, were allied after the First World War to the Scots Guards, and King George VI had become their Colonel-in-Chief by the time they mobilized in September 1939. The Grenadiers served in Jamaica and Bermuda for 17 months before being assigned for special service to Hong Kong.[22]

The Training and Equipment of the Expeditionary Force

The War Office had stated, on 11 October 1941, that first-line reinforcements should accompany the Canadians to Hong Kong, amounting to six officers and 150 other ranks for each battalion. At the time the units were selected, the Royal Rifles were at full strength and, in addition, had three officers and 59 other ranks surplus to establishment. The Winnipeg Grenadiers, on the other hand, were well below their war establishment of 807. Subsequently, some 80 men of the Grenadiers and 71 of the Rifles were struck off strength for medical or other reasons. To bring the battalions up to strength and to provide them with first reinforcements, approximately 440 new men in all were required and had to be provided within 14 to 16 days. The additional men were found by combing the training establishments; more than 100 of the men had not yet completed their 16 weeks of basic training.[23]

The two battalions clearly had not reached the advanced state of training that one would wish troops to attain before confronting the enemy. But to suggest that they were sent into battle untrained is misleading. Both British and Canadian authorities believed that the troops were going to Hong Kong for garrison duty, and there was some reason to believe that training deficiencies could be remedied there.[24]

The related question that needs to be answered, though, has been hotly debated by US historians in connection with the attack on Pearl Harbor: was the Allied leadership culpable in thinking, as late as the end of September 1941, that Japan would not attack in the immediate future? The Canadian government and its military hierarchy knew that the Royal Rifles and the Grenadiers were not combat-ready. Was there in fact any realistic hope that they would have an opportunity to complete training before combat began? In the event, of course, they did not have such good fortune.

Galen Perras recently provided an appropriately balanced assessment of the case, indicating that the reinforcement of Hong Kong in 1941 was a mistake. Adding 1,975 soldiers

> obviously did not deter a Japanese assault, nor did the extra troops make a difference once war began. But it is far too easy to look back at the events of 1941 (and what happened to the British and Canadian survivors in Japanese prison camps) and say the bolstering of Hong Kong was folly and a calamity that could and should have been avoided. Unfortunately, fixating on the consequences of a military defeat, only natural given the human costs involved, does little to illuminate properly the reasons behind the decision to ask Canada to provide "C" Force.[25]

On 27 October the bulk of the Force embarked from Vancouver on the *Awatea*, a New Zealand transport ship provided for the expedition. In addition, four officers and 105 Other Ranks of the Royal Rifles were carried on the escort ship HMCS *Prince Robert*, an armed merchant cruiser.[26] Both ships sailed that night. Under the command of Brigadier John K. Lawson (1890-1941),[27] the actual strength of the force was 96 officers (plus two Auxiliary Services supervisors) and 1,877 Other Ranks. This included four medical officers and two nursing sisters, two officers of the Canadian Dental Corps with their assistants, three chaplains,[28] and detachments of the Canadian Postal Corps and the Royal Canadian Corps of Signals.[29]

The medical personnel were Maj. John N.B. Crawford, Captains Stanley Martin Banfill, Gordon Cameron Gray, and John A.G. Reid, all Royal Canadian Army Medical Corps (RCAMC); Captains Winston R. Cunningham and James C.M. Spence, both Canadian Dental Corps (CDC);[30] and Kathleen G. Christie and May Waters, nursing sisters.[31]

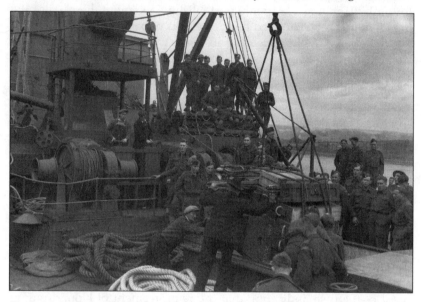

Figure 1.3. Loading of Canadian military equipment aboard HMT *Awatea*, in Vancouver, en route to Hong Kong, 27 October 1941. (National Archives of Canada, National Photographic Collection, PA.116789.)

On 16 November the Canadians docked at Holt's Wharf, Kowloon. Their numbers had shrunk by one; Rifleman Schrage had hidden his severe diabetes mellitus from his medical officer. While at sea he developed hyperinsulinism after over-treating himself, and died.[32] This self-sacrificing (and sometimes suicidal) determination to serve was not uncommon early in World War Two.

At the Hong Kong docks they were greeted by Sir Mark Young, new Governor of Hong Kong, and by large numbers of the local inhabitants. The latter applauded vigorously. Many made the unfortunate assumption that, with two additional battalions, the garrison was now capable of withstanding a Japanese attack.

The Grenadiers and the Royal Rifles were given quarters in Sham Shui Po Camp on the edge of the mainland city of Kowloon.[33] They found these quarters a revelation, as were most aspects of life in the Far East for these young, often naive, and largely untravelled Canadians. One soldier reported to his parents that the barracks were simply beautiful, "all made of cement with gardens and grass...you can eat off the sidewalks."[34]

The task of the Hong Kong garrison was to defend the Colony against external attack and to deny the use of the harbour and dry dock to the enemy. Thus mechanical transport would be essential for the movement of troops and supplies. Canada was to provide this transport, amounting to 212 vehicles, 20 of which were to be placed aboard the *Awatea*. However, the vehicles for the *Awatea* did not reach Vancouver until 28 and 29 October, and by that time the ship had already sailed.

As a result, no transport went with the Canadian forces, and the 212 vehicles intended for it were loaded on the American freighter *Don Jose*, which sailed from Vancouver on 4 November, one week after "C" Force. Normally the freighter would have reached Hong Kong about 6 December. However, the ship was rerouted under orders from United States naval authorities via Honolulu and Manila, reaching the latter only on 12 December, after the outbreak of war with Japan. On 19 December, the War Committee of the Canadian Cabinet approved diverting the vehicles to the use of the US forces in the Philippines.[35]

Eight days before war began, the Royal Scots loaned the Grenadiers an old Bren gun carrier so that the men could receive some instruction—in hopes, presumably, of the vehicles arriving later. "Some of our driver mechanics are working on the old carrier hoping it will hold together so we can practice with it." Two days later, during training sessions, sections of men were marched about pretending to be Bren Gun carriers.[36]

After the Canadians arrived there was, as it turned out, only a disastrously short period for acclimatization. This fact would seriously impede their efforts to carry out their role in the fighting, since they seldom had the necessary detailed knowledge of the terrain over which they had to fight. The area abounds with steep hills, often blanketed with bushes and trees, although the slopes nearest the cities of Kowloon and Victoria were being denuded by the enormous numbers of refugees scrabbling for firewood. Nevertheless the hills still contained wild boars and miniature deer, called "barking deer," preyed upon by packs of wild dogs.[37]

A British soldier in the Royal Scots noted in his diary of the Canadians: "Poor devils! Straight from guard duties in the West Indies & Canada they had not a clue about H.K. terrain and were pitch forked into battle almost before they knew which was the Island and which was mainland. They suffered heavy losses and were indeed a burnt offering."[38]

On arrival, the physical condition of the Canadians was good though inevitably somewhat reduced by their long sea voyage. In Hong Kong the significant medical conditions involving the Canadians during the next three weeks were an epidemic of food poisoning[39] and the expected outbreak of venereal disease as these vigorous young men encountered the exotic, entrancing, but frequently diseased prostitutes of this teeming port city. About 90,000 prostitutes worked the city, some of them frequenting a dance hall known to the men as Gonorrhea Racetrack.[40] Another favourite spot was the Sun Sun Café in Wanchai. By the end of November the incidence of venereal disease had reached "alarming proportions," despite efforts at prophylaxis by the medical team.[41] According to one of the Canadian medical officers, the first night the men were given leave, the supply of condoms gave out in a couple of hours.[42] The consequence was predictable; many Canadians, as well as British and Indians, went into battle while struggling with the distressing though not incapacitating symptoms of acute gonorrhea. It is also possible that they gave as well as got. Certainly the Royal Rifles, having been posted to Newfoundland, had opportunity to acquire venereal diseases there. Some evidence suggests that "a large proportion of unmarried Newfoundland women" had "no effective inhibitions relative to non-marital sexual intercourse" in the early 1940s, and an eyewitness saw couples copulating along the roadside as he drove by.[43] Maj. Donald Bowie, the chief surgeon at Bowen Road Hospital before the war, and later Senior British Medical Officer (SBMO), noted that a high proportion of the Asian prostitutes in Hong Kong were infected. In an effort to avoid gonorrhea and syphilis, "some men sought satisfaction in their own sex. Alas, this did not safeguard them from infection."[44]

The senior medical officer with the Canadian troops, Maj. John N.B. Crawford, RCAMC, arrived in Hong Kong as Medical Officer, Winnipeg Grenadiers. On 3 December he was posted as second in command, Hong Kong Field Ambulance, a unit under the command of Lt.-Col. (later Sir) Lindsay T. Ride. The Hong Kong Field Ambulance comprised regular RAMC personnel, members of the medical company of the Hong Kong Volunteer Defence Corps, and members of the St. John's Ambulance Brigade. The duties of the Field Ambulance were to provide preliminary treatment of battle casualties and then to transport them to hospitals in the rear.[45] Five days after taking up his post, Crawford and all of Hong Kong were at war with Japan.

In the days immediately before war began, Hong Kong attempted to carry on as if the axe would not fall. Dances were held, the bars and cafes did a roaring business, and inter-service sporting events continued. One Canadian soldier remembered the pain of "drilling with murderous hangovers."[46]

War hovered near. Perhaps fortunately, no one could have predicted the magnitude of the catastrophe that would begin on 8 December 1941.

Chapter 2

The Eighteen-Day War:

8-25 December 1941

Death is not an adventure to those who stand face to face with it.
—Erich Maria Remarque

*T*he defence of Hong Kong fell into two successive phases: a delaying action in the mainland territories, followed by a prolonged defence of Hong Kong Island. The latter, Imperial authorities hoped, would last at least six months.

Two infantry brigades were created out of three battalions. The Mainland Brigade, under the command of Brigadier C. Wallis, consisted of the Royal Scots on the left of the Gin Drinkers' Line, covering the slopes of Tai Mo Shan Mountain and the Shingmun Redoubt; 2/14 Punjab Regiment, which was assigned to cover the center of the mainland area; and 5/7 Rajput Regiment on its right.

Brigadier J.K. Lawson was appointed to command the second Brigade on the Island, which included his two Canadian battalions and 1st Middlesex Regiment. Such was the defence scheme in which the Canadians took their places.[1]

The role of the Hong Kong Volunteer Defence Corps (HKVDC) was not spelled out in this plan, though the addition of their numbers was significant, consisting of 94 officers and 1,665 men, plus 14 officers and 860 men of the Hong Kong and Singapore Royal Artillery, and three officers and 250 men in the Hong Kong Mule Corps.[2] There was also a contingent of the Hong Kong Royal Naval Volunteer Reserve. Thus the total contribution from Hong Kong itself amounted to almost 2,800 men.

Notes to Chapter 2 are on pp. 331-35.

On 6 December, as the threat of war escalated, military units were called into readiness. The Hong Kong Field Ambulance was recalled from the New Territories and, on the 7th, it took up its battle positions.[3] The Japanese attack on Hong Kong began on 8 December (7 December on the North American side of the International Date Line) with a damaging air raid, and continued relentlessly for the next 17½ days. On Christmas Day 1941, the Colony was forced to surrender.

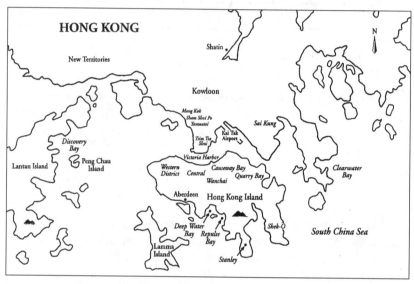

Figure 2.1. Map showing outline of Hong Kong and New Territories. (Faculty of Health Sciences, McMaster University, Hamilton, ON.)

Misinformation had clouded the preparations for war. Supposedly the Japanese were inadequate soldiers of poor physique and stature, short-sighted, and unable to see—and therefore fight—at night. Allied soldiers quickly discovered that these were lethally wrong predictions. Within a few days, a nurse in Kowloon, already in captivity, observed Japanese troops training for the assault on Hong Kong Island. The men's physical fitness and stamina was "depressingly first-class," she noted.[4]

During hostilities at least a dozen hospitals on the Island took in military casualties. These included: Bowen Road Military Hospital; Tung Wah East (the Indian military hospital); St. Albert's Convent; St. Stephen's College, Stanley; Stanley Prison Hospital; the Royal Naval Hospital; Queen Mary Hospital, Pokfulam; University Hospital in various University buildings; the Hong Kong Hotel; War Memorial Hospital, The Peak; Matilda Hospital, The Peak[5]; and the Happy Valley Racetrack, where a temporary hospital was set up by 12 December. On the mainland there were several military and civilian hospitals, including St. Teresa's Hospital, the Kowloon Military Hospital, the Indian Hospital in Whitfield Barracks, and Kwong Wah Hospital, as well as a number of emergency hospitals located in suitable large buildings: for example, the Peninsula Hotel, the Magistracy, Central British School, and La Salle College. Several other hospitals handled civilian casualties exclusively, such as the French Hospital on the Island. This institution was prepared to hold as many as 600 patients. The Sisters were retained and, in addition, European and Chinese physicians and nurses were added when war broke out. All these men and women were under the overall direction of Dr. Dean Smith.[6]

As fighting began, the light sick were discharged to their units and casualties began to flow in. Arrangements often were makeshift, as medical officers and nurses who found their way to assigned posts struggled to cope with large numbers of injured and, in many instances, were seriously overworked because other medical personnel did not arrive. Dr. J.J. Woodward's experiences epitomize this difficulty: a member of the Indian Medical Service, he was first stationed at a Modified Casualty Clearing Station in the old Kowloon Military Hospital, 8-10 December 1941; then he was evacuated to the Indian General Hospital in Whitfield Barracks. A number of civilian medical officers (MOs) were to work there but most did not appear. He was the only surgeon. Nursing arrangements fell through but four Sisters volunteered from the Italian Carnossa Convent. They handled between 300 and 400 patients, mostly Indians.[7]

Mainland Hospitals in Kowloon

The work of these hospitals will be described first since they were closest to the fighting when it began and thus tended to see casualties early. Unfortunately, official records of these hospitals are lacking. As a result, the reconstructions here are of necessity anecdotal and fragmentary, depending heavily on the recollections and observations of harried participants, sometimes recorded at the time, often later. Indeed, of all the many hospitals, permanent and temporary, functioning during December 1941, only the activities at Bowen Road Military Hospital have been detailed in an adequate historical record.

Kowloon Hospital

A number of Chinese non-government doctors had been assigned to Kowloon Hospital. Most of them became disaffected early on and also caused much trouble by sowing dissension among the Chinese labourers at the hospital. By 12 December, the Chinese staff, both the menial staff and most of the Chinese medical practitioners, had either disappeared or had become singularly uncooperative. The nurses, however, and two loyal Chinese physicians—Doctors Yeo and Yu—were praised as admirable by Dr. K.H. Uttley (a civilian doctor who had a practice in Hong Kong before the war).

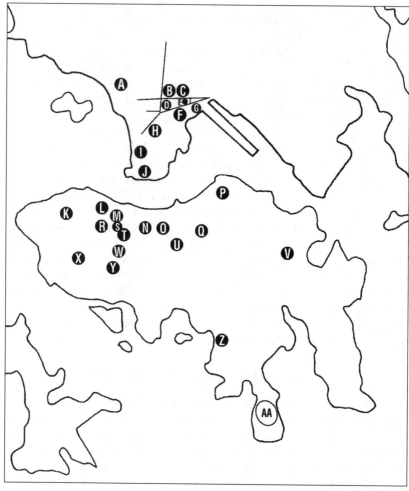

Figure 2.2. Map showing Hong Kong Island and Kowloon with sites of military hospitals, both permanent and temporary, and other sites, marked. Legend: A: Sham Shui Po POW Camp; B: Maryknoll School; C: La Salle School; D: Kowloon Hospital; E. Argyle Street POW Camp; F. Central British School (now King George V School); G. Ma Tau Chung POW Camp (Indian troops); H. Kwong Wah Hospital; I. Whitfield Barracks; J. Peninsula Hotel; K. St. Stephen's School Emergency Hospital; L. Hong Kong Hotel; M. Murray Barracks; N. St. Frances Hospital; O. Royal Naval Hospital (now Ruttonjee Sanatorium); P: North Point POW Camp; Q. Tung Wah Eastern Hospital; R. Hong Kong Volunteer Defence Corps Headquarters; S. Nethersole Hospital; T. Bowen Road Military Hospital; U. Happy Valley Temporary Hospital; V. Shau Kei Wan Medical Stores; W. Canossa Hospital; X. Queen Mary Hospital; Y. War Memorial Hospital; Z. Repulse Bay Hotel; AA. St. Stephen's College Temporary Hospital and (later) Stanley Civilian Internment Camp. (Faculty of Health Science, McMaster University, Hamilton, ON.)

On 12 December, the situation obviously hopeless, Uttley sent a note to the Japanese Commander offering to surrender the hospital. They were ordered to hoist the Japanese flag. Later, a Japanese medical officer appeared who had, as Uttley expressed it, the "usual superficial friendliness characteristic of the Japanese official."[8] Not only the Chinese feared the arrival of the Japanese. Everyone had heard about the atrocities in China. Some were more frightened than others, such as a woman "well known in Hong Kong society" who wanted Dr. Uttley to have her and some of her fellow ANS nurses taken over to Hong Kong, and not to be left in the hands of Japanese soldiers. When he pointed out that their orders were to stay put, she gave him "the most complete and most voluble ticking off I have ever had in my life or am ever likely to have."[9] Nevertheless, the initial treatment of the various medical establishments by the Japanese seems to have been unexceptionable.

Dr. Isaac Newton, also working out of the Kowloon Hospital, kept a diary that tells us much that otherwise apparently went unrecorded. On 15 December 1941, while under Imperial Japanese Army (IJA) guard in Kowloon, Newton reported that they had a visit from Japanese officers, who came with an interpreter and, Dr. Newton noted, were pleasant and asked what they could do for them. They brought the medical prisoners a sack of rice, some sugar and vegetables, and a few cigars, but no water.[10]

The last being needed urgently because the city water mains had failed,[11] Newton decided to risk a foray into newly occupied Kowloon. He handed a note written in Chinese to the sentry. After reading it, "he pretended to percuss my chest so I nodded and felt his pulse, he laughed and pointed in the direction of the wells and I nodded and left." Newton felt that none of them could complain of the way they had been treated till then. Later, he told a Japanese officer about two sick persons in the POW group. The officer arranged for a car to take them to a functioning hospital and allowed Newton to go with them, take messages, and collect belongings.

> It was the most terrifying drive I have ever experienced, we started by going in reverse twice, then we shot forward full speed in bottom gear straight across Nathan Road and managed to [stop] just before we reached the curb....Along Nathan Road we swerved from side to side across the whole middle of the road, fortunately there was practically no traffic.[12]

By 15 December the entire medical staff was incarcerated. Several physicians, some of their families, and a strangely varied group of others were confined together. The Sisters and ANS nurses cooked and kept their quarters in order. They contributed greatly to morale. And morale sorely needed support at times. One doctor, whom Uttley did not name, had brought in a large quantity of food; he and his family consumed it behind the backs of the others for several days. He "made no attempt to share it with the others who were almost starving."[13]

On 22 December 1941, the IJA moved the party of 83 men and women, mostly doctors, nurses, and other hospital staff, to the first floor of the luxurious Kowloon Hotel.[14] There the group, minus Dr. Fehily (an Irish doctor eventually released because of his nationality and therefore neutral status) who had been returned to run Kowloon Hospital, were joined by Drs. Hargreaves, Gozano, and Yaroogsky.[15]

Early the next day a Japanese doctor arrived to collect Drs. Newton, Hargreaves, Gosano, and Uttley to "look after the British Army." They went first to the Kowloon Hospital, where they found all nurses and medical staff had been removed the day before to the Chinese YMCA. As additional survivors came in, they heard news of friends and were surprised and delighted at how few casualties there had been among them. Dr. Dean Smith had a gunshot wound of the arm, the only serious injury. Of course, they would not have learned about the slaughter at Shau Kei Wan, and the St Stephen's atrocity had not yet occurred.

Peninsula Hotel Temporary Hospital

Mrs. Day Joyce had been in the Auxiliary Nursing Service in Britain, and joined the Hong Kong organization when she moved there. She had one month's training in a hospital each year, mostly in casualty departments or operating rooms where, in the summer heat, "[m]y amateur perspiration would drip into the poor patients' sores."[16] The ANS personnel assigned to the Peninsula Hotel were a mixed lot of nearly 50 volunteers representing at least a dozen nationalities. The day fighting began, Mrs. Joyce tried (and failed because of downed telephone lines) to reach her group. In a final act of normality and habit, her "coolie" had run a bath. "One has to try to live up to calm devotion to duty like that." She bathed and put on her grey cotton uniform.[17] Her world was changing forever.

Although she hadn't been able to telephone the nurses they began to trickle in to the Peninsula Hotel:

> Of course I did not think of it at the time, but now one's heart is torn by the thought of the partings that took place on that Monday morning—from husbands, lovers, children, needy ones, from homes and animals, even from jewels and books....The Indian girl came, the Japanese woman with the English name and the just-grown-up son, the large Turkish lady (we lost her again), the Portuguese and many Eurasians, and the handful of Europeans like myself; I am English. Gradually they all turned up. A wife and mistress came together, having said goodbye to their man.[18]

Dr. Uttley's job on the outbreak of hostilities was to take medical charge of the hotel in Kowloon, and to turn the first two floors into an emergency hospital. He ate what breakfast he could, though "I frankly admit it was all I could do to get down a piece of fried bacon and an egg."[19]

Handing over Kowloon Hospital to Dr. Newton, who was to be the chief medical officer there, he set off for the Peninsula Hotel in his Austin car, a slow journey because of damage from the air raid. When Uttley finally arrived at the hotel he told the manager, Mr. Nixon, that he was there to open a hospital as had been previously arranged. Nixon was cooperative and helpful. "I then saw Miss Dickson, the Hotel Nursing Sister, and by 11 a.m. all our nurses, ANS nurses and Sisters had turned up. I thought that this was very good but no Doctors (all Chinese) nor any Chinese subordinate staff put in an appearance all the day."[20]

They took over the ground floor, the mezzanine, and the first floor. By mid-afternoon the manager had cleared hotel property from the areas to be converted into a hospital; the staff started setting up camp beds and unpacking the hospital equipment that had been stored in the hotel garage in preparation for the emergency.[21] During the afternoon of 8 December he allocated rooms to the nurses on the mezzanine floor. Uttley was impressed with the hard-working and helpful team of ANS nurses, who were either former Nursing Sisters who had married or were young women who had had a short period of training in the ANS at Kowloon or Queen Mary Hospitals, such as Mrs. Joyce.[22]

No patients arrived at the hotel that first day. Nor was any food sent to them. The logistical arrangements failed almost totally in the first few confused and disastrous days. Dr. Uttley confirmed the failure of the logistical arrangements: "No food came to us on this or any other day from the Medical Department; the commissariat broke down completely in Kowloon so I had to fix up with Mr. Nixon to feed us at his expense for the time being."[23]

On 10 December Uttley expressed relief that no patients had arrived as yet. Casualties had been light, so their services were not yet required. The Peninsula Hotel was intended to be an overflow hospital for the Kowloon Hospital and the Central British School emergency hospital. All major cases went in the first instance to Kowloon Hospital, which was very busy. Dr. Isaac Newton and his Chinese colleagues there operated on 150 patients injured in bombing raids in these early days. The lack of patients at the hotel was fortunate for another reason. A serious problem had arisen because "every relative of every coolie, boy or amah of the hotel has flocked here for safety in the bomb-proof basement."[24] Uttley estimated that about 1,500 persons had camped there, and the medical staff were unable to squeeze into the so-called shelter during a raid. The conditions were almost indescribable. The floor was covered with excreta and there was no ventilation.

Uttley had tried for days to reach Dr. Gray, the Medical Officer of Health, but had been unsuccessful. "I heard later that he had bolted and was hidden in the Hong Kong Hotel, permanently drunk." He was found by Dr. Selwyn-Clarke, brought over by him personally to Kowloon, and told to get on with his wartime duties, but he apparently bolted again and was back in Hong Kong before Selwyn-Clarke himself had returned.[25] Lacking Gray's assistance, Dr. Uttley secured the services of two Sanitary Inspectors who got things better organized. Then, in mid-afternoon, he received an urgent phone call from Dr. Newton telling him to close down the hospital and remove all the nurses and all the food as quickly as possible to the hospital at La Salle College.

La Salle College Temporary Hospital

This site was much closer to the fighting than was the hotel. Alarmingly close. La Salle College was a Roman Catholic boys' school, almost in the foothills of the New Territories. A truck was purloined for the hospital staff—seconded from the inactive Peninsula Hotel—and their baggage. Mrs. Joyce herself went a little later. "Every single one of the volunteer nurses climbed aboard without demur. Great hearts. In the terrible hours to come there was not a single failure of that quiet and lonely courage."[26] This is an exaggeration. As will become evident, there was some perhaps understandable failure of courage as surrender loomed.

At the college they organized a guard to patrol the hospital and consequently had a quiet and unmolested night. The guard consisted of Chinese soldiers who had been interned in the Argyle Street Camp after they escaped mainland China to Hong Kong; they were released on the outbreak of the war with Japan. Efficient at their job, they stayed with the medical group to the end.

More than a year later, while struggling to cope in Stanley internment camp, another internee heard what he described as a "believe or not story." A Mrs. Sheldon, who was working in the La Salle hospital during the war, remembered the Japanese entering the place. They saw a box of Kotex. The officer in charge immediately exclaimed, "For face, yes?" Then he tied one of these objects over his mouth and nose, after stretching it to fit, tying it at the back of his head. The rest of his group followed suit, and continued their inspection of the hospital "appropriately" masked.[27]

One or two doctors had, apparently, behaved in unheroic fashion. As described, Dr. Gray seems to have hidden himself away throughout the war. "Dr. Tomlinson also did a bunk from Aberdeen FAP [First

Aid Post] when a shell exploded rather nearer to him than he liked and he hid himself in the Peak Hospital with a self-made diagnosis of 'shell-shock' until things were quiet again. Here, however, I blame Dr. Kirk, who was in charge there, for letting the man get away with it so easily. Apart from these two discreditable performances, the medical department did very well in the war."[28]

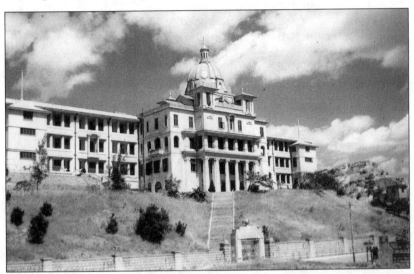

Figure 2.3. LaSalle College, Kowloon, used as temporary hospital briefly in December 1941. Photograph September 1945; the building no longer exists. (Reproduced by permission of the Urban Council of Hong Kong, collection of the Hong Kong Museum of History P94.750.)

Meanwhile, the Japanese were fighting a vigorous and successful war. If casualties were somewhat lighter than anticipated, this was because rapid advances required equally rapid retreats by the Allies, with few long-term confrontations. Kowloon fell on 13 December after only five days of battle.

The Island Attacked

Just a week until Christmas and the news was all bad. Hong Kong had already been heavily battered. The Japanese attack on 8 December had succeeded spectacularly. British, Indian, and Volunteer troops, and a few Canadian elements had suffered major losses while being driven from fixed positions with discouraging speed. As early as 13 December, only the Island of Hong Kong itself flew the British flag. Sure of themselves, the Japanese took a few days to rest and reorganize their army while the artillery pounded the Island.

A chill rain rattled on windows throughout the black night of 18-19 December, an ideal situation for invasion. The moon was hidden as heavy clouds lowered the sky, and burning oil from damaged storage tanks added roiling clouds of acrid smoke.

The inevitable invasion occurred that night. The Japanese advanced rapidly after landing on the northeast corner of the island, and fighting grew bitter as small-scale battles were fought, often at the level of hand-to-hand combat. The situation was confused, and worsened by inadequate methods of communication and, for the Canadians, a general lack of knowledge of the terrain where they fought. Late in the battle, small groups of men often were cut off from their units, with no idea of what was expected of them, other than to struggle for survival. Remarkable escapes preserved a few. One group of Volunteers were close to enemy troops for hours: "The Japanese were within short stone-throw—they were throwing clods at a dog which was whining at the door of the shelter and hit Winch twice."[29] Ultimately, the Japanese moved on and Winch and the rest of the Volunteers survived to fight again.

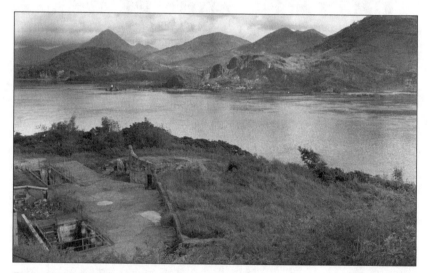

Figure 2.4. Lye Mun Passage separating mainland (background) and Hong Kong Island. Japanese troops invaded here 19-20 December 1941. (National Archives of Canada, National Photographic Collection, PA. 1555-28.)

On 19 December, local radio station ZBW made its last broadcast. John Stericker crouched in an auxiliary power station and gave the BBC news by thrusting a small radio tuned to London in front of the only microphone. After the news ended, Stericker "with no confidence in myself or the future wished everybody the good night which they knew they were not going to get."[30] ZBW went off the air.

Before detailing the medical activities in the various Island hospitals, it must be said that the majority of casualties were treated first—and, in the case of minor and of lethal wounds, only—in the field. Medical staff, and persons with little or no medical training, coped with the increasing flow of wounded men in largely unrecorded fashion. H/Capt. Uriah Laite, attached to "D" Company, Winnipeg Grenadiers, found himself on 19 December giving first aid to a severely wounded man within an hour of joining the company. By 21 December Laite had been placed in charge of all the wounded, no medical officer being available at that time.[31]

Hospitals on Hong Kong Island

The work of the Island hospitals continued without serious interference until the Japanese completed their invasion of the New Territories and Kowloon by occupying Kowloon in mid-December. After that date, supplies of anesthetic gases, water,[32] and electricity were cut off,[33] and some of the hospitals came under enemy artillery fire.

Bowen Road Military Hospital

Bowen Road Hospital, a large building occupying a conspicuous place high on a hillside overlooking Kowloon, could scarcely have expected to be spared, and it was not. Shell fire and bombs did much damage and the upper two floors became unsafe for use. All surgery thereafter was carried out in the basement operating theatres.[34]

Nor was shell fire the only hazard. On 19 December 1941, Col. Shackleton, chief at Bowen Road, issued Hospital Order No. 298: "Owing to danger from snipers, personnel will not proceed above the ground floor of this hospital."[35] The uniform for the Volunteer Aid Detachment nurses (VADs) consisted of white overalls and caps. The women had no other clothes to wear because they had been unable to return to their homes. White overalls were the worst colour to wear when crawling about in air-raid shelters. Moreover, Bowen Road Hospital was situated half-way up the Peak and could be seen by the enemy through binoculars. The nurses feared that their white overalls made them conspicuous.[36] A full description of the work of Bowen Road Hospital appears in a later chapter, as most of its existence was as a POW hospital.

Queen Mary Hospital

This multistoried institution was located on the west side of Hong Kong Island and was the main hospital caring for the European inhabitants of the colony during peacetime. At one point during hostilities, more than 100 casualties were being admitted each day. Eventually, late in December, the press of patients was so great that the upper-floor wards, closed because of fear of injury from enemy fire, had to be reopened.[37]

Happy Valley Racetrack Emergency Hospital

Barbara Redwood wrote at the end of November 1941: "Mum was on duty at Jockey Club—they had real patients dragged out from hospitals—in this cold weather!"[38] Training was thus as realistic as possible for those assigned to this temporary hospital.

The matron at the Jockey Club emergency hospital in December 1941 was Miss Amy Williams. Her staff included three trained nurses plus 15 European and about 30 Chinese nursing assistants (ANSs). The patients were largely Chinese women and children, with a handful of Indian soldiers.

Mrs. Redwood has left a detailed account of these dangerous times. The nursing staff were billeted in a Chinese hotel not far from the racetrack; the nurses, mostly quite young women or girls, were told to book themselves for a bed and meals. But many of them lived nearby and they decided that it was as easy to get home and have the comfort of a hot bath, sparing themselves the annoyance of queuing for it. "We still intended to have a comfortable war."[39]

One day, Japanese cavalry were seen on the racetrack. Alert troops let loose a rain of machine gun fire, only to discover too late that the "cavalry" were riderless racehorses that had broken out of the stables. The chief asset of the Jockey Club had met with a gruesome end. One horrified officer described the sight: "Blood on their silky coats, streaks of blood in their wide staring eyes, heads high in panic, they ran a futile race with death."[40] Dead animals littered the course and the surrounding streets. The effect over the next few days must have been grossly unpleasant, though the locals almost certainly would have butchered the carcasses for their own use.

As fighting raged on, many of the volunteer nurses set up camp beds in the betting booths. Artillery shells were landing all around the area. The doctor in charge at Happy Valley did not think that the Japanese would deliberately shell a hospital. They were, he maintained, fighting a "Gentlemen's War." He claimed that they were shelling the guns on the hills behind. That was obvious, but the hospital itself had been hit more than once, the operating theatre wrecked.

> Maybe it was bad marksmanship, but we had no Red Cross flag to denote that we were a hospital, and after all the Japs were aware of the military post next door....The doctor suggested that they make and display a flag without delay. Two of the nurses created one from a sheet and strips of red blanket. It proved difficult to get it hung, given the amount of shooting in the neighbourhood. At last a couple of the men, braver than the rest, managed to attach it to some posts that usually bore the names of the horses and jockeys in each race.[41]

Sanitation presented a major problem. The flush toilets had stopped functioning, and there was no water even to clean the bedpans. Two large reserve tanks were inexplicably locked. Since washing wasn't possible, one of the nurses produced a large bottle of eau-de-cologne: "we each had a drop or two...to freshen our faces."[42] The perfume would have been helpful for another reason. The corpses in the garage were beginning to make their presence felt.[43] All this was on 24 December 1941.

The morning of the next day, that grotesquely memorable Christmas, some of the staff stood chatting outside when a nurse noticed a group approaching. A man seemed to be leading Japanese soldiers on a rope. However, a second look showed that the man on the rope had his hands tied. The Japanese used him as a hostage or as a human bomb detector. He was a well-known elderly Anglo-Indian doctor.[44]

Suddenly the Japanese soldiers were in their midst. The soldiers looked at them with "toothy grins. A more repulsive mob one could not imagine. Dirty and unkempt and unshaven for days by the looks of them. But I suppose their condition was excusable as they had been fighting heavily for days."[45] There were several such visitations during the morning of Christmas Day, but without any untoward happenings. Then one of the staff ran up to tell the matron that soldiers had taken some of the young Chinese girls away, members of the St John's Ambulance: "they must have hidden somewhere and the Japs had found them. Soon they came from upstairs crying their hearts out. They had been badly used. We comforted them as best we could, they were not more than about 15 years old."[46]

That night the situation deteriorated. The first inkling the worried women had of what lay ahead for some of them came when a flash-light lit up their room:

[O]ur place was pushed open. There stood a group of Japanese soldiers. The one who held the torch (which had a beam like a car headlight) flashed around, showing us all huddled beneath our blankets. They advanced. "Get up all" one commanded. We in the beds all scrambled out. Rather undignified we must have looked, as climbing out of a camp bed by the end, could not be done with dignity....They scrutinized each one in turn, almost blinding us as they shone the torch in our faces one by one. It was a terrible ordeal, as we did not know what was to happen, and when they selected about four, we feared the worst. As they selected each one the spokesman said "Go Jap. No come kill all." Then turning to the rest he said "Sleep," and we again climbed to our beds. They went away, taking the girls with them....I could not say how long it was before we heard running light footsteps, and one of the girls rushed in sobbing. Very soon the others followed, and almost before we could get them quieted, the torch reappeared...they looked under the table, and found those who had taken refuge there. They made them come out and ordered some of them to go with them. The same threat, "No come kill all."[47]

The unfortunate women returned, one by one, terrified, dishevelled, some of them badly injured. Then the flashlight shone again and more unhappy victims were hauled away. The ordeal continued.

Mrs. Redwood was one of the more elderly women in the group and, happily for her, failed the flashlight test. All the nurses were in uniform. During Christmas Day most of the Chinese staff had slipped away. Eventually, a total of six Europeans, as well as at least six Chinese women, were raped.[48]

One woman escaped during the night. She fled to Bowen Road Hospital, where she told the senior medical officer what had happened. He asked the Japanese for the immediate evacuation of the nurses. About noon on the 26 December, a Japanese soldier once again entered the area. He began to drag a woman away with him; then a Japanese officer appeared at the end of the room. The soldier left hurriedly. This grim period finally was over.[49] The nurses were evacuated to Queen Mary Hospital.[50]

According to one report, a full-scale massacre was prevented by Dr. J.A. Selby, who opened the liquor stores to the Japanese troops, many of whom drank themselves into a stupor.[51] The strategy apparently succeeded in this instance, though in general its wisdom might be debated. Drunkenness usually fuelled savagery.

Hong Kong Hotel

This hotel on the Island, long since demolished, was a leading establishment before the war. Like many other large and centrally located buildings, the Hong Kong Hotel was designated as an emergency hospital, and soon after the war began was used largely for the care of lightly wounded soldiers.

Two days before the surrender, Barbara Redwood heard that an old boyfriend had been wounded and was at the hotel. He phoned her and said he was convalescing on the first floor. "I careered down to the hotel, plus 6 packets of cigarettes from Mrs. Boulton, and found Sid lying on a 'biscuit' on floor with hundreds of others. He looked a bit wild and woolly."[52]

Unfortunately, other than these few words, no participant in the medical activities that took place at the Hong Kong Hotel seems to have left a record.

St. Albert's Convent

The story of the temporary hospital in St. Albert's Convent during December 1941 began on 12 December when four nursing Sisters, including Sister D. Van Wart, 40 VADs, and several voluntary trained staff, were sent to open a relief hospital in this large Spanish institution. Initially, most of their patients had malaria as there was an epidemic at the time.[53]

One day the Chinese house where the nurses lived took a direct hit on the dining room just at lunch time. Fortunately, the cooking stove was temperamental and lunch was late, or many of the nurses would have been injured or killed. The acting matron was seriously wounded, and one Sister killed as they went out to rescue a pet dog. The dead woman had just become engaged to a young officer. When he heard of her death he unnecessarily and deliberately exposed himself to enemy fire and was killed. After the war his remains were identified by his fiancée's hospital badge that she had given him as a keepsake.[54] St. Albert's itself was bombed 19 times, but fortunately only one patient was killed.[55]

Muriel McCaw, then in her early twenties, was one of many young women who joined the nursing section of the HKVDC before the war. Their training was minimal: evening classes in first aid and in home nursing, plus an annual one-week course at Bowen Road Hospital, where they did little nursing; rather, they observed the routine of the hospital and, "of course, we were ogled by the Military patients which was rather unnerving." When war began, Miss McCaw was also assigned to St. Albert's Convent. Among their early patients were a few Canadians with malaria and several with wounds. There was also a Japanese prisoner/patient:

> Our Drs. did what they could for this Japanese soldier but he had a very serious buttock wound and it was thought he did not have long to live. I was told the Drs. were merciful and gave him a shot of their precious supplies of morphine much to the disgust of some on the staff. A friend of mine, Betty and I were on night duty and…we spent the small hours of the night in the little room off our ward watching the face of the enemy. He looked like a porcelain doll with close cropped hair and long spiky eyelashes. The smell of gangrene was so strong we had to douse our handkerchieves [sic] with disinfectant. Towards dawn he became very restless and plucked continuously at his waist. We noticed he had a cloth round his body and discovered it was a Japanese flag. So we respected his wishes to leave it when he pushed our hands away.[56]

Their patient died soon afterwards. The hospital was captured on 23 December. Their hands tied behind their backs with wire, the matron and the commanding officer were dragged outside and a machine gun trained on them. The nurses and up-patients were herded into a room and a Japanese soldier, "camouflaged with small branches sticking out of his helmet like a Christmas tree," guarded them. After a long time one patient fainted and finally the captives were allowed to sit. "I remember thinking, Fancy ending my life like this, and kept praying that I would be shot outright."[57]

There was much ominous threatening, but this suddenly dissipated when the troops discovered that their dead comrade had been decently cared for. There were no atrocities at St. Albert's.

After the surrender of Hong Kong the Japanese wouldn't allow the medical orderlies captured at St. Albert's to search for their wounded comrades on the hillside behind the hospital. The staff knew that they could have saved more lives if they had been allowed to look for casualties. "One was reminded that the bodies were there by the vultures circling above the skyline."[58]

The Japanese interfered only occasionally with the running of the hospital. All POWs, medical or not, had to bow to all Japanese officers; otherwise they were liable to be beaten up. The wounded Indians and personnel from the Naval Hospital were brought to St. Albert's, which made conditions crowded. As the patients recovered they were given new clothes and two army blankets from the hospital stores and sent off to the mens' camp in Kowloon.[59]

Dr. K.H. Uttley arrived at Stanley Camp 23 January 1942. The Japanese sent him and three colleagues to St. Albert's Hospital, where they told the colonel in charge that they had been told to take what drugs they needed. "The poor chap was nearly distracted. His hospital was full of British and Indians (I think about 400 patients) and he had heard nothing about this arrangement."[60] This was not surprising; the Japanese were not good at communication and informing the hospital beforehand was the sort of thing that happened only rarely. This was the first that the military medical officers had heard that they had to go to Sham Shui Po. The Japanese had told Uttley that the move was to take place but it had not occurred to them to inform the St. Albert's Hospital staff. They were moved a few days later, without any stores.[61]

Nethersole Hospital

Founded in 1886 as the Alice Memorial Hospital, this institution moved to newly constructed quarters in Bonham Road in 1893. At the same time, the hospital was renamed the Nethersole Hospital. The London Missionary Society sponsored and staffed the hospital, with generous financial contributions by Dr. Ho Kai, whose English wife, Alice, had been memorialized in the first building.[62]

Little information seems to have been preserved of the work done in December 1941 at Nethersole Hospital. The sole record discovered to date is by an anesthetist there, Dr. Annie Sydenham. However, her wartime station was the Casualty Clearing Station at War Memorial Hospital.

War Memorial Casualty Clearing Station

On 8 December, the staff of the Nethersole Hospital had to take up their wartime duties. Dr. Sydenham's were not in her own hospital but as an anesthetist at the War Memorial Casualty Clearing Station on The Peak.[63] As well as civilian patients they had British, Canadian, and Indian military casualties. The second anesthetist, a Chinese doctor, left. Then a Canadian medical unit was billeted in the hospital. "We benefited from the assistance of a Canadian Doctor as the second anesthetist in place of the Chinese Doctor, as he knew his own men and was able to give them confidence and cheer."[64] Within a few days both the water supply and the electrical system ceased to function. However, engineers from a scuttled ship produced electricity for the operating room from a small dynamo. The staff used basins of water over and over again in the operating room; the only sterilizing available was achieved by wringing out towels in disinfectant and using them wet on wounds.[65]

After Hong Kong surrendered, Dr. Sydenham continued to work at War Memorial until 30 December 1941. They were visited by the Japanese but were allowed to carry on treating their patients. No new patients came in after the surrender, and "one can only guess what happened to those wounded and left on the hillsides." Nearly all those left in the hospital at the end of 1941 were soldiers, and as there were three male doctors to care for them, Dr. Sydenham decided to return to Nethersole Hospital, which was full of Chinese civilian casualties. She walked back down The Peak.[66]

Tung Wah Hospital

This institution was erected by the wealthier Chinese in Hong Kong and was opened in 1872 in Po Yan Street.[67] Again, as with several other hospitals, no record seems to exist of its activities during the fighting in December 1941. The hospital continues to serve Hong Kong to this day.

Other Locations

All registered medical practitioners, plus otherwise unassigned medical officers, were assigned to duty either in a first-aid post or a hospital in time of emergency. When war broke out on 8 December these individuals, or most of them, went to their posts. For example, one man's home was situated opposite the university, so he was appointed to the nearest first-aid post, which was at the St. Louis Institute on Pokfulam Road. On the second floor there was an operating theatre where accident patients were seen, bullets extracted, wounds dressed, and first aid assistance provided. Medical residents, nurses, and Sisters were all mobilized and were on rotating duty day or night. Because all first-aid posts were run in essence as out-patient clinics, all patients who required hospitalization were sent on to the Queen Mary Hospital.[68]

Atrocities

Though previous atrocities such as the Rape of Nanking were widely known, nevertheless, the men and women of Hong Kong would have been shaken had they understood the nonchalant attitude of the invading IJA troops towards what the rest of the world termed "atrocities." One Japanese soldier, Tominaga Shozo, recalled his time in China in a recent interview: "Most of us thought then that murdering, raping, and setting fire to villages were unavoidable acts in war, nothing particularly wrong."[69]

Even the text designed to guide a Japanese soldier's actions could be interpreted to excuse, if not condone, violence towards prisoners, at least in the heat of battle. The relevant passage reads, in translation: "When within the surroundings of the battlefield, one is apt to be absorbed by what is immediately before one's eyes and stray from principles and occasionally these acts may be contrary to one's duty as a soldier. Much discretion is needed."[70]

Despite the civilized treatment experienced by Dr. Newton and his party in Kowloon, there were many shocking atrocities committed by Japanese troops during and after the attack on Hong Kong. A number of these centred on wounded Canadian, British, Hong Kong, or Indian soldiers and on their medical attendants.

In many cases uniforms or other signs of medical responsibilities were ignored by the Japanese. L/Cpl. Williamson, Winnipeg Grenadiers, stated in a deposition that he was marched to North Point Camp on 22 December 1941. His party passed through the outskirts of Victoria, where he saw eight or nine decapitated St. John's Ambulance personnel." Some of these bodies were still in a kneeling position with hands tied behind their backs. They were dressed in the St. John's uniform and the St. John's hats were lying on the ground."[71] Almost certainly, these men would have been Chinese or Portuguese.

The incidents of brutality against prisoners at the time of capture by the Japanese may have many explanations. Amongst these are drunkenness, so-called battle lust or blood lust, perception of continuing resistance from within a group purportedly surrendering, confusion because of propinquity of combatant and non-combatant formations, apparently official orders to kill prisoners, and implicit or explicit sanction to celebrate victory and expiate the death of friends by means of theft, brutality, rape, and murder. All of these excuses were put forward at Hong Kong at the time of the events, and also at war crimes trials held after the war and in more recent writings.

Three atrocities of particular seriousness took place on Hong Kong Island on 19 and on 25 December 1941. One was the murder of Royal Army Medical Corps and other personnel near the Salesian Mission at Shau Kei Wan, early on the morning of 19 December 1941. The second were the bloody episodes of murder and rape at the temporary hospital in St. Stephen's College on 25 December 1941.[72] And the third was the previously discussed rampage of rape committed against nurses at the Happy Valley Racetrack emergency hospital on 25-26 December.

Shau Kei Wan

In October 1941, the Salesian Mission, located in the district of Shau Kei Wan in the northeast section of Hong Kong Island, was the recently designated site of the Army Medical Store. Its stores included a year's supply of medical equipment and stores of all kinds for two military hospitals, plus full equipment to stock Regimental Aid Posts, Advanced Dressing Stations, and Advanced Surgical Centres.[73]

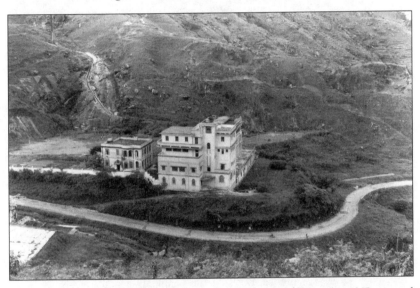

Figure 2.5. Salesian Mission near Shau Kei Wan, Hong Kong, September 1945; scene of Japanese atrocities, 19–20 December 1941. (Photographer J. Hawes; National Archives of Canada, National Photographic Collection, PA116804.)

By 14 December, Allied forces had concentrated on Hong Kong Island. Thus, on the night of 18-19 December, the Japanese landed across the Lei Mun Straits onto the northeast sector of the Island. A short distance from North Point is the district known as Shau Kei Wan. There, the 5/7 Rajputs along the north shore of the Island and the Royal Rifles of Canada on the eastern shore opposed the attackers, consisting of two battalions of the 229th Regiment, the Tanaka Butai, under command of Col. Tanaka Ryosaburo.[74] The 228th and 230th Regiments landed at the same time, but somewhat further west along the north shore.[75]

The staff of the Medical Store at Shau Kei Wan comprised 12 RAMC personnel.[76] In addition, a Medical Collecting Post (Military) was located there under the command of Capt. S. Martin Banfill, RCAMC, with 2nd/Lt. Osler Lister Thomas, HKVDC, a most memorably named medical student, second in command; the other members were Rfmn. Raymond J. Oakley and L/Cpl. Argyll C. Harrison, RRC, and Driver Kelly, RASC. Civilians attached were Mrs. Tinson, a captain in the St. John's Ambulance Brigade; ANS nurses Lois Fearon and Mary Suffiad, and six St. John's Ambulance nurses (one European, one Indian, four Chinese); Dr. Orloff, a Russian doctor; Dr. Tsang Fook Chor and Dr. Chau, Chinese physicians; and eight Chinese stretcher-bearers of the St. John's Ambulance Brigade.[77] Total personnel were thus about 40.

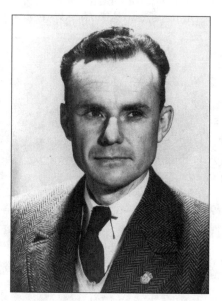

Figure 2.6. Dr. S. Martin Banfill, 1946 or 1947.

Early on 19 December, unaware that the enemy had landed, three men left the Mission in an ambulance to take two wounded British officers of the Rajputs to hospital. They had gone only a few yards when they were firedon by machine guns. The driver and Oakley, who was wounded in the thigh, leapt out. Lt. Thomas backed the vehicle up to the Mission and gave the warning.[78]

At about 7:50 am[79] on 19 December 1941, a chilly, drizzling day, Japanese troops entered the Salesian Mission and captured all Allied personnel there. No shots were fired by anyone in the Mission, nor was resistance offered. The Mission building was flying a Red Cross flag and all equipment, such as stretchers, were plainly marked with large red crosses.[80] Dr. Banfill believes the flag may have been shot down and therefore not visible when the Japanese arrived; there had been much shelling and bombing in the days preceding the 19th.[81]

Somewhat surprisingly, given other events that would occur in Hong Kong over the next week, the women were all released unharmed.[82] A Japanese medical officer and two men accompanied the women's party away from the Mission and then released them after about a two-hour delay. Mrs. Tinson wrote out some of the details in a letter in 1946:

> Dr. Tsang [Chinese] was taken into the Fort and made to give injections to about 100 Japanese wounded, after this he was set free, and I and my girls were also told that we could go. I managed to get the girls to safety in a Chinese house, and after some trouble...Miss Fearon and I found refuge with a Chinese Priest and two Chinese nuns, who sheltered us until January 2nd, 1942, when we were rescued by British Red Cross men.[83]

The fate of the men was tragically different. They were ordered to remove boots or shoes and tunics. Pte. Oakley, who had been shot in the thigh and was unable to walk, was presumably bayoneted by the Japanese.[84] The RAMC personnel had Red Cross identification cards but the Japanese trampled these into the ground; neither Capt. Banfill nor the Royal Rifles men had these cards and none of the men had Red Cross armbands because they had been unable to obtain them. The civilian doctors had no markings of any kind; all St. John's Ambulance personnel wore a distinctive uniform with Red Cross badges on the sleeve.[85]

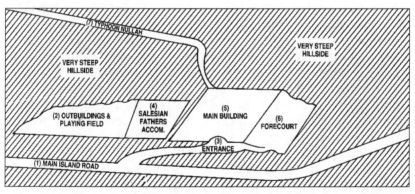

Figure 2.7. Drawing of Salesian Mission and area, based on a sketch made by Norman Leath for the author in 1988. Key: 1: main Island road, here running roughly north-south, north on right; 2: outbuildings and playing fields; 3: entrance to main building; 4: smaller building, in 1941 occupied by the Salesian fathers; 5: main Mission building occupied by Army Medical Store; the Collecting Post (Military) commanded by Capt. Banfill was located in the basement; 6: forecourt where Allied staff was assembled by the Japanese; 7: typhoon nullah up which the men were marched and, shortly, executed except for three who were wounded but escaped, and also excepting Capt. Banfill, who was spared. (Reproduced by permission from C.G. Roland, "Massacre and Rape at Hong Kong: Two Case Studies Involving Medical Personnel and Patients," *Journal of Contemporary History* 32: 43-61, 1997)

After having had some of their valuables confiscated, they were marched away from the Mission and into the hills behind.[86] Here the women were sent away. They saw the bodies of the two wounded officers who had been in the ambulance.

At a small clearing the captives were halted facing a nullah, or drainage ditch. Capt. Banfill was moved away from the men and tied, his arms behind his back and a loop of rope around the neck.[87] The Japanese soldiers began to bayonet their prisoners. The bodies were kicked into the nullah. Then, as a survivor noted later, "panic must have broken loose as a number of those on the lower end of the line broke and ran and these were shot."[88] The party of women was still in sight and observed these killings.[89] The Japanese attempted to behead some of their prisoners with swords.

One of the latter group was Cpl. Norman Leath, miraculously a survivor, who reported feeling a terrific blow on the back of his neck. Feigning death, he was later able to wriggle away and roll into the nullah where he saw the bloody bodies of some of his colleagues. Further away, he came across Lt. Thomas, who had managed to jump into the nullah and hide, partially covered by the bodies of the dead and dying.[90] Both men survived.

Eight days later, after many hardships, Leath managed to make his own way to North Point POW Camp, where he gave himself up. He received some treatment, then was taken to Queen Mary Hospital where there were more adequate facilities. However, his condition was so serious that, given the press of other casualties, he was left in a bed "apparently to die in due course."[91] Then, on 3 January 1942, an RAMC corporal found him there and took him to Bowen Road Military Hospital.[92] Finally, 18 days after his potentially fatal wound, Leath received definitive treatment. Maj. James Anderson, RAMC, operated on him on 6 January 1942. Leath recalled being told that the wound was infested by maggots which had prevented the wound from becoming seriously infected.[93]

On recovery, Leath worked as chief clerk at the hospitals at Bowen Road. Remarkably, apart from some considerable stiffness in his neck, which he noted was also "a little sore," he did not feel any major effect from his injuries.[94] He continued vigorous and healthy until not long before his death in 1999. Half a century after the event, the scar on his neck remained impressive.

Second Lt. Osler Thomas, a member of the HKVDC Field Ambulance, was a medical student in 1941. Somehow, in the melee once the slaughter began, Thomas managed to fall untouched into the nullah. The bodies of two other victims fell on him and protected him from "the orgy of shooting and bayoneting that followed."[95] He escaped to mainland China where he worked with the British Army Aid Group (BAAG), supporting escapes from the Japanese and conducting a significant Intelligence activity throughout the war.[96] Thomas completed his education after the war. He now practises medicine in Australia.

A third survivor of execution was Ah Tim, a Chinese member of the St. John's Ambulance group which, separated from the Banfill-

Thomas-Leath group, were also executed. About to be shot, he ran, rolled down a hill, and was left for dead.[97]

While these grisly and barbaric murders took place, Capt. Banfill was made to lie down and told that he would experience the same fate as his men, but only after he had been interrogated.[98] He heard the sounds of Japanese conversation and laughter mingled with blows and shots and with the cries and screams of dying men; even though a Japanese had a foot on his face, Banfill had a clear view of the massacre. Then he was forced to his feet and marched away from the scene. Some days later, with at least encouragement and perhaps direct aid from a Japanese officer or interpreter named Honda, he was sent off to a prison camp, uninjured except for the appalling mental strain. By late February he rejoined the remnants of his regiment in North Point POW Camp. He had been given up for dead and his "death" was reported officially. In a grim twist of fate his wife, in Quebec, was so distraught at hearing of his supposed death that she took her own life.[99]

These actions by members of the 229th Regiment were not only brutal but blatantly illegal. Although Japan never ratified the 1929 Geneva Convention on Prisoners of War,[100] the murder of surrendered military personnel was a practice officially abandoned by all civilized countries by the twentieth century and interdicted formally by the Hague Conventions of 1899 and 1907, and by the Geneva Convention of 1929 Relative to Sick and Wounded in the field; all of these Conventions Japan had formally ratified.[101] Moreover, the protection due to medical personnel was laid down explicitly in the Hague Convention of 1907.

Although the 229th Regiment had made a night landing and was in combat on 19 December, there had been no fighting at the Salesian Mission, staffed entirely by Protected Personnel and nurses. No justification of "the heat of battle" or of "revenge for hostile actions" could be sustained in behalf of the Japanese troops.

The commanding officer of the 229th Regiment, or Tanaka Butai, was Tanaka Ryusaburo, a colonel in 1941. At his trial six years later, Tanaka claimed to have issued "caution addresses" to his men through the regimental officers. The gist of the purported caution was:

> No unnecessary killings and ill treatment should be allowed. The purpose of an operation is to break down the fighting streng an enemy and as a surrendered personnel or a sick or wounded enemy is not a fighting strength, unnecessary killing and ill treatment should not be allowed. If such treatment is allowed it is not only inhumane, but it is a crime.[102]

Such testimony might seem predictable from someone on trial for his life. One can only conclude that Tanaka lied about giving such cautions, or his cautions were not transmitted by his officers, or the

Tanaka Butai was grossly insubordinate and undisciplined. The English-speaking officer who took charge of Dr. Banfill after the remainder of the men had been killed, told Banfill, "Order is, all captives must die."[103]

Tanaka was found guilty and sentenced to 20 years' hard labour, but on the charges specifically related to the incident described at Shau Kei Wan, he was adjudged not guilty. No men of his battalion were brought to trial in connection with these murders.

St. Stephen's College

In the second major atrocity involving medical personnel, the antecedents are more equivocal. These barbarous murders and rapes were perpetrated at St. Stephen's College on 25 December. This institution is located on pleasant grassy slopes just above the neck of land that connects the main portion of Hong Kong Island to the Stanley Peninsula on the southeastern side. Supplies and equipment appropriate to permit the establishment of a 400-bed emergency military hospital were moved to St. Stephens just before the fighting began.[104]

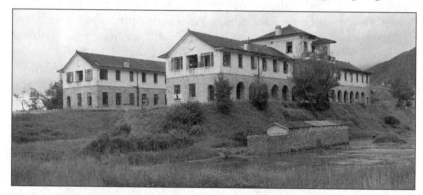

Figure 2.8. St. Stephen's College, Hong Kong, September 1945. (Photographer Jack Howes; National Archives of Canada, National Photographic Collection, PA. 145352.)

The main building of St. Stephen's College was being used as an emergency hospital. In the hall on Christmas morning were about 65 patients, with at least 40 more in the adjoining classrooms. The medical staff comprised Lt.-Col. G.D.R. Black (HKVDC), Capt. P.N. Whitney (RAMC), two Nursing Sisters from Bowen Road Military Hospital (Miss A.F. Gordon and Miss Elizabeth A. Fidoe), six VADs (including Miss Andrews-Levinge, Mrs. A. Buxton, Mrs. E.M. Begg, and Mrs. W.J.L. Smith), five Chinese nurses of St. John's Ambulance, and a number of hospital orderlies.

At 5:30 a.m. on Christmas morning, while the fighting was still continuing along the adjacent ridge, about 150 to 200 Japanese broke into the hospital. Col. Black went forward and endeavoured to stop them. He was shot through the head and bayoneted "dozens of times" as he lay on the ground. The Japanese troops then began attacking the bed patients, driving their bayonets through bodies and mattresses.

One can visualize the mental state of these men, one of whom subsequently recorded, "I clearly saw the intention of the Japanese troops who had reached the hospital and had already commenced bayoneting every bed they encountered."[105] This man and his wife, a nurse, got under the bed and escaped injury, though a Japanese private bayoneted the empty bed several times. The massacre continued until more than 50 of the patients in the hall, which had only a single entrance, had been stabbed to death. The others concealed themselves under beds and in dark corners.[106]

All the women were wearing nurses' uniforms and Red Cross armbands. Nevertheless, their treatment was atrocious. They were confined first in a small upstairs room in the College. The Chinese nurses were raped repeatedly by Japanese soldiers, then taken away and were not seen again. Three of the British nurses were also taken away at intervals, and their mutilated bodies were found next day. The other four were raped again and again throughout the morning and afternoon, but survived.[107] In the evening a Japanese officer told them that they were lucky that Hong Kong had surrendered; in another hour they also would have been dead.[108] Several of the women had been sexually mutilated during or after the rapes took place.[109] The dead British nurses were Mrs. A. Buxton, Mrs. E.M. Begg (wife of then Sgt. Maj. Stewart Duncan Begg), and Mrs. W.J.L. Smith, all members of the Nursing Detachment of the HKVDC.[110] The names of the Chinese nurses seem to be unrecorded. Here is one woman's post-war testimony:

> We were left in peace for a short time only—three soldiers came in and took me to a small adjacent bathroom, knocked me down and all raped me, one after the other, and then let me return. Mrs. Fidoe was then taken and underwent a similar experience. Both Mrs. Fidoe and I were taken out a second time and raped as before.[111]

Word of these atrocities had somehow been conveyed to the newly captured Allied POWs elsewhere on the island. Officers among them immediately reported the outrage to the Japanese Headquarters, which "allowed us to send a truck to get the [surviving] nurses to the main hospital for treatment."[112]

While the rape and murder of the women was underway, the captured men were being killed systematically. Crowded together into small rooms, one or two of their number would be selected arbitrarily and forced to leave the room. After the door was locked again the remaining prisoners would hear screams and shouts followed by shots; then silence until the next selection in half an hour or an hour.

When the slaughter ended, survivors were put to work cleaning up after the massacre. On the 26th prisoners had to carry bodies, blood-stained mattresses, clothing, and other debris outside. There an enormous fire consumed some of the gory evidence. At this time, Sgt. Maj. Begg had the shock of seeing and identifying the naked and mutilated bodies of his wife and two other nurses.[113]

Later, just after the surrender, an Allied officer asked an IJA colonel if it was the practice of the Imperial Japanese Army to rape hospital nurses and shoot and bayonet the wounded in their beds, as had happened at Stanley. The colonel replied that, if this allegation were true, the culprits would be found and shot in accordance with Japanese military law. Apparently, some such sentence was carried out a few days later. One survivor recorded that the Japanese "took some of our officers to witness the shooting of 14 Jap soldiers for going in the hospital and doing the killing."[114]

Nevertheless, the Japanese claimed that the shooting of the wounded at Stanley was justified because firing had come from the school which was being used as a hospital and armed men were found inside; "they could not know who were wounded men or who were shamming and waiting to shoot any Japanese who approached."[115]

In statements prepared in July 1942, two eyewitnesses to these events recorded some details that may explain, though not condone, the violence that occurred. The statements were made by Sgts. H. Peasegood and J.H. Anderson, RAMC.

First, Peasegood noted that a machine gun post had been sited about 100 yards from the hospital; later, several additional machine gun posts were placed even nearer to the hospital. On the night of 24 December machine guns began firing from the College hospital verandah and continued to do so throughout the night.[116] Sgt. Anderson provided further information about this obviously improper placement of machine guns in immediate proximity to a hospital:

> Towards midnight on 24 December machine gun and mortar fire increased and numerous machine gun posts were set up in the grounds of the hospital. Later on these posts actually used bales of hospital blankets and mattresses from the linen stores to build machine gun nests within six yards of the entrance to the hospital reception hall. Guns were also set up on the rising ground behind the cookhouse and another within arm's reach of the flagpole carrying the red cross. The machine gun outside Brigade HQ actually had to fire over the top of a large St. George Cross flag (the only other red cross available) which had been hoisted over the end of the tennis courts.[117]

Recognition that there was some provocation because of the combining of combatant and hospital roles seems to have been widespread among the POWs. For example, in 1945, Capt. John Reid, RCAMC, in an affidavit about war crimes observed in Hong Kong and Japan, stressed that he had not been at St. Stephen's but that it was his understanding that the Japanese attacking in the area had driven Allied troops back to "or actually within the grounds of this hospital. The British troops from these positions had taken a toll of the Japanese so that when they were overcome the Japanese in full lust of battle continued on into the hospital and committed the above crimes."[118]

Rfn. Randolph Steele, RRC, was not captured until 26 December. He was near St. Stephen's College with a small group of other Canadians, afraid to surrender after finding some British soldiers tied together with wire and bayoneted. One of these unfortunates had lived long enough to tell the Canadians what had happened. Finally they had to surrender, and were taken to the St. Stephen's tennis court. Lined up, they expected to be shot but a Japanese officer came along and "he shouted to the gun crew and he slapped the Jap Sergeant's face and made them take the gun out of the court."[119] The officer found water and food for them. "He also gave us a record player and about 50 opera records that didn't do too much good for our nerves."[120] They were put to work piling up bodies, which the Japanese soaked with gasoline and burned. This grim task would not have helped their nerves.

Nor was the disposal of bodies complete. A month later, St. Stephen's College was within the area set aside for Stanley Internment Camp. Wenzell Brown was one of a group assigned to the St. Stephen's science laboratory. In the first room they found, face downward in a corner, the body of a Canadian soldier; on the floor above, a dead Canadian and an Indian shared one room. The internees could find no identification on the men, but they prepared shallow graves for the decomposing bodies and buried them as reverently as they could.[121] This burial had to be carried out quickly for health reasons. The Japanese had carefully cremated their own dead but not the British or their Allies. Soon, graves dotted the camp grounds as more and more bodies were discovered. If a body did not lie within the wire, the Japanese refused permission for burial, and Brown relates a poignant account of a young woman who watched daily with morbid despair while her brother's body gradually disintegrated before her eyes, a few yards outside the barbed wire enclosure.[122]

Nurses of the Hong Kong Volunteer Defence Corps

These women, chiefly Chinese and some Portuguese, were also subjected to sexual outrages by the victorious Japanese. At least, that seems a reasonable assumption. A member of the Volunteers, Arthur Gomes, recalls seeing a group of these nurses being marched towards a nearby public building when he and his comrades were in turn being marched into Sham Shui Po Camp on the mainland, shortly after the capitulation. Screams and cries were heard repeatedly throughout that night, and it seems plausible to infer that multiple rapes were committed.[123] Given the inbred reticence and modesty of women from many eastern cultures, it is not surprising that this event has failed to be documented. No record in English has been found.

To provide a context for what happened at St. Stephen's, it must be kept in mind that at least 10,000 girls and women in Hong Kong were raped in the month following the Japanese victory. The number may have been much higher, but modesty led to a reluctance to disclose at least the less violent and bloody instances and probably kept many victims from identifying themselves or reporting their ill treatment to authorities. The estimate of at least 10,000 was put forward by a Chinese physician who was in active practice in Hong Kong during 1941 and 1942.[124] In autumn, 1942, he and other practitioners were dealing with the "deluge" of babies resulting from this orgy of rape.

Zia, also a civilian physician in Hong Kong, states that the rapes were all committed during the first two weeks after the invasion.[125] This same writer cites several accounts of rape, including one of a physician who killed a Japanese soldier in the act of raping his wife.[126]

The ubiquity of rape during wartime has been amply described. Brownmiller has summarized at least some of the reasons, both immediate and political:

> When a victorious army rapes, the sheer intoxication of the triumph is only part of the act. After the fact, the rape may be viewed as part of a recognizable pattern of national terror and subjugation. I say "after the fact" because the original impulse to rape does not need a sophisticated political motivation beyond a general disregard for the bodily integrity of women. But rape in warfare has a military effect as well as an impulse. And the effect is indubitably one of intimidation and demoralization for the victims' side.[127]

Perhaps the most convincing accounts of the ubiquity and the permissiveness connected with rape by the Japanese armed forces come from statements published in the past 15 years by Japanese participants in such events. Variously motivated by guilt and by a perceived need to set the record straight, these former soldiers and sailors have documented the banal nature of various acts of brutality, including rape.[128]

The recollections of one man will demonstrate the tenor of these recollections. Yomisu Omae served in China in the late 1930s. He wrote of two instances of gang rape of Chinese women, attempting to indicate what his state of mind might have been:

> At another house, however, some soldiers kicked in a door to find a married couple and their three children huddled together on a bed under an old mosquito net. They had been unable to escape. Ripping the

net away, we dragged the woman out and raped her—all of us. Somewhere in the back of our minds we probably felt that this little extra pleasure was totally deserved, since we were laying down our lives for our country.[129]

As well as Brownmiller, other observers also have described the culture-destroying effects of rape, whether in China in the 1930s, in Berlin in 1945, or in Bosnia-Herzegovina in the 1990s. Seifert refers to evidence suggesting that rape has always been a part of warfare, and that "the mass rapes that accompany all wars take on new meaning: by no means acts of senseless brutality, they are rather culture-destroying actions with a strategic rationale."[130] There is every reason to believe that Japanese troops became accustomed to raping, owing to the commonness of that crime throughout the war against the Chinese. The outrage that became known collectively as the Rape of Nanking is only the most widely known among many such occurrences during these years, most frequently at the individual level as described by Omae.[131] But Peking, Shanghai, Hankow, and Canton suffered in similar ways.

In addition to these crimes against women, Japanese troops committed many other brutalities, frequently ending in physical injury and in many cases death of the victim. Thus the events at Shau Kei Wan, St. Stephen's, and the emergency hospital at the Jockey Club are a microcosm selected out of the violence that swept over Hong Kong after the capitulation, and which had of course begun 10 days earlier in Kowloon when that city was abandoned by the British troops.

There was no evidence of compassion towards wounded men by the Japanese at Hong Kong. Incapacitated casualties were killed routinely; their bodies, often tied hand and foot, were found all over the island during and after the fighting. Though undoubtedly an exaggeration in detail, one historian has claimed that there was only a single case of the Japanese caring for a wounded British soldier. This man had been raised in Japan and spoke fluent Japanese. But though he was cared for, the Japanese refused his requests for aid to his compatriots.[132]

Frequently, captured British, Indian, Canadian, and Hong Kong soldiers were butchered. Some able-bodied men, often with hands bound, or tied in groups of two or three, but not evidently otherwise incapacitated, were bayoneted or shot. Their bodies were found by Allied observers in the days immediately after the fighting ended.

On 19 December, several Canadian soldiers of "A" Company, Winnipeg Grenadiers, were captured at Jardine's Lookout. They were bound together in groups, and one group of four ultimately was bayoneted to death. But the circumstances in at least this one incident clearly exonerate the Japanese. Another member of the larger group of 36 or 37, L/Cpl. Charles Bradbury, attested in an affidavit after the war: "I personally saw Pte. Roy Land (end man in one of the bound groups) remove a Grenade from his pocket, draw the pin, and throw the Grenade toward where a group of seven (7) Japanese soldiers were visible. The Grenade exploded killing at least four (4) Japanese soldiers." Not surprisingly, the remaining captors immediately bayoneted to death all four Grenadiers. No army in the world would have behaved differently. The truly remarkable fact was that the remaining 32 POWs were not killed or mistreated, but instead were ultimately marched off into imprisonment.[133]

Cpl. Les Canivet, a Canadian soldier, had a horrendous experience. He sustained a serious wound to his face and jaw just before Christmas Day. Trying to escape, he and some companions swam across Repulse Bay, several drowning in the attempt. On the other side the survivors hid amongst some beach cottages but eventually they were found by Japanese troops:

> The four of us were led to a ravine and were tied together and shot. I got shot in the shoulder and the hip and the right hand; the first shot hit me in the shoulder and knocked me down. I sort of played dead. When I came to, or when the Japanese had disappeared, and I felt it was safe to sit up again, my buddies were dead, but I was still tied up and we were still tied to one another.[134]

Soon after, he saw a Chinese man whom he knew, a houseboy to a local family that had Canadian connections. Canivet was still tied; for the privilege of stripping the other bodies, the Chinese man untied him, taking as well Canivet's ring and watch. After that, the Canadian corporal wandered into the hills, wearing only his army underwear and shoes, plus some shorts he had found in the shed.

Eventually he was picked up by a patrol and sent to Bowen Road Hospital. There, doctors found his extensive facial wounds swarming with maggots and free of infection. He was hospitalized for months but eventually healed completely.

Where violence against captives did not occur, as at Bowen Road Military Hospital, sheer good luck is a probable explanation. Col. Bowie recalled that at the time of the surrender, the front line was only about 400 yards away. Long columns of Japanese troops were seen from the hospital. "I believe that it was the fact that we were not overrun in battle that saved patients and staff from the rape and murder which disfigured the campaign in Stanley, Happy Valley and elsewhere."[135] Thus combatant troops never had a reason to invade the hospital and no atrocities occurred.

At Hong Kong, the key to survival as a newly captured prisoner apparently rested most substantially on two factors: whether or not resistance of any kind was made after surrender (for example, struggling to prevent the theft of valuables), and whether or not one was prevented from walking because of wounds or injuries. Resistance or immobility almost guaranteed death. The Japanese captors would not tolerate interference with their "right" to loot, and they made no humanitarian allowances for the severely disabled. To these generalizations, Shau Kei Wan seems to be the exception; the unfortunates captured there had done nothing to bring on their fate. They seem to have been doomed from the beginning. Why this was so remains a mystery that has probably gone to the grave.

Much violence was still in store for those who survived to become prisoners of war, but it was of a different kind, calculated to humiliate the POW and exalt the Japanese or Korean guard. Rarely did this routine brutality escalate to murder.

Capitulation

At varying times from mid-December till the massive denouement on Christmas Day, the troops had to surrender. None of them had been trained in how to do so. And everything they had heard of the Japanese sharply emphasized the potential risks when their turn came. One Canadian rifleman recalled his sensations:

> Lay down your arms? I couldn't! It was all wrong. But the others *were actually doing it*. "Pile them here!" My precious Lee-Enfield? My security? My protector through all the mad chaotic events, my faithful friend, the only thing I didn't discard. Without it I was half a man, helpless." The others were laying theirs down, man after man. Slowly I followed suit, overcome by a terrible, alien sensation of nakedness, of being totally helpless, an act of ritual self-destruction.[136]

Another POW found it ironic that, perhaps to emphasize the indignity, for the first few days the Japanese simply ignored those captured on Stanley Peninsula. They cordoned off the peninsula and established a system of sea patrols. Then the POWs were left to their own devices while the Japanese gathered and cremated their dead. They dragged iron bed frames from houses in Stanley village and improvised an open-air crematorium. For a day and a night the macabre fires blazed. Japanese casualties at Stanley had run into thousands. This single engagement, they told the prisoners later, cost them more than any other part of the Hong Kong fighting.

> As the flames died, special corpsmen moved down the line with steel chopsticks picking a few fragments of bone and ash from each smoldering pile. These were placed in small urns, and the urns in uniform white boxes inscribed with the names of the victims. And soon the white boxes would start on the long journey back to Japan....Only when all this was finished and the mass memorial services for the Japanese dead had been

held were we allowed to send out our own burial parties on a task that by then had become a nameless horror.[137]

Eventually, the Chinese civilian dead and the dead Allied servicemen could be collected and buried. The university football field on Pokfulam Road was turned into a public cemetery.[138]

At Singapore, another Canadian, Maj. Benjamin Wheeler, a medical officer in the Indian Medical Service, expressed the fears of many. Singapore surrendered on 15 February 1942. At medical headquarters they knew that when the Japanese had captured the main hospital, they shot more than 200 patients and staff. As far as they knew only one man survived. Added to this, Allied propaganda had stressed the Japanese practice of taking no prisoners. Thus, "though it seemed hardly likely they would slaughter a whole army, one could hardly feel certain of a long life, when we watched General Percival go out to make the final surrender."[139]

Such fears were widespread. Nevertheless, this sort of general slaughter did not occur at Hong Kong. Instead, the survivors of the fighting were forced into an experience that would alter their lives forever. They became prisoners of war. The following chapters attempt to reconstruct what their lives were like for the many long years remaining in the war.

Chapter 3

The Prisoner-of-War Camps

and Hospitals

The problem remained for every Japanese POW throughout the war.
How could you best behave and yet maintain some dignity?[1]

*O*n 25 December 1941, the Hong Kong garrison capitulated and
all surviving Allied troops became prisoners of war. The
remainder of this book will be devoted to telling what happened to
these unfortunate men. The main groups of prisoners were the survivors of the two British, two Indian, and two Canadian battalions,
and the Hong Kong Volunteer Defence Corps. There were also prisoners from the Royal Navy, the Royal Air Force, engineers, ordnance and
supply units plus, of course, the various medical detachments.

Several nursing sisters remained at Bowen Road Hospital for the
first half of 1942. Then they were removed from the hospital and sent
to the civilian internment camp on the Stanley Peninsula. They were
no less incarcerated there, but in general the Japanese treated internees somewhat less badly than they did POWs. Moreover, for the
Canadians, Nursing Sisters Kay Christie and May Waters, though
they had no way of knowing it in 1942, the following year would be
repatriated home.

For the men, those last days of 1941 and the first days of 1942 have
survived in memory as a confusing and intensely worrisome time of
frightening chaos. Frequently they have difficulty remembering the
events just after the capitulation. A Canadian lieutenant was "very
hazy about what happened after that. We sort of wandered around.
Told to go here, go there, do this, do that for the next couple of days. I

don't even remember where we ended up. I can't remember whether my first internment camp was Sham Shui Po, or whether it was North Point,"[2] though these camps were several miles apart, one on the mainland and one on the Island.

The Imperial Japanese Army suddenly found itself with a Christmas present of more than 8,000 prisoners to be accommodated and fed. Even though the IJA officially declared that Japanese troops should never be taken prisoner, they also knew that few other modern nations—perhaps only the Soviet Union under Stalin—subscribed to the same belief. Thus they would have known that when they went to war there would be prisoners taken and, since they confidently expected to defeat their opponents, they must have made some plans for the management of POWs. But the dominant motif of the early days after the surrender on Christmas Day remains one of confused milling about by the Japanese as well as by the POWs. Nevertheless, the Japanese were in fact organizing the means of their prisoners' future existence.

There were many itineraries for captured Allied troops during this time of great uncertainty. This state lasted for weeks while the Japanese struggled to accommodate these thousands of POWs and to decide what to do with large numbers of civilian foreign nationals. To give some flavour to this confusion and the gradually evolving order, here are brief summaries of the varied movements enforced on three Canadian POWs late in December 1941 and early in January.

L/Cpl. Francis D.F. Martyn, Winnipeg Grenadiers, became a prisoner on Christmas Day. He was sent immediately to Mount Austin Barracks on Hong Kong Island, where he arrived at about 7 pm; the next day he was moved to Peak Mansions; then, on the 27th, about noon, to the University of Hong Kong. Late the next morning, Martyn was marched to Victoria Barracks, where he remained for two days. All these sites are on Hong Kong Island. On 30 December he was marched to the docks and ferried to Nanking Barracks at Sham Shui Po Camp, in Kowloon, arriving about 4:30 pm; from there he later became part of the large group of Canadian POWs transferred to North Point Camp, back on Hong Kong Island, on 23 January 1942. Thereafter his movements paralleled the Canadians' generally.[3] But in less than a month he saw six different sites of imprisonment. Martyn ended up in Oeyama Camp, Japan, in January 1944, where he remained until the war ended.

Cpl. Sydney Hiscox became a POW on the Island before the general capitulation. He was captured after the Japanese invasion from the mainland, on 19 or 20 December. After surviving the ordeal of the first minutes and hours, when some of his comrades were killed (chiefly the seriously wounded), Hiscox's group of 30 to 40 was marched to North Point, in use as a POW Camp at least by 20 December, the day

Hiscox arrived. On 21 December they were taken to Argyle Street Camp in Kowloon. Two weeks later they were moved to Sham Shui Po, and late in January 1942, Hiscox, like Martyn, was among the large body of Canadians sent to North Point Camp.[4]

Another Canadian, Samuel Kravinchuk, was in a group moved from North Point on 21 December to Maryknoll School, in Kowloon.[5] There they sought medical attention for the more than 40 members of the group of 61 Canadians who had injuries. Ultimately the Japanese gave the wounded first aid. Later that day, they were moved to Argyle Street, near Maryknoll School, and subsequently followed the common path to Sham Shui Po, North Point, and ultimately back to Sham Shui Po.

The surviving members of the Hong Kong Volunteer Defence Corps had a somewhat less tumultuous time. Gathered together as the war wound down, the men were first held in the Alhambra Theatre opposite the Kowloon Magistracy Building. On Christmas Day the Japanese moved them to their pre-war headquarters at Garden Road, on the Island. There they occupied huts at St. John's Place until 28 or 29 December. At that point they plodded to the Star Ferry, were transported back to Kowloon, and made the final humiliating march through the streets to Sham Shui Po. There many of them were to wait out the war.[6]

These itineraries, though unusual, were not unique. On the morning of 30 December the bulk of the Canadian prisoners were assembled, removed from the Island, and marched through Kowloon to Sham Shui Po Camp. The route was anything but direct. A Chinese woman missionary saw the dispirited column that day and followed the men for a long time, out of sympathy. They shambled along to Argyle Street Camp, northeast of downtown Kowloon. After a brief rest there they were then marched directly west to their ultimate goal, Sham Shui Po. Those familiar with Hong Kong will know that this route was a circuitous triangle. No one was left at Argyle Street nor was anyone added.[7] But the dog-leg extended the journey by two hours. Presumably the Japanese chose the route both to weaken and to further humiliate their captives by displaying them in defeat to the Chinese citizens of Hong Kong.

Sham Shui Po had been a large, permanent British army camp on the edge of the harbour on the west side of Kowloon. The Canadians knew this camp—it had been their living quarters after their arrival in Hong Kong. Then, towards the end of January 1942, all Canadians moved from Sham Shui Po to North Point Camp on Hong Kong Island, where there were already substantial numbers of their countrymen. At the same time, Indian POWs were consolidated at Ma Tau Chung Camp in Kowloon near Argyle Street Camp, and Sham Shui Po became the chief place of imprisonment for the British battalions and the HKVDC survivors. But consolidation remained incomplete for months; as late as 18 April, 80 Canadians came into North Point Camp from Sham Shui Po and Argyle Street.[8]

Relatively little information seems to have survived about the experiences of these men in the first month of imprisonment. There is no reason to suppose that they did not work, have entertainments, encounter diseases, and suffer all the miseries of POW life. During the short time that the men of the several different nationalities remained intermixed, some antagonisms arose, often on racial rounds: "Several truck loads of army stuff came in camp. The Indians nearly mobbed it. Had to be driven off, a near riot between whites and Indians. Pickets out all night patrolling between the lines."[9] What is known about the incarceration of Indian nationals, including the efforts of the Japanese to persuade these men to join the Indian National Army and to fight against the Allies, will be discussed later.

While this re-grouping began, there were many unresolved questions to be answered, the most distressing being the whereabouts and condition of hundreds of missing men. When the fighting ended, wounded and ill men were scattered all over Hong Kong, mainland and Island, in various official and makeshift hospitals. Many more were hidden away, languishing in culverts and huts, under bushes or in nullahs. During and immediately after the fighting, such men were usually executed on the spot by the Japanese.

After the capitulation, however, the Japanese in some areas permitted their charges to search for survivors and bring them into camps and hospitals. Three senior medical officers, Col. C.O. Shackleton, RAMC; Col. Lindsay Ride, RAM; and Maj. John Crawford, RCAMC were given passes permitting them to tour the battle sites and to collect any wounded still surviving. Their findings make grim reading.

> My commanding officer (I was second-in-command of the field ambulance) was a man named Lindsay Ride who was later knighted, but at that time was professor of physiology at the University of Hong Kong. Lindsay knew the country like the back of his hand. He and I started off (got a pass from some Japanese officer) and we tramped around the island looking for casualties. We must have walked about 20 miles that day. It was a long tiring day and a very traumatic one, because we found masses of dead who had been butchered—hands tied and bayoneted and so on—very rough.[10]

At the same time, the Japanese required hospitals for their own casualties. The interrogation report of an escaped naval officer recorded that early in 1942, the Japanese cleared the Naval Hospital in which he was a patient. "At 0900 hrs, a lorry load of naval ratings drove into the yard, and these were quickly posted round the grounds and in the building. An officer then read an order stating that the Japanese authorities required the hospital, and that it had to be evacuated by 1700 hrs that day." The sickest patients went to Bowen Road and the remainder to St. Albert's Convent.[11]

Meanwhile, conditions in Hong Kong itself began to deteriorate badly. Despite what would seem to be an obvious vested interest in keeping the city functioning as efficiently as possible, in fact Hong Kong worked badly under Japanese rule. A civilian physician reported that malignant malaria, cholera, and other diseases broke out quickly. Hong Kong's government anti-malarial squads stopped work, of course, and "the scavenging coolies abandoned their rounds. Garbage and filth, accumulated in heaps everywhere, bred an unprecedented number of flies; and the thousands of decaying bodies scattered on the hillsides were additional breeding grounds."[12]

Japanese Camp Administration

On 20 February 1942, Lt.-Gen Isogai Rensuke arrived in Hong Kong to assume the post of Governor of the Japanese colony of Hong Kong.[13] Isogai replaced Sakai Takashi, commander of the 23rd Japanese Army that had assaulted and captured Hong Kong. In 1945, Isogai was in turn replaced by Gen. Tanaka Hisakichi.[14] The POW administration was conducted out of a house on Forfar Road, quite near the sites of the Argyle Street and Ma Tau Chung POW Camps.

A succession of Japanese officers functioned as camp commandants. The first of these at Sham Shui Po was known to most of the POWs only as "George," though his name was Lt. Saikanu.[15] One man noted in April 1942 that he looked "slightly oiled." He added a note long after the war: "'George' was the name given to the then camp Commandant. He was tall for a Jap, with a humorous grin (at times). Like all Jap officers at work he looked terribly scruffy, with crinkled clothes and a long sword dragging behind him. He used to advance with a scuffling jingling sound. At times he 'hit the bottle' and the result was amusing, a sight best observed from a distance."[16]

By September 1942, "George" had been replaced by a Captain Wada. He appeared to be "an inoffensive little fellow, not too bad really. Always smiling and promising the sun, but nothing comes of it."[17] Lewis Bush had a more flattering memory of Wada as a camp commandant:

> He seemed a good man....We had an excellent example of this in the case of the discovery of a radio in the room occupied by a Dutch submarine officer and some of his crew. It was quite obvious that the camp informers had located this instrument through information supplied by one of the Indonesian members of the submarine crew. Now, had Wada reported this matter to the "kempei," it is certain that the Dutch naval lieutenant would have lost his head. It was settled with a beating, which

seemed brutal at the time…but I am sure it was light compared to what might have been if Wada had not been a decent man.[18]

A Canadian NCO seemed to concur. In January 1943 Wada returned from Japan and was in charge of the camp: "There should be less slapping now."[19] Another commandant, a man named Honda, also created a favourable attitude. In April 1944, Les Fisher made an entry in his secret diary about a group of 200 POWs leaving Sham Shui Po. "As it left the lads gave three cheers for the camp commandant Honda, because he is the only one we have had who has been decent to us."[20]

Bowen Road Military Hospital

Bowen Road was a classic example of a tropical-zone hospital, constructed with outside stairwells and wide verandas protected by overhanging eaves and floors. In less parlous times, when there was no need to be concerned with the potentially lethal effects of shrapnel or small-arms fire, the spacious verandas made ideal locations for convalescing patients to be uplifted by the splendid view of Hong Kong Harbour. There were no elevators.

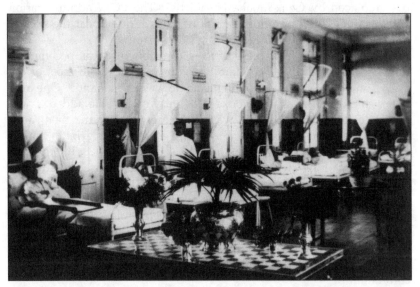

Figure 3.1. Ward in British Military Hospital, Bowen Road, Hong Kong Island, 1930s. (Hong Kong Museum of History P94.260.)

Col. Shackleton, Senior British Medical Officer (SBMO) at Bowen Road when war began, continued in this position under the Japanese in the first months of captivity. However, on 7 August 1942 he was moved to Argyle Street Camp with the other senior officers of the garrison, and Maj. Donald C. Bowie took over as SBMO. Fortunately for our understanding of the history of the hospital, Bowie kept detailed notes, most of which he was able to preserve. In 1975 he published a lengthy, detailed, and precise account of his superintendency.[21]

The opportunity to operate Bowen Road Hospital from the time of the surrender in 1941 until April 1945 displays an apparently co-operative approach by the Japanese. Bowie was in the ideal position to see these matters from the inside: "The Japanese obviously decided as an article of policy to leave our hospital with its own staff to look after allied sick and wounded prisoners of war....They did not interfere with the treatment of our patients nor did they remove anything other than minor quantities of drugs and equipment from our stores."[22] In May 1945, the site was changed to the Central British School, in Kowloon, where the uprooted hospital continued to function.

Permitting Bowen Road Hospital to function provided the Japanese, Bowie contended, with a propagandistically useful instance of conformance with the Geneva Conventions. Doing so was not effected without cost to the Japanese. It must have been a substantial administrative inconvenience because, from September 1942 on, the staff and patients at Bowen Road were the only POWs on the Island, all others being in Sham Shui Po, Ma Tau Chung, or Argyle Street Camps in Kowloon.[23]

While internal control at Bowen Road rested with the POW med-ical officers, their activities were governed by Japanese regulation of the number of patients permitted, as well as the intake and discharge of particular patients; moreover, they sent in rations and fuel accord-ing to a scale that they established.[24]

The intensity of official scrutiny varied. Routine discipline contin-ued to be wielded by the Japanese. Regardless of the weather, daily parades were held—the much-loathed lengthy *tenko* so familiar to POWs throughout the Far East. The parades were probably less rigor-ous than in ordinary camps, but nevertheless everyone except the unequivocally bedridden had to appear and be counted. Some were able to take an ironic view of the enforced *tenko* at Bowen Road: "Each day a roll call established that none of the amputees or TB cases or can-cer patients had escaped during the night."[25] But the routine could be brutal. One patient wrote, on 12 February 1942: "Absolutely freezing, or so it seems....Parade for Japs at 4 pm. Impossible to stand still, everyone double marks time. Off after $1^1/_2$ hours of agony."[26] Fortunately there were other occasions when "the Japs work smartly and have us off in 10 mins."[27]

On 15 January 1942, all the wounded and ill men at Bowen Road who were able to stand were paraded with their belongings in front of the hospital. From there, they were marched to the docks in Victoria, transported across the harbour in lighters, then marched the two miles to Sham Shui Po Camp.[28] Six days after these transfers, all sick and wounded Allied troops in War Memorial Hospital, near The Peak, were removed to Bowen Road Hospital. The civilian medical staff at War Memorial, St. Teresa's, and also the temporary hospitals were sent into internment camp at Stanley Point on Hong Kong Island, where civilians from the Allied powers were segregated.[29] Civilian internees were administered separately from the POWs.

Late in May 1942, the hospital experienced a major problem. As they did at POW camps throughout their jurisdiction, the Japanese demanded that all prisoners, including patients, sign a warranty not to escape. As happened at most other camps, the patients and staff at Bowen Road refused to endorse such a document. The consequences promptly became evident:

SPECIAL ORDER by Lt. Colonel C.O. SHACKLETON, RAMC. Wednesday 20th May 1942. The Japanese Authorities have forbidden until further notice the playing of tennis, Mahjong, or any card game (involving more than two persons) by either patients or members of the Staff. Similarly, Music, Concerts, Dancing and Singing is prohibited. The Concert and Dance arranged for the 22nd and 28th are hereby cancelled as well as all other forms of recreation and amusement. This order is a reprisal for the refusal by RAMC Officers and Other Ranks and Members of the Nursing Staff to sign blindly an Affidavit stating that they will in no circumstance make any attempt to escape. The Japanese Guard have received orders to deal with any offenders.[30]

Ultimately, all signed, having been assured by their officers that a promise extorted under duress would not be viewed, after the war, as "collaboration" with the enemy, nor as dereliction of duty. Some escapes did take place, as will be discussed.

The medical staff, here as in other POW medical institutions, wrestled with the question of how much opposition to the enemy could be permitted. Early in captivity a prisoner named Carter operated a radio hidden behind a wall in the X-Ray Department.[31] Perhaps reluctantly, Col. Bowie ordered that the radio be dismantled. It was a mortal danger to Carter, and its discovery could possibly have led to the hospital being closed and everyone moved to the main camp.

Fortunately, all was not gloom and despondency at Bowen Road. Many irrepressible members of the RAMC staff worked hard to maintain morale in the face of the apparently implacable enemy. For example, the anonymous editor of *The Snake and Staff,* a typewritten newsletter, reported in the first issue, in January 1942, that the publication had, at "enormous expense," been printed on edible vanilla-flavoured paper. But "do not be misled and think that the colour of next month's issue will be flavoured with Chocolate." Light-hearted advertisements appear, and numerous amusing or wry anecdotes of events during the recent fighting. Several poems, often with shaky metre, were featured:

> Twinkle, twinkle, little star,
> How I wonder if there are
> Men upon your world so high
> Half as hungry as am I?

Not deathless material, but it must have uplifted the spirits of patients and staff alike. Apparently only the first number has survived—possibly only one appeared.[32]

Once the men were incarcerated in their regular camps it became almost impossible to have a sick man transferred to Bowen Road. This is yet another example of the apparently senseless inconsistencies that tormented the prisoners. Common sense would seem to dictate that if a hospital was left intact and functioning, it should treat all seriously ill POWs in the immediate area. Yet medical officers in the regular camps remember, with frustration and anger, how difficult it was to persuade the Japanese that a patient needed the more specialized care available at Bowen Road.

Frequently, surgery had to be performed in primitive surroundings at Sham Shui Po because the patient seemed likely to die due to the inordinate delay.[33] Major Crawford found it fairly easy (though often there were delays) to have men sent from North Point Camp—also on the Island—to Bowen Road; but once the Canadians were moved to Sham Shui Po this possibility vanished.[34] Bowie stated: "I recall only about four occasions in two and a half years in Bowen Road when special admissions for consultations were arranged, and of these two were for non-urgent eye conditions."[35]

Given the lack of inter-service cooperation among the Japanese, it may be possible to explain at least partially these failures to move sick men promptly, on the basis of logistical problems. It seems likely that the POW Administration had few vehicles under its control. If they had to requisition one from a reluctant military unit in Hong Kong, it is entirely believable that the requisitioned vehicle might arrive days later, or not at all. But other, less charitable, explanations are not only possible but probable—as the example of Maj. Hook shows.

As late as July 1945, Maj. Henry W. Hook, Winnipeg Grenadiers, died at Central British School. He had been ill in Sham Shui Po Camp "N" since 18 May with fever that was found to be caused by spinal meningitis. He was under the care of Capt. Arthur Strahan, IMS, who noted signs of meningeal irritation shortly after Hook became ill. A sample of cerebrospinal fluid was found to be cloudy, suggesting that the normally clear fluid was already infected. The Japanese medical officer, Saito, was told; he saw Hook and said the diagnosis was mistaken—the officer, Saito stated, had malaria.

Strahan smuggled a sample of fluid into the other camp, where there was a microscope. Later the same day he managed to slip through himself and "actually saw the organisms of meningococcal meningitis with three other doctors." Despite this information, Saito remained adamant. Strachan requested sulfapyridine to treat Hook. Saito sent an ounce of potassium permanganate.[36] Hook developed pneumonia. The medical officers tried for two weeks to get the Japanese to provide a truck to take him to Bowen Road. At the time they were using three trucks to move some paper stocks they had in camp. "They finally did give us a truck two days before he died."[37]

The medical officers at Bowen Road were forbidden to send drugs to the POW camps, though in fact much smuggling was done.[38] But inside the hospital, the medical staff had a free hand.

Fortunately, equipment for a second operating theatre at Bowen Road, in addition to a resuscitation unit, x-ray film, and a large supply of splints and surgical dressings, was transferred to the hospital just before hostilities began.[39] But Bowen Road was far from being adequately supplied, at least by North American standards. A nursing sister remembered vividly some of the deficits, many items being in short supply even before the war. One was the lowly tongue depressor. According to Kay Christie, a Canadian nursing sister who accompanied "C" Force to Hong Kong:

> They had four tongue depressors, four wooden tongue depressors, and one metal one for a whole ward. All of our boys had a sort of flu, and this was before hostilities began. The Medical Officer was going around looking at their throats and then he'd put the tongue depressor down and I'd take it and break it. After I'd broken three, the orderly, the British Army orderly said, "Sister, you don't break those....We boil them and use them again. That's a ward allotment."[40]

The chief Japanese medical officer, Capt. Saito, never established any sort of professional relationship with Bowie. The latter nevertheless believed that Saito gave them "that to which he or his commander considered we were entitled under the Geneva Convention so far as lay within his power, though he showed no tendency to do more than he need."[41]

Though Bowen Road British Military Hospital was an imperfect institution, its continued existence was a great boon to those fortunate enough to be treated there. In a picture varying between overall grey with many splashes of solid black, representing Japanese handling of POWs at Hong Kong, their action in permitting Bowen Road to continue operation is at least one substantial bright patch. A lieutenant in the Middlesex Regiment voiced, in imperfect verse, the majority opinion among the prisoners. The poem is entitled "A Prisoner's Prayer at Bowen Road":

> Lord, do not suffer me to go
> Back to the gloom of Shamshuipo

> Nor yet direct my stumbling feet
> Within the wire of Argyle Street
> Grant, Lord, that I may pack my grip
> And go aboard some friendly ship
> Bound for London or Southampton
> But, Lord, if this prayer is stamped on
> Then, I pray, make light my load
> And let me stay at Bowen Road.[42]

Bowen Road Hospital operated at its Island site until March 1945. Then the patients and a reduced medical staff were moved to Kowloon, going first to Sham Shui Po, where they remained about a month, segregated from the rest of the camp. The Bowen Road staff were told originally that they would take over Heep Yun School, which would have been unsatisfactory as a hospital; but this location was soon changed to the Central British School, near Argyle Street Camp. "This was a quite modern and airy building and was ideal as a hospital."[43] Indeed, the Central British School had been used as a hospital during December 1941, and afterwards by the Japanese. In mid-April 1945, staff and patients moved to this site and established a makeshift hospital that functioned until the end of the war. A POW in Sham Shui Po recorded the date of the move as 12 April 1945, when "there was a big shuffle in camp. All the amputees were moved to the new 'Bowen Road' at Central British School."[44]

Much detail about conditions treated at Bowen Road, medications used, and related matters, will appear in later chapters.

St Teresa's Hospital, Kowloon

St. Teresa's Hospital, Kowloon, was a new and fully equipped French Mission Hospital of 80 beds that had served usefully during the fighting. On 27 February 1942, the Japanese sent there a team of POW medical officers, medical staff, and nurses. The resident nuns had to vacate the hospital so that it could accommodate sick from Sham Shui Po and Argyle Street Officers' Camps. A Nursing Sister in the party recalled: "One day in February we were told the hospital was to be moved in an hour. We could take what we could carry and a bedding roll....We were herded into lorries and sent to Kowloon to a French hospital, St. Theresa's....We arrived in the dark and our bedding rolls were thrown out onto the pavement in the rain."[45]

The medical officers were Maj. J. Officer, RAMC; SurgLt. C.A. Jackson, RNVR; SurgLtCmdr. W.D. Gunn, RN; and SurgLtCmdr. J.A. Page, RN. A request was made for a Roman Catholic priest and a Church of England padre. The priest arrived at 6 a.m. and Catholic personnel were woken up and told to go to confession and mass. The padre arrived that evening and was ordered to stay, as he would be useful for funerals. Some Japanese did attempt to be helpful. A pay-master arrived and announced that he had brought the matron a pres-ent for Easter, but she must return it after use. "She opened the parcel which proved to contain a number of prayer books written in Norwegian, taken from the Church at the end of the road."[46]

Most of the patients came from Sham Shui Po Camp, the early ones suffering from malaria; then came terrible cases of dysentery "and we nurses were busy emptying the large commodes filled with blood and urine from those patients able to stagger out of bed."[47] Treatment meant being given rice water to drink. Later in 1942, diph-theria broke out in Sham Shui Po. There was little serum, tra-cheotomies were performed, and there were many deaths. This epi-demic is described in Chapter Six.

In August 1942 St. Teresa's was closed and the patients sent to Bowen Road (severe cases) or Sham Shui Po (lesser severity).[48] Sister Van Wart, who wrote about their precipitate arrival at St. Teresa's, found their departure even more trying: "Another ghastly moment in my life was when we were told the women were to pack and go to Stanley Civilian Internment Camp, so we had just to walk out of the hospital and leave those sick men to be nursed by mostly conscripted orderlies who were quite untrained. I learnt at the end of the war that nearly all the patients died."[49]

When a patient died at St. Teresa's, orderlies became pall bearers, and several nurses formed an honour guard to the burial site, a bare piece of ground not far from the hospital.[50] Miss McCaw recalled that they felt sorry for the deceased, but still they "could not help feeling excited" at being able to get away from the hospital briefly.

> We had some difficult times in St. Teresa's. The strutting Japanese Officer in charge of our Hospital hated the idea of being in charge of a bunch of prisoners. It was a disgrace, he felt, not being able to fight for the Emperor. He got drunk one day and came into the hospital grounds, his bandy legs encased in shiny brown boots, and being short, his long sword scraped along the ground. But of course we didn't dare show our amusement and contempt when he was around. He pulled out his razor sharp sword, and slashing at some nearby bushes, spat out 'Doctors!' then another slash and this time 'Sisters,' and yet another slash, 'Nurses.' It was most unnerving and we wondered how it would all end. Then our RAMC Sergeant Foster did a very brave thing. He walked up to the Japanese Officer, spoke softly to him, and put his arm around his shoulders and asked him to go and have a drink! To our surprise the Japanese Officer was led away and we all heaved a sigh of relief.[51]

North Point Camp

North Point Camp was situated on the Island of Hong Kong, on the northern waterfront about two miles to the west of Lye Mun Gap.

It functioned as a POW camp from 20 December 1941 until 26 September 1942. The camp comprised a number of wooden huts originally built to house the Chinese refugees who flooded into Hong Kong while escaping the war zone on mainland China.

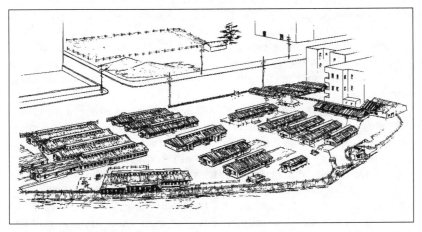

Figure 3.2. Plan of North Point POW Camp in 1942, based on exhibit from war crimes trial. (Original source: PRO WO 235/1012, Pt. 2, Exhibit L3.)

The Japanese landing on Hong Kong Island occurred near here and, as a result, the huts and other buildings were considerably damaged by shell fire. Sanitary conditions were appalling. The area had been used as a garbage dump first by the British, and later by the Japanese during the battle. The largest dump, to the west of the camp, was the garbage heap for the city of Victoria.[52] Moreover, the Japanese seem to have used portions of the camp as a stable for horses or mules, perhaps as a horse hospital, and "[b]lood-stained pads, dung and putrefying carcasses had to be cleaned away."[53] The area was thick with millions of flies, and the latrines were awash with human excrement when the first POWs arrived. They had to transform this shambles into a livable camp, with essentially no assistance from Japanese sources.

One former inmate of the camp recalled several details while being debriefed after the war:

> The camp at North Point was surrounded by a barbed wire fence about seven feet high. Some time during the Spring or early Summer of 1942, an electric fence was constructed about eighteen inches outside the barbed wire fence and was made approximately the same height as the barbed wire fence. This electric fence was about the same distance outside the barbed wire fence all the way around the camp....This fence completely encircled North Point Camp except for the area directly behind the hospital where there was no fence, the fence being anchored at both ends of the hospital building.[54]

This architectural fact played a role in a tragic escape attempt from the camp in the summer of 1942, described later.

Bugs and parasites of many kinds populated North Point Camp. The flies swarm through every man's recollections. One veteran had the smothering, nauseating sensation of almost breathing flies. They settled on every forkful of food before it could reach the mouth. Men spent their days swatting flies. At night, when flies swarmed in their millions on the rafters in the roofs of the huts, "parties would climb up, squash thick black layers of them and scrape the mess into buckets, but all efforts made not the slightest difference."[55] And this was in January, during the cold season.

In addition to flies, lice, fleas, and bedbugs were ubiquitous plagues at North Point Camp. Wherever the former residents, Chinese refugees, had gone by January 1942, they had left many millions of their travelling companions behind, waiting ravenously for their next involuntary hosts. Lt. Harry White, Winnipeg Grenadiers, noted his disgust when, just four days after arriving in North Point Camp, he found lice on his underclothing for the first time in his life.[56]

Bedbugs were especially hated. The men were unable to sleep because the bedbugs would bite all night, and in the morning one would look like a person with the measles.[57] In addition, bedbugs have a foul odour much intensified by squashing them. George Orwell recorded a method used against these pests when he encountered them in Paris in the 1930s: "Mario had told me of a sure remedy for them, namely pepper, strewed thick over the bedclothes. It made me sneeze, but the bugs all hated it, and emigrated to other rooms."[58]

Ultimately, fly-catching was ordered by the Japanese, an order that some POWs looked upon as quaint or stupid. This began as early as 6 February 1942, when it was ordered that everyone must kill his quota of flies each day.[59] The idea was not stupid, for eliminating tens of thousands of flies had to have some effect. But it may have seemed like déjà vu, at least to those older Canadians POWs who had long memories. Before World War One, about 30 years before the events chronicled here, at least three Canadian cities conducted fly-catching contests among their citizens, all with the same hygienic goal that activated the Japanese.

Edmonton, Hamilton, and Toronto all proclaimed this an official municipal activity. The Toronto *Star* co-sponsored the Fly-Catching Contest of 1912, for children under 16. By the end of the contest—terminated when it was found that some enterprising children were breeding their own flies[60]—3,367,680 squashed flies, weighing 2,758 pounds, had been counted carefully and stored in bottles in the Department of Health office. "A teen named Beatrice White was crowned the Queen of Swat after personally downing 543,360 flies. For her troubles, White won $50."[61]

At North Point Camp in Hong Kong, only some modest prizes of cigarettes were awarded. But at least the Japanese did become concerned about sanitation. They offered a packet of cigarettes for every 100 dead flies collected. They counted the flies, or made the POWs count them at first; then they decided that they would weigh them. The prisoners, predictably, started tying little weights to the flies' feet; some men bred flies in their mess tins in order to get cigarettes. Eventually the Japanese discovered this scam. The offer of cigarettes ended.

> I remember in my room, there were five of us in the room, and we had a lot of flies of course, and the chaps used to come in and say, "I will give you two cigarettes, sir, for the fly rights of this room once a week." So I said, "You come in whenever you like." He said, "While we have the fly rights, you're not to let anyone else kill any flies in this room. And you're not to kill any yourselves." I said, "No, I promise I'll do that. I'll only kill mosquitoes." They didn't like mosquitoes. They got the fly rights in payment for a couple of fags. It shows you the lengths people will go to get a cigarette. Absolutely daft![62]

Many of the men acquired parasites. Patients having anesthetics often regurgitated masses of worms, perhaps irritated by the chloroform.

The men who faced the prodigious task of making North Point livable included Canadians, British, Indians, and members of the multinational and multiracial Hong Kong Volunteer Defence Corps. Men of the Royal Engineers cleared a well so that some water was available for bathing. It would be weeks before proper latrines were functioning and, until then, 2,000 men hung their British, or Canadian, or Indian, or Chinese, or Portuguese behinds over the sea wall to empty their bowels—something almost everyone had to do with accelerating frequency as disease struck.

Soon dysentery struck, exacerbating the routine existence of dietary diarrhea. The sea itself continued to be their latrine. Ken Cambon had his first bout of bacillary dysentery at this time: "I had lots of cramps and I was holding on the fence over the wall and I looked down and there was still quite a few bodies floating by...and I thought, 'God, what's happened here!'"[63] The contrast with his relatively sheltered youth in Montreal was shocking. Some men were so weak that they had to crawl to the sea wall and tie themselves to a post to keep from vanishing into the befouled bay.

Huts with a "maximum" capacity of 50 soon held 175. Double-decker wooden bunks made it just possible for everyone to lie down at the same time. "The bunks were pushed together in pairs, and in this way seven could sleep in the floor space otherwise occupied by three—two on the top bunk, three below and two on the floor."[64]

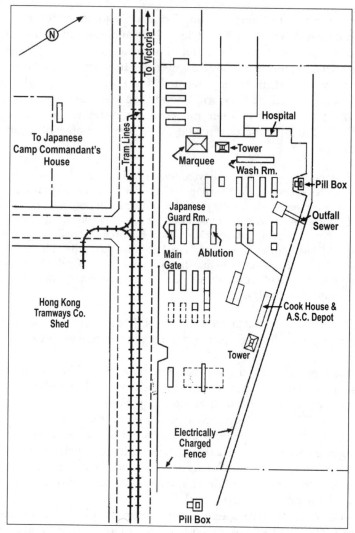

Figure 3.3. Plan of North Point POW Camp, 1942. (Derived from war crimes trial transcript, WO 235, File 1012 Part 2, Exhibit B2.)

The rations at North Point consisted of white rice, vegetables, and occasionally a little fish. Sanitary conditions and overcrowding were perhaps the worst features of the camp, while the low-vitamin, low-protein diet began to give rise to a host of deficiency diseases. Of these, the most dramatic was the so-called "happy feet" or "electric feet." Beriberi and pellagra were common.

During January 1942, the Japanese ordered that a hospital be set up in North Point itself, rather than relying on Bowen Road.[65] The need for medical facilities was obvious and urgent. A small decrepit warehouse about 30 by 40 feet was made the camp hospital. There were 12 beds, though the number of patients rose as high as 42. The roof leaked, and during rainy weather it was not uncommon to find an inch of water on the floor, with large numbers of patients lying in the water because there were not enough beds.[66] By mid-February, when one might have expected that the hospital would be functioning effectively, a patient described it in depressing terms:

> So-called hospital was an old warehouse, no windows in east or south, dank concrete walls and floor, roof supported by six huge stone columns. It reminds me of Byron's description of the prison of Chillon. There is a makeshift stove here but it will not draw, giving more smoke than heat.[67]

At first there were some medicines in the camp, but the drugs at North Point were not replenished. One medical officer noted the contents of the almost bare cupboard: magnesium sulphate in fair quantity, sulfapyridine (about 500 tablets), and sulfanilamide (about 3,000 tablets).[68] Nothing more. There were in the camp at this time more than 2,000 men, many with wounds of various kinds and most sick. No diagnostic or laboratory facilities were available.

The patients in North Point Camp hospital represented a group at some ill-defined mid-point with respect to degree of illness. Early in 1942 it was still possible to send the seriously ill to Bowen Road Hospital, while the least severely ill were, so far as possible, kept in their own barracks because of the limited number of beds available in the camp hospital.

After breakfast on 21 January 1942, all the Indian POWs were sent to Ma Tau Chung Camp in Kowloon. Two days later, POWs from the Middlesex, Royal Scots, and HKVDC were marched to the ferry, en route to Sham Shui Po. The Canadians in North Point remained there, and when the Volunteers reached the ferry wharf they saw Canadians arriving from the mainland, obviously headed for North Point.[69] On 18 April 1942, the Royal Navy POWs were moved out of North Point Camp. From this date, only the Canadians and a few Dutch mariners were left there.[70]

A major advance in camp civilization occurred on 2 February 1942: two Asian-style toilets were repaired and working.[71] Two days later, another sign of civilization appeared: classes were started. These covered a wide range of topics, including mathematics, civics, French, and many others.[72]

Nevertheless, the camp was not a happy one, even by POW standards. On 25 February 1942, R.B. Goodwin was moved from an outside hospital to North Point Camp. He was stunned at what he found:

> What had happened? Who were these broken, spiritless, dirty, slovenly, unshaven, gaunt-looking spectres who stared at us with unfriendly,

unwelcoming eyes? Could these be those same officers who had so recently looked so immaculate on the dance floor of the Hongkong hotel? Two months had passed since the last guns boomed, and that scene of demoralisation made us wonder with trepidation what conditions in the camp would be.[73]

Definitely, all was not well at North Point. Treatment by the Japanese was not especially bad, but there was increasing unrest because of what was described as the "utter selfishness" of some of the officers, who had wired themselves off in a separate compound where they enjoyed better food than the other ranks, and seemed "to care for little else than playing bridge and making petty complaints to the Japanese. There was one group which demanded gin!"[74] An RAMC officer who experienced all the Hong Kong camps wrote the following account of North Point:

> The effect of defeat and hardship on the morale of men inadequately acclimatized, whose brief military career prior to the Hong Kong campaign had been eighteen months garrison duty in the West Indies, was dramatic. For the first month demoralization was complete. There was no open insubordination but a sullen apathy, shown particularly in disregard of personal cleanliness and appearance....At this stage there were no working parties for the Japanese, and the men would spend their days lounging around the corners of huts, the only subject of conversation being food.[75]

Because of the reference to garrison duty in the West Indies, this passage must refer to the Winnipeg Grenadiers. Happily, that regiment gradually regained its morale. Nor, as will become evident, was it the only unit coping with demoralization.

Despite these problems, one young Canadian rifleman found North Point Camp relatively congenial. He discovered a spirit of cooperation and discipline that did not exist in later camps, particularly in Japan, where he encountered a "dog eat dog" attitude.[76] Perhaps his memory of North Point is from a time later than that of the demoralization described here.

The negative view the POWs had of the Japanese, initiated by the then routine anti-Asian prejudice and pre-war and wartime propaganda, was accentuated, often ineradicably, in these early days in the camps. Most hadn't seen their comrades butchered in the hills of Hong Kong Island or at St. Stephen's College, nor the brutal rape of nurses, but they had all heard of these atrocities.

The more thoughtful among them might have been able to understand, if not excuse, some of these atrocities as battlefield excesses. But at North Point their education in Japanese callous brutality continued. Allister has written how, one cold night, he watched a naked Chinese woman die slowly after being raped in the guardroom.[77] This was not the rage of battle; it was lust and brutality indulged in weeks after the fighting ended. Another Canadian at North Point saw similar cruelties:

> One night I was looking through a crack in the wall and I saw the guards beating a man. Then they tied him up and continued beating him. Then they untied him and stuck a bayonet through him and threw the body into the harbour....Then the two guards took turns taking shots at the body and clapped each other on the back when they hit it. That's how much life was valued by them.[78]

Similarly, at Sham Shui Po, one member of the HKVDC watched a Formosan guard shoot a Chinese girl who came too near the camp, searching for shellfish along the beach. She lay "twitching in the mud for nearly half an hour before he put another bullet through her head."[79]

Sham Shui Po

Sham Shui Po[80] (which means Deep Water Market) is a district in northwestern Kowloon as well as the name of a permanent British military encampment and, from the last days of 1941 till August 1945, a POW camp.

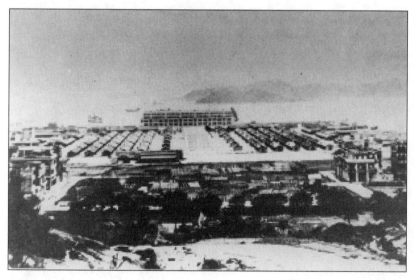

Figure 3.4. Aerial view of Sham Shui Po Camp, Jubilee Buildings in the background. (Frank Evans, *Roll Call at Oeyama*, 1985.)

James Bertram described Sham Shui Po as it was just before the war began at the end of 1941:

> The camp lay between the hills and the sea, on a reclaimed harbor flat scored by deep typhoon drains. The whole area had formerly been used

as a British military barracks. There was room for several thousand men; and the general design of the camp was not bad—two large gravel parade grounds at either end, and two broad surfaced avenues shaped in cruciform. Everything reflected the sort of military mind that delights in chessboard uniformity—the barrack huts, spaced as rigidly as tent lines, were long low affairs with concrete floors. A freak amid all this severity was a fantastic four-storey block of flats that rose like a mirage along the water front. Known as Jubilee Buildings, it had originally been built by an enterprising Indian speculator, who had sold it (at a good profit) to the army for use as officers' quarters.[81]

Actually, the builder of the Jubilee Buildings was Sir Thomas Ho Tung, the project being part of a housing development begun in 1925.[82] The Jubilee Buildings were the best-made structures at Sham Shui Po. The buildings were large, relatively modern, three-storied (by the European style which numbers floors above the main or ground floor), made of concrete, and with wide verandas.

The huts were wooden but built to withstand the high winds and stresses of typhoons. The rafters were trusses of Oregon timber. Soon, the POWs removed every second rafter. The timber split easily and made excellent fuel.[83]

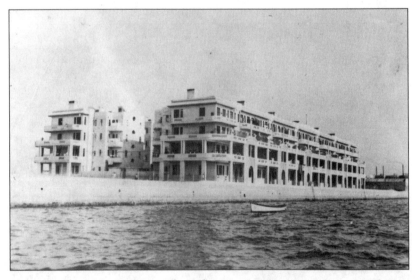

Figure 3.5. The Jubilee Buildings, Sham Shui Po, taken in 1941 just before war began. (Courtesy of Mr. Peter Kifford, Crawley, UK.)

The initial impression the men had as they approached Sham Shui Po for the first time as POWs was of space and order. The buildings appeared substantial, and grass and trees had survived. But as they came closer the picture changed abruptly. The barracks had been an early target of the Japanese air force, and bombs had perforated the

Jubilee Buildings from corner to corner. Many of the huts had been gutted. As numerous diarists attest, the ravages of looters, who had swarmed into the camp after the British garrison withdrew from Kowloon, were unbelievable. The prisoners found only the brick or timber shells of buildings. They had to improvise doors and windows as best they could, and they slept on the concrete floors.

Maj. H.G.G. Robertson, RAMC, who arrived as a POW at Sham Shui Po on 30 December 1941, adds more detail: "All the windows and doors, taps, and electrical fittings had been torn off. There were no latrines, nor any means of digging them, and the only water source was a tap on one side of the parade ground."[84]

Lt. Harry White was at Sham Shui Po immediately after the surrender, before being sent to North Point Camp. He recorded in his diary for 30 December 1941 some of the concerns that affected many groups of newly captured POWs, presaging the depressed state of the men already referred to at North Point:

> We are working hard to get things organized but a lot of the men are letting go—their morale has broken and discipline is difficult to enforce. With the Canadians it's not too bad as we Platoon Officers are working pretty close with our men and on the whole getting cooperation. There is a little mutinous talk but we shall bring them round. It's quite a job trying to make some men realize they must do certain things for their own good.[85]

Two days later, the Japanese brought 30 pigs into the camp, producing a positive if temporary impact on morale.[86]

The daily schedule at Sham Shui Po called for reveille at 6:30, 7:00, or 7:30 a.m., depending on the season. Morning muster parade was at 8:00 a.m., breakfast at 8:30, and medical examination at 10:00 a.m. Dinner was served at 12:30 p.m., "Conveyance of Order" at 4:00, supper (again depending on season of year) at 5:30, 6:00, or 6:30. Evening muster parade was held one hour after supper. Lights Out was at 9:30 or 10:00 p.m.[87]

By late January, when the Canadians had been moved to North Point Camp and the HKVDC and the British consolidated in Sham Shui Po, some order had begun to appear. But self-preservation was a major drive, and for some men this meant survival at the expense of others. Bosanquet was one of those who moved into camp from North Point. The first night in Sham Shui Po was a nightmare: "I had almost everything I possessed stolen. When you have almost nothing, it is very precious....It cast me into depths of despair. It was that act that sparked in me the first seeds of the need to get out."[88] Ultimately he was one of the few Europeans who escaped successfully.

Theft within the camp was all too common, especially in the early weeks. It became the practice to assign two men to look after each hut.

These men would rush to the huts at the end of the Japanese roll call, before the remainder of the POWs, who had to march off. This was done to discourage men from other huts taking short-cuts through, stealing blankets and other belongings on the way.[89]

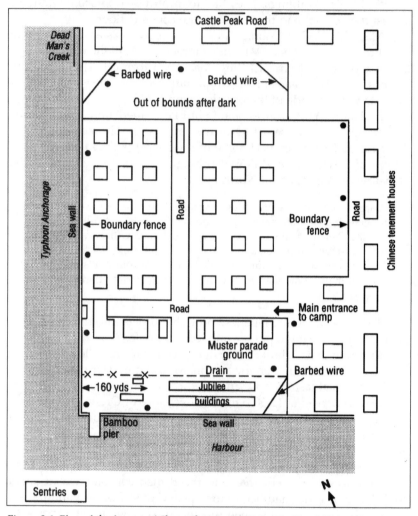

Figure 3.6. Plan of the layout of Sham Shui Po POW Camp, Hong Kong. (Based on a sketch in David Bosanquet, *Escape Through China* (London: Robert Hale, 1983).

Some officers stole, setting a demeaning example for the men. A few officers took articles to sell, and one or two, Goodwin thought, may have been court-martialled at Sham Shui Po for stealing watches.[90] No additional documentation seems to have survived about these events. But this is by no means the only instance of stealing by officers. Dr. Isaac Newton noted, at Argyle Street Camp, that after a group of officers left the camp he checked the store of tinned food and found that three tins had been taken, plus a packet of darning needles that they had brought from Queen Mary Hospital. "The IMS Major says that in his hospital the British soldiers actually stole the ward sister's tea when she was away."[91]

Just as at North Point Camp, at Sham Shui Po poor morale was a major problem. One British POW remembered vividly a stern lecture, late in January 1942, by the senior officer to the officers and NCOs; it became an embarrassingly "frantic appeal for unity, discipline, regard for sanity and respectfulness." It would be a scandal, the officer concluded, if he had to turn men over to the Japanese for punishment.[92]

One problem that occurred occasionally was that some POWs literally could not understand each other. Accents often grated against the unaccustomed ear. Not all took it as philosophically as an Aussie in Japan: "Ian Doherty remarked: 'George Keil (Royal Scots) has been very friendly with the Australians. A happy and welcome diversion. It is difficult to interpret some of his remarks, but, if we can learn Japanese surely we should soon learn Scottish.'"[93]

Ingenious and sometimes bizarre rumours proliferated fantastically, and inevitably they affected morale also. In May 1942, the reigning rumour was that Queen Elizabeth had had a son and heir.[94] This happy event did not occur then, or ever. Bugs interested in a diet of human flesh and blood were not limited to North Point Camp. At Sham Shui Po a Royal Navy POW had his worst night ever; the bugs attacked in thousands. "Had no sleep before reveille at 0600 and used a whole box of matches trying to burn them off. As soon as bed was clear and I lay down they would start again. All huts affected in the same way."[95]

In April 1942, medical inspection revealed that some of the Royal Scots were lousy.[96] They were not alone in their affliction, which was routine in camps throughout the Far East; washing facilities and the supply of soap were almost invariably insufficient.

Interpreter Watanabe Kiyoshi, a sympathetic Japanese throughout the long years of imprisonment, was acutely aware of the need for a delousing centre at Sham Shui Po. He told his biographer that the worst of those who were infested often had lumps of living matter hanging in such places as under the armpits. "Other men," he said, "got sick at the sight of the flesh sagging from the weight of the heaving lice."[97]

Later, in Senryo Camp in Japan, at Nagasaki, POWs discovered an ecological fact that served them well: fleas eliminate lice. Fleas suck the blood of lice, thus killing them, before going on to attack their human host.[98]

Because the electrical system at Sham Shui Po had been destroyed, at least as much by Chinese looters removing electrical wiring and fixtures as by bombing and shelling, electricity was a rare luxury. Indeed, no power whatever was available until 10 March 1942, when the electricity finally became marginally operative.[99] Once rough wiring had been restored for widely spaced low-wattage bulbs, ingenious POWs fashioned water heaters from bared wires, on occasion short-circuiting the entire camp system. The apparatus was ingenious but potentially dangerous:

> A wooden frame, some 24" by 18" of 2" by 1" was covered on one face by an asbestos sheet scrounged from the hut walls. Old heavy gauge wire netting was unraveled, straightened and formed into coils around a broomstick or thinner rod. The requisite number of coils, found by trial and error, were connected in series across nails spaced about 2" apart along the long side of the frames, the two ends hooked into the mains. Accompanied by flashes and weird humming noises the system would warm up as the zinc from the galvanising burnt off the wire with pretty green flames. Soon the coils would be red-hot—in places—and cooking could begin. Sometimes a pot would accidentally fall or 'short' the coils; with the result that the whole apparatus would become a welded mass.[100]

One POW recognized how annoying these gadgets were for the Japanese. As fast as they were confiscated, the POWs made others. "I feel that the Japanese were really most patient in this regard."[101] They might well have made the inevitable power failures reason for brutal retribution; they did not.

In March 1942, the Japanese gave permission for a canteen to be opened. Once the limited supply of money in camp was used up, the canteen was viewed as unhelpful, for the items seemed largely useless and expensive. It did, however, sell cigarettes; once the men began to labour for the Japanese, outside the camp, and thus earn small sums, much of the money apparently was spent on cigarettes.[102] For most, the smokes were a small comfort and solace. But for a few they became a menace, as we will see in Chapter Five.

Once, a senior Japanese officer inspected the camp. The POWs formed up, and three hours later he arrived. By then, many had fainted from fatigue and hunger. After the inspection the men were issued with soap, a razor-blade, a tooth-brush, and a small towel, all free of charge,[103] items needed desperately because most POWs had lost their personal kit. The tedious wait had been worthwhile.

After the closing of St. Teresa's Hospital, patients requiring hospitalization at Sham Shui Po had to be treated within the camp. Rarely could a patient be sent to Bowen Road Hospital on the Island. Though the barracks at Sham Shui Po were built long before the war, there had never been a hospital on site.[104] Space had to be found within Sham Shui Po for this vital activity, further overcrowding the camp.

In September 1942, when the Canadians returned to their pre-war barracks area at Sham Shui Po, they brought with them their own medical system, which functioned largely independently of the existing arrangement that provided care for the two British regiments and for the HKVDC. Indian Medical Service personnel cared for the Indian POWs at Ma Tau Chung Camp.

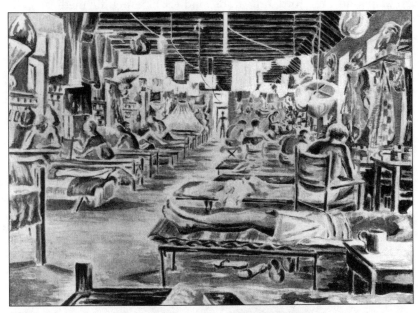

Figure 3.7. Interior of barracks at Sham Shui Po POW Camp, 1944. (From A.V. Skvorzov, *Chinese Ink and Brush Sketches of Prisoner of War Camp Life in Hong Kong, 25 December 1941-30 August 1945*, A.V. Skvorzov, 1945.)

Six weeks after they were moved to Sham Shui Po, Harry White was appalled at the state of the new Canadian "hospital" there, which he thought was no better than the ramshackle affair at North Point. "Just one of the huts, makeshift doors and windows, blanket up for blackout, two small lights. It's a hell of a place. Filthy, no room to work on the patients—two or three may be lying dead for hours. All cases in the same building, Dysentery as well. The stench in the place is terrific from sores, dysentery, sweaty bodies, etc."[105] But this was no worse than the "hospital" used by the British.

So poorly supplied and so overcrowded were the hospitals that the men quickly adopted attitudes combining resignation, cynicism, and despair. Some fatalistically minded POWs began to avoid the hospital early in captivity, resulting in an official statement recorded in May 1942, by W.T. Carden: "An order issued today says that men must not refrain from reporting sick because they know there are no medicines and therefore can get no treatment, as they may have an illness which may spread an epidemic through the camp and therefore must be isolated from their fellows."[106]

Saito Shunkishi was the senior Japanese medical officer for the Hong Kong POW camps. He failed to provide appropriate medical attention, as will be detailed in regard to the epidemic of diphtheria that ravaged the camp during 1942. He was notorious for having beaten Maj. John Crawford, on parade, and for blaming the medical staff, doctors, and orderlies, for the high rates of illness and death.

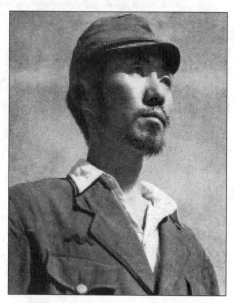

Figure 3.8. Capt. Saito Shunkishi, IJA, formerly senior medical officer at POW headquarters, Hong Kong, ca. 1946. (Photo loaned by Norman Leath.)

Dr. Saito graduated from the Kyoto Prefectural Medical School in spring 1940. He joined the army on 15 May 1940 with the rank of sergeant. On 28 January 1942 he arrived in Hong Kong as the senior medical officer in the prisoner-of-war camps there.[107] Saito was then a full lieutenant and in medical charge of some 10,000 prisoners of war. He called at the various camps perhaps once every three months. Customarily he stayed for about 10 minutes, or just long enough to refuse all requests—whichever was the shorter time—according to Capt. Woodward, IMS.

> It was hazardous to insist on any points with him as he was prone to slap one in the face and leave in a huff which resulted in some further privations for the sick. He had been subdued and partly trained by Ashton-Rose and as a result regarded Evans and me [Woodward] with a slightly less jaundiced eye due to our association with Ashton at the Lower 'Hospital' and to us fell the rather delicate task of dealing with this savage creature, on the rare occasion of his visit.[108]

Woodward saw "the good Dr. Saito" for the last time on 29 April 1944, the day Woodward embarked for Japan. Saito laughed heartily when Woodward pleaded with him to return his copy of Boyd's Pathology, which he had found and removed from Woodward's kit.

> He said I would have no time for study when I got to Japan where every-one must work. When I told him that I was most concerned to have Medical books to study so that my years of imprisonment would not be entirely wasted he pointed out that I need not concern myself about it as we should all be kept as slaves till we died after Japan had won the war.[109]

Saito was sentenced to death after his war crimes trial in 1946–47, for crimes allegedly carried out in all the camps at Hong Kong. Ultimately, his sentence was commuted to 20 years at hard labour and, given the general commutations that took place in the early 1950s, he probably served little of that term.

Saito's reputation was bad, but some of his staff were capable of human gestures:

> He had a corporal, Dolyama, I remember quite well, who was very kind to me personally. He was quite a stickler over things, but he used to buy me tobacco outside and bring it in occasionally. I gave him money for it of course; he was very good like that, and quite an amusing little man....He used to come in and tell you when you were going to be inspected, and said, "Oh you must splash around with lysol and every-thing around the door, put soap in it and all this, to show the people we are very clean and good." You know, put on a bit of a show. But he never whacked you or anything like that, where Saito was quite prepared to give you a sharp slap.[110]

By mid-1942, drafts of men began leaving for Japan to help offset the critical labour shortage there, caused by massive inductions into the armed forces. In September a draft was ordered. After these men departed there was then room for all the Canadians to be moved to Sham Shui Po on 26 September. North Point Camp was closed.

One event, on 25 October 1942, gave the Hong Kong POWs great joy. On this Sunday afternoon Allied bombers attacked targets in Hong Kong for the first time. The effect on the Japanese was uncertain, though high casualties were rumoured. The effect on the POWs was dramatic. Morale soared. At last the war was being carried to the enemy before their very eyes.[111] Hong Kong had not been forgotten.

What they could not have known and, cynically, might have dis-believed if they had, was that the Canadian government had not for-gotten them either. Vance has suggested that Canada devoted as much effort to the problems of its Far Eastern POW nationals as it did to those in Europe.[112] But dealing with the Japanese was far more difficult that dealing with Germany. For example, it was not until June 1943 that the Canadian government, after many diplomatic exchanges, obtained a presumably complete list of the names of its Hong Kong POWs.[113]

Throughout the last half of 1942, medical problems in Sham Shui Po became progressively worse. The diphtheria epidemic was still severe (see Chapter Six). More and more men were dying of dysentery and the complications of malnutrition and starvation (see Chapter Five). On 22 November 1942, a Canadian officer wrote: "The deaths in camp are terrible, very bad for morale. Stopped blowing Last Post in camp. The poor lads in hospital lie and wonder if their turn will be next."[114]

One month later, on 21 December 1942, the International Committee for the Red Cross (ICRC) was permitted to visit the camp for the first time. Afterwards the Delegate, C.A. Kengelbacher, described Sham Shui Po in rather more neutral terms than the POWs might have used. This camp, situated on the Kowloon peninsula facing the bay opposite Hong Kong Island, with mountains at the rear, "consists of 132 [*sic*] stone/mortar buildings, mostly single storied, on level ground, very sunny location, plenty of light. It includes kitchen, bakery, canteen and storehouse. Most of this site was formerly used by the British army."[115] It is only fair to note that this was only a small portion of his report. Moreover, outspoken criticism by the Red Cross was counterproductive. The Japanese read all ICRC reports, so the Swiss had to be circumspect; if they were not, access could, and probably would, be denied in the future and thus they would be unable to do anything whatever to aid the prisoners.

The sufferings of Far Eastern POWs were intensified by the failure of the Japanese to permit individual Red Cross food parcels to be delivered to the prisoners. Unlike the camps in Europe, where, except for the last months of the war, parcels were received almost weekly, most of the men at Hong Kong and the other areas held by Japan saw no more than at most, five or six parcels throughout the entire period of captivity.[116]

The few Red Cross parcels that were received made a real difference in the lives of the men. One shipment arrived 4 September 1944: "We got two more parcels and part of one. The distribution has been well-handled this time. Maj. Crawford, Cndn. Sr. MO, in charge."[117] On 27 February 1945, all Canadians received packages that included large quantities of cigarettes. These were a much sought-after substitute for money, and diary entries for some time after were filled with the dietary and morale-building benefits of having the extra food they could now trade for.[118]

But some of the Red Cross material was diverted to other, illegal, uses. This became a significant factor in several of the war crimes trials held in 1946 and 1947. For example, on 27 May 1943, a diarist recorded:

"The Compradore told us that Red Cross bacon was selling down in town at 5.00 Yen a small tin—the bastards, where is it coming from?"[119]

Within the camp, conditions worsened slowly and inexorably. Everyone was ill to some degree, many severely. And brave men attempted to alleviate the condition of their fellow prisoners, often at deadly risk. One of these was F/L Hector Gray, RAF. Imprisoned in Sham Shui Po Camp until removed by the Japanese, Gray died in Stanley Prison, Hong Kong, 18 December 1943. He was awarded the George Cross posthumously, and this citation was promulgated:

> Flight Lieutenant Gray was taken prisoner in Hong Kong in December 1941 and while in captivity he did all he could to sustain the morale of his fellow prisoners. He smuggled much-needed drugs into the camp and distributed them to those who were seriously ill, and he also ran a news service on information he received from people outside the camp. He was tortured continually over a period of nearly six months to make him divulge the names of his informants, but he disclosed nothing, and was finally executed by the Japanese.[120]

On 20 August 1943, all remaining officers above the rank of major incarcerated in Sham Shui Po (including some medical officers) were moved to the Argyle Street Camp.[121] (The most senior officers had been moved to Argyle Street Camp in 1942.) Presumably, one reason was to prevent further attempts such as Gray's to provide a focus of leadership. At Argyle Street they joined the large contingent of fellow officers who had been moved there months earlier.

For those who had relatives or friends among the civilian population in Hong Kong, some improvement in supplies of food and clothing was possible. The Japanese appointed a day each week on which gift parcels could be delivered to individual POWs. The arrangement could be cancelled, and often was, in retaliation for offences real or suspected. When the system worked it did much to sustain those fortunate enough to obtain such parcels. But the Canadians had been in the colony for only three weeks before the fighting began. Dr. Selwyn Selwyn-Clarke managed to obtain the names of all six thousand POWs in Sham Shui Po Camp, including the survivors of the two Canadian regiments. The solution worked out by Selwyn-Clarke was to arrange contacts for the Canadians by proxy among his numerous helpers. "Supplies of food, vitamins, soap and other articles for the camps in Kowloon were stored for me nearby by Dr. T.J. Hua, in charge of the Kwong Wah Hospital, who was to be repaid for his staunch co-operation by a spell of imprisonment."[122]

The Japanese permitted a system of weekly parcel deliveries, so that many of the men were supplied with extra food throughout the war. Some members of the British and Indian regiments who had been in Hong Kong for substantial periods of time had established liaisons or marriages with local women, including often "Wan Chai girls" of possibly malleable virtue, and thus had the same advantages. Many of these liaisons were formalized by proxy marriages, ceremonies that must have had at least two motivations, one being genuine emotional attachment, the other a recognition that invaluable food parcels could result. Some of the marriages were conducted by Captain the Reverend Eric John Green, a padre imprisoned with the men.[123]

Once the Japanese approved the principle that individually addressed parcels could enter the camp, a system was established. Periodically, deliveries were suspended temporarily as retaliation for some POW transgression, but in general a woman could bring her man a parcel once a month.

On the appointed day, Chinese and mixed-race women carried parcels in sacks to the Sham Shui Po and Argyle Street camps. Similar groups trudged with the precious supplies up the hillside to Bowen Road Military Hospital on the Island. Public transport had vanished, so the women had to walk to the camp. For those living on the Island, it is about three miles from the Star Ferry Terminal to Sham Shui Po. Hard work, carrying a parcel of any size and, often, trailing children. Favoured items were brown sugar, and almost anything that would not spoil and that might convey some palatable flavour to the endless, insipid boiled rice. Clothing was much valued also. These volunteers were organized and accompanied by Mrs. Selwyn-Clarke, widely known as "Red Hilda," both because of her hair colour and her politics.

Here the name of Helen Ho must be mentioned also, for she played a major role in organizing parcels of food and clothing—both openly and clandestinely—for POWs in the Hong Kong camps. Miss Ho had been a kindergarten teacher until the war began. After the capitulation the Japanese closed the schools. During the fighting she had done some nursing at LaSalle College temporary hospital. There she met Dr. Selwyn-Clarke, who later persuaded her to become involved in aiding POWs once it became apparent that their life was going to be extremely difficult. Once the Japanese decided to permit it, food parcels were sent in to Sham Shui Po, 12 each week. If the intended recipient did not pick up the parcel, usually because he had died, it came back and then would be sent to another name on a list of Allied POWs. This list included names of Canadians.

Helen Ho's involvement became major and, should the Japanese have found out, probably lethal. Drugs had to be smuggled in. They were put in 555 cigarette tins, which were flat. She or others gave them to Rev. "Uncle Jon" Watanabe, IJA interpreter, who carried them into the camps. After the war, Miss Ho was awarded the MBE for her bravery and determination. Later she went to England, studied social work, and followed that profession as her post-war career. She died in the 1990s.

Another woman who assisted in these efforts was the flamboyant Emily "Mickie" Hahn, who had a daughter by Maj. Charles Boxer just before the war began, and who remained in Hong Kong until 1943, trying to find ways to help her wounded lover, by then a POW. Hahn was recruited by the Selwyn-Clarkes. Though terrified of the potential for disaster and its likely impact on her infant daughter, the American journalist helped to carry black market items into internment camps.[124] After the war, Mickie Hahn Boxer received a certificate from Hong Kong recognizing her efforts.[125]

In late January 1943, the Canadian hospital was moved to different huts in Sham Shui Po. This was part of a reshuffling within the camp after the dispatch of a large draft to Japan, including 663 Canadians, on 19 January. The new hospital was in huts on the north west side of the camp. The patients had more room, though it was depressingly dark. Three weeks later the Japanese finally provided some glass for windows,[126] which until then had been boarded up against the winter chill and rain.

On a quite different theme, we have one brief fashion note from this camp. On 7 April 1943, Harry White wrote in his diary: "Had my hair all off, common practice here, cool and clean. We look like hell though."[127]

Questionable Behaviour by Allied Pows

There is voluminous evidence of cooperative and helpful behaviour among the inmates of Allied POW camps in the Far East. The closest ties were within combines of two to six men who banded together for mutual support; often these combines comprised men from the same military unit. On a larger scale there was inevitably inter-regimental rivalry, sometimes intense and even destructive, and equally inevitably there were inter-racial and inter-national antagonisms. But in large measure the POWs united, with varying degrees of cohesion, against the common enemy.

In a few instances, however, Allied POWs acted to the real detriment of other POWs. As noted, theft occurred among the POWs. Stealing from their captors was considered desirable, necessary, and even patriotic. But theft from other POWs was regarded as particularly heinous. Yet petty theft, both from their fellows and from the Japanese, was common.[128]

More sinister were instances of collaboration with the enemy, sometimes unquestionably real and deliberate, sometimes unintended or thoughtless and largely innocent, and sometimes unproven. Informers were a remarkably common problem. A Royal Navy POW wrote a withering comment on one type of collaborator, adding a post-war observation to his diary entry for 1 March 1944:

Unfortunately we did not know all informers; they were mostly Imperial troops who had done at least one tour of duty in H.K. and married local girls. Their object to be allowed to remain in H.K. was to receive food parcels and thus survive. There was nothing sacred to these warped bastards and good men died as a result of their treachery. They were organised as a H.Q. group under Major Boon, R.A.S.C., who ran the camp for the Japs.[129]

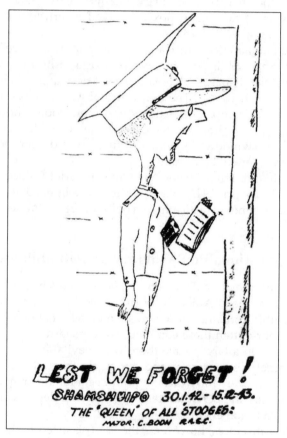

Figure 3.9. Cartoon-style drawing of Maj. Cecil Boon, RASC. Caption: "Lest we forget! Shamshuipo 30.1.42-15.12.43. The 'Queen' of all 'Stooges.' Maj. C. Boon R.A.S.C." (Imperial War Museum MS 85/42/1, Papers of CSM R.A. Edwards.)

On 18 April 1942, the Japanese gave orders for all officers to move within an hour. Almost all officers except MOs were sent to Argyle Street Camp. Boon was left in charge of the camp.[130] Some weeks later, Alsey, an NCO in the Royal Scots, took charge of a work detail under Maj. "Cissy" Boon, as he was known among the POWs. Alsey thought Boon acted and looked like a stage-hall English officer, and had to leave him "ere I spewed my disgust up."[131] In September Alsey reported, in continuing disgust, that a naval Petty Officer had been confined to quarters for 10 days for not saluting Boon.[132]

Maj. Cecil Boon, according to a fellow officer, had been an army dancing champion before the war, an avocation that might not have raised his status among the troops. At Sham Shui Po, Boon was suspected of being more or less a self-appointed liaison officer with the Japanese. Most of the POWs despised him. He was remembered as a dapper figure, well dressed, invariably wearing dark glasses. During the early days he appeared to have a generous supply of dollars. [133]

Dr. Coombes didn't think that Boon was a vicious man, or working against the POWs deliberately, or that he was particularly pro-Japanese. He was merely a mouthpiece for them, apparently agreeing immediately to follow their orders and passing them on to the men. "He didn't make a fuss about it, which a lot of people thought he ought to have done, he ought to have stood up to the Japanese and refused. He'd only have been beaten up, mind you. But he was not a great character at all, a forceful character in any way."[134]

The Japanese transmitted all their orders through Boon. If there was to be a parade and search, the purpose being to get everybody out on the parade ground while they searched all the huts, Boon gave those orders. "I suppose he couldn't avoid having to do that, but he had a very thin time after the war, I believe. I think there was some prosecution."[135] In fact, Boon was court-martialled—and exonerated.

Some of the friction in the camp related less to collaboration than to corruption. The kitchen and anything to do with food handling was the source of many complaints. Billings recorded a row in camp in the middle of August 1944: "Fish came in to-day; they smacked it into a boiler and made fish soup as a way out. One of the stooges, however, saw the staff frying their own. Case going to Japs."[136] Lt. Harry White commented on the same sorry event, with the cooks having "a little feast on their own."[137] Everyone knew that this had happened and it was bitterly resented by all.

Two weeks later, one of the kitchen workers was caught selling rice to the Japanese. At least one 220-lb (100 kg) sack had disappeared, "to say nothing of oil, M & V, bully and beans over the last six months. He was fined ¥ 200 by Japs. Money was paid out of amenities fund to which we were asked to contribute ¥ 2 each last week. He was not even placed on a charge, because so many, including officers, were involved. What a camp!"[138] Obviously, discontent seethed in Sham Shui Po, where unhappiness and suspicion constantly surrounded the acquisition and distribution of food.

Another source of dissension, sometimes implicit, often explicit in many writings about this period, has to do with the different treatment accorded officers compared to the enlisted men. Much bitterness marks some of the writings, and it positively resonates throughout

Will Allister's novel, *A Handful of Rice*, based upon his experiences at Hong Kong.[139]

How wide was the gap? Sheer survival is perhaps the most fundamental measure. And some figures are available. For example, in the Royal Australian Navy, 39 officers and 342 ratings were captured, the vast majority in the Far East. Of these, 6 officers and 113 ratings died in captivity (5 officers and 4 ratings executed) and 33 officers and 229 ratings came home. This works out to a mortality among officers, excluding those executed, of $1/34$ (2.9%); in the ratings, $109/338$ (35%). Including those executed the figures are $6/39$ (15%), and $113/342$ (33%). These data suggest that being an officer enhanced one's likelihood of survival.[140] One possible contributory reason is that, in general, officers did not have to work.

Joan Beaumont has compiled similar data with respect to the Australians of "Gull Force." The survivors of this group were imprisoned on the islands of Ambon and Hainan between early 1942 and the end of the war. Of 21 captains and lieutenants, 4 died in captivity (19%); of 103 NCOs, 64 died (62%); and of 404 privates, 304 died (75.2%!). Among those sent to Hainan, no officers died, 6 of 43 NCOs, and 56 of 204 privates.[141] One message at least seems clear from reading these figures.

Similar computations can be made for the Canadians at Hong Kong. Of 94 officers, 27 had died by 1945, or 29 percent; of 1879 Other Ranks, 530 died, or 28 percent. This seems democratic enough. But if the deaths are broken down into deaths by or as a result of battle and deaths in POW camps, the figures change dramatically. Twenty-four percent of all Canadian officers died in battle or of wounds, 5.6 percent of the survivors died while POWs. For the men these figures are 14 percent and 16 percent. Thus the officers had high fatality rates in battle but low rates afterwards, suggesting that as prisoners they fared significantly better than their men.[142] And this finding would reinforce the bitterness that continues to be felt by many ex-POWs, half a century after the war and their imprisonment ended.

One source of discontent among Other Ranks related to their understanding as to how Allied POWs *ought* to behave while in captivity. Carden wrote in his diary in February 1942 that the POWs were being smartened up, under orders purporting to come from the Japanese but which the men suspected originated with their own officers. These related to conduct on parade, general bearing, dress, and saluting. He admitted that parades had become better "as the chaps stand still and do not talk or wander about so much. This, of course, is contrary to what prisoners should do as we understood it was our duty to cause the enemy as much trouble as possible." But the orders were given by their own officers, who awarded punishments for infringements of discipline on these parades. One of their captains was "more than the usual type of pig, and that the vast majority of our offi-cers are either boys, old men or bloody fools."[143] Later that spring Alsey recorded that the CO of the Royal Scots attended drill parade and "nattered" all the time. "He wants pukka depot stuff, and in these circumstances. I reiterate—he's a doddering old twat."[144]

Some inmates of the camp were disappointed that the great majority accepted their prison life and appeared to be contented with it; most seem never to have entertained serious thoughts of attempting escape or to have wished to take part in further hostilities. "No doubt this was largely, if not in many cases entirely, due to the lead set by the senior officers, who were so strong in their determination that no one should attempt to escape."[145]

One officer's mind-set about escaping comes through in a diary entry from 1944: "Awful trouble on Monday as one fellow, quite with-out consultation etc I think—walked out on Sunday night and has apparently got away with it....It has had a lot of repercussions—no newspapers!! a sad blow...it has lead [sic] to a lot of difficulties with sentries and we have to have an officer on duty all night in each hut, and several odd counts up during the night."[146] Personal inconven-ience seems the dominant concern here. Lt.Cmdr. R.B. Goodwin, RNZNVR, escaped the night of 16–17 July, 1944.[147]

Periodically, goods were brought in for the so-called "canteen," largely benefiting the officers because only they had money. When cheese, jam, or chocolate came in, these items were snapped up by the officers. One NCO observed that he had yet to see an officer with beriberi or pellagra like the other ranks had.[148] It was clear that some officers did use their status to assure themselves better living condi-tions than those endured by their men, as would be affirmed by the man whose iron bed was taken from him for an officer who had entered the camp.[149] Other instances of real or apparent inequality will be cited throughout these pages.

Argyle Street Camp

The former Nationalist Chinese Soldiers' Internment Camp in Argyle Street became Argyle Street POW Camp at the end of 1941. It was located in Kowloon, on the land between Argyle Street and Prince Edward Road West, abutting on Lomond Street to the west. At that time the area was largely open country. Forfar Road, where the IJA Prisoner-Of-War Headquarters was located, is one block further west. The camp is 600 metres east of Kai Tak Airport. Argyle Street Camp still existed, though unoccupied, as recently as 1995. Three kilometres east was Sham Shui Po camp.

It is necessary to return to the time of the fighting in December 1941, to provide a chronological account of this camp. On Christmas Eve 1941, Dr. Isaac Newton and three colleagues—Drs. Uttley,

Hargreaves, and Gozano—apparently the first captured medical officers, were moved to this camp. About 950 British, Canadian, and Indian troops were there already, about 150 wounded. The medical officers had no operating theatre, no instruments, little in the way of wound dressings, few drugs, and no nurses. They dressed wounds as best they could, carrying on at night by candlelight.[150]

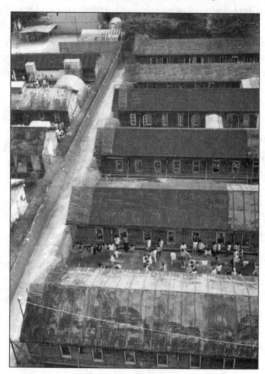

Figure 3.10. The former Argyle Street POW Camp, Kowloon, Hong Kong, still in use when this photograph was taken, 8 September 1987. (Photograph by the author.)

In the next few days, Captains S. Martin Banfill, RCAMC, and L.W. Ashton-Rose, IMS, arrived.[151] For Banfill this was a significant event, an exchange from a state of constantly pending but regularly deferred execution to the profoundly more desirable status of just another imprisoned medical officer.

Most of their patients had been wounded a week or more before and still had their original dressings. The MOs were amazed at how well the majority of them were doing. Fortunately most injuries were from rifle bullets and hand grenades, with few bomb and shell splinters.[152] The latter injuries were much more destructive of human tissue and therefore more difficult to treat, even with adequate medical facilities.

Newton was forced by the appalling conditions and scanty supplies to go back to fundamental methods and practices:

> The suffering is awful and we can do hardly anything to relieve it, it is a most awful feeling of helplessness and there is so much to be done that we can't do it all or anything like all. We have no nurses....You can't walk through the ward without men calling out to you for one thing or another but they never complain and some of them must be suffering terrible pain. Tomorrow we are going to start operating on them but it will be pretty primitive surgery I'm afraid....We had another batch of about 60 prisoners brought in today so we must total very nearly a thousand men in barracks built for 300 Chinese.[153]

Gradually, some order was introduced by the Japanese. On 28 December 1941, 200 relatively fit soldiers were taken from Argyle Street Camp to work at Sham Shui Po, with the idea of moving the remainder of the POWs there soon.[154] By 31 December there were 5,000 men and officers confined at Sham Shui Po Camp.[155]

Nevertheless, on 3 January 1942, Argyle Street Camp still contained more than 1,000 men. About half had blankets, some had overcoats, but many had only the clothes they were captured in. At night they slept on boards or on the concrete floor. The dysentery cases and wounded men were no better off. Inadvertently soiling their clothing and bedding, they created a serious problem because there was nowhere clean to put them while the floor and their clothes were being washed. There were few drugs. On one occasion a dead man couldn't be buried for 48 hours because there were no spades to dig a grave. For the same reason they were unable to dig proper latrines, "and with 700 undisciplined Indian soldiers you can imagine what a hopeless task it has been. The food also is none too good and apt to be quite revolting when it gets cold as it frequently did if there was a lot of work for us to do. Finally the whole place is crawling with flies because the Japanese had horse lines near the camp."[156]

On 8 January, Newton recorded that although 169 dysentery patients had been sent off two days before, there were 70 new cases (13 European, 57 Indian). The epidemic was out of control. Fortunately, on 16 January 1942, Dr. Selwyn-Clarke was able to provide 500 grams of Dagenan, an anti-dysentery drug.[157] Thus they were able to treat at least the worst cases. Gradually, more elaborate medical services became available. For example, on 20 January 1942, Newton was permitted to take a patient needing to have one eye removed, and a metal fragment removed from the other, to the Queen Mary Hospital, where they had an electromagnet.[158]

In April 1942, Argyle Street Camp was transformed into an officers' POW camp. Until then non-Indian officers were scattered among the other camps; in January 1942, the Indian officers had been moved to Ma Tau Chung Camp.

The early and essentially complete segregation of the Indians paralleled Japanese practice in Singapore and elsewhere. Every effort was made to persuade the Indians to volunteer for the Indian National Army; separation from the influence of their British officers was an essential first step in the process. Thus, excepting most of the medical officers and some subalterns, all non-Indian officers captured by the Japanese, about 600 in number, were eventually incarcerated at Argyle Street Camp.

The first commandant at Argyle Street Camp was Lt. Sawamori, until July 1942, when he was succeeded by Lt. Tanaka Hitochi. Tanaka was tried in 1946–1947 for his actions while in charge there, found guilty, and sentenced to three years at hard labour.[159] From December 1943 to April 1944, Lt. Hara was in charge, followed by WO Ichiki in May 1944. The officers were moved to Sham Shui Po on 21 May 1944.[160]

Maj. Gen. Maltby, GOC Hong Kong, was transferred to Argyle Street Camp from Sham Shui Po. He had destroyed his official papers before the capitulation but retained a diary. The general and his staff distributed the pages of the diary among themselves, fastening the papers to their legs with adhesive tape. At Argyle Street Camp the papers were sealed in a jar that was buried in concrete. The position was marked and, after the war, the papers were recovered intact.[161] Presumably they helped convict some of the Japanese POW personnel at war crimes trials.

In Argyle Street Camp the officers were not forced to work, but their own administration made gardening compulsory.[162] There were at least three dozen medical officers in the camp—far more than were needed to care for their fellow officers. Thus, of the IMS medical officers, only Capt. J.J. Woodward, being a certified surgeon, did medical work at Argyle Street in the first months.[163]

For the first five months of the camp's existence the Japanese refused to provide facilities for a camp hospital. The sick had to be treated in their own huts.[164] However, an operating room of sorts was available in Ma Tau Chung Camp, a short distance away, and some surgery was done there. On those few occasions when this was permitted by the Japanese, the surgeon and the anesthetist first functioned as stretcher-bearers, carrying the patient the 300 to 400 metres between camps. "The Surgeon stated that his surgical technique was hardly improved by his having to undertake the preliminary carriage of the patient."[165] Woodward explained the apparent Japanese rationale for this order: "Stretcher parties were forbidden for fear of communication with the Indians and it usually fell to the lot of Surgeon Commander Cleave, RN, the Navy Surgical specialist and myself to carry the case down a distance of about half a mile and to operate on it if we could still stand up on arrival."[166] On one occasion, permission to move a patient having been denied, his perforated ulcer was operated on in the Argyle Street Camp dental room—successfully.

Finally, in October 1942, an outbreak of acute gastroenteritis occurred, apparently due to fish poisoning. Four cases showed symptoms resembling those of cholera, and the diagnosis of that disease was made bacteriologically by the Japanese. This outbreak disturbed them sufficiently to order the opening of a camp hospital.[167]

Capt. Strahan, IMS, had had some experience of cholera in India so it was arranged that Strahan and Woodward would be isolated with the patients in a separate hut that the Japanese allowed them to use.[168] After this disease (almost certainly not cholera) was cleared up, the Argyle Street Camp hospital was staffed by IMS Capts. Evans (physician), Strahan (dysentery and skin), and Woodward (surgical and OC). Through a Japanese medical sergeant they were able to get iron beds and mattresses. This success they thought was chiefly due to the reflected merit of their previous association with Maj. (A) Ashton-Rose, of whom the Japanese approved.

According to Woodward, RAMC orderlies were found unwilling or incapable of doing the hospital work. They were replaced by volunteer officers "who worked hard for 3 years at this work and made a great success of it."[169]

Dr. Saito, then a full lieutenant and in complete medical charge of some 10,000 POWs, called at the camp on an average of about once in three months. One of Saito's duties was to select cases for transfer to Bowen Road British Military Hospital. "He seldom proceeded farther than the main gate, however, where he might state that perhaps four cases out of the seven suggested to him might go." In the case of one sick medical officer, Saito's refusal to allow a transfer to hospital was immediate and firm, unimpeded by any examination of the patient. His attitude to sick men was that of complete indifference to their well-being. "No opportunity was given to assess his skill as a medical officer, as he avoided at all times any contact with the sick.[170]

A common criticism made by POW medical officers was the lack of medical involvement by Japanese medical officers. Their attitude seems usually to have been that they were in full administrative control but they would not accept clinical jurisdiction or risk expressing medical opinions. In at least a few instances, these men seem not to have been the best products of Japanese medical education; their noninvolvement may have been a positive factor for the POWs.

Capt. A.J.N. Warrack, RAMC, was at Argyle Street from April 1942 till he was sent to Japan in April 1944. He judged this camp to be significantly better than the other Hong Kong and mainland Japanese camps that he experienced.[171] Among other matters, his official report included information on the medical organization. Lt. Col. Shackleton, RAMC, acted as SMO Argyle Street Camp and organized a medical committee of 12 of the medical officers in the camp. This committee received reports on the state of the camp health from MOs in charge of personnel and hospital, and made recommendations and suggestions to the administrative authorities.[172]

The diet at Argyle Street Camp was poor. The principal food was white rice, with the quantity varying from about 375 to 700 grams a day.[173] But the officers, who were paid regularly, were able to supplement this ration. In addition to buying food for themselves, the officers sent money to the Other Ranks camp at Sham Shui Po, where malnutrition was severe and food supplies even more restricted.[174]

According to Warrack, in most months the Japanese issued a small but inadequate quantity of medicine. But no drugs at all were issued from July to September 1942. When medicines were issued, they included iodine, aspirin, magnesium sulphate, sodium bicarbonate, small amounts of sulfanilamide or sulfapyridine, and some vitamin B.[175] Fortunately, the indefatigable Dr. Selwyn-Clarke was able to send many valuable drugs into the camp during 1942.

R.B. Goodwin was debriefed after his escape from Hong Kong in 1944. Among other things, he stated that from the end of May 1942 until early in 1944, the Japanese gave POWs a regular monthly supply of tooth powder, washing soap, and toilet paper. During that period they also received "a sufficient supply" of toothbrushes and small face towels. This must have been while Goodwin was in Argyle Street Camp, where officers unquestionably were better supplied than were the men in Sham Shui Po. Again, the unconscious arrogance of the officer appears; the phrase "gave POWs" obviously is capable of being read as "all POWs" rather than "POW officers," though the latter is what was meant.[176] Whether the bias was Goodwin's or his interrogators' is unknown.

The caloric intake for the officers at Argyle Street was estimated to vary from 1,400 per day (only Japanese rations available) to 2,000 per day (canteen purchases and Red Cross supplies included). The men in Sham Shui Po received roughly the same caloric intake, but unlike the officers they had to work. Thus the gap between caloric needs and caloric supplies was much greater for the men than for their officers.

For the two-year period Warrack was at Argyle Street Camp the POWs were living, he stated, "on the verge of deficiency disease."[177] Nothing expresses more clearly the difference between this officers' camp and camps like Sham Shui Po that were maintained for the Other Ranks, where that verge had been passed long before and where vitamin deficiency diseases of numerous complicated kinds were the chief medical complaints. While Sham Shui Po was haunted at night by wraiths seeking ways to stop or diminish the agony of "electric feet," at Argyle Street only a few cases of painful feet were seen, and results of treatment in these mild cases were good.[178]

Another measure of the profound difference comes through in the distressed tone of an officer of the Royal Artillery, in Argyle Street Camp, when he discovered that a stray dog had mounted his bitch, Sheila.[179] By this time, October 1942, any dog in Sham Shui Po would have been eaten, not petted. In January 1943, the Other Ranks at Sham Shui Po or Ma Tau Chung would have been disgusted and infuriated to hear that "Sheila's pup is being fed on a pint of milk and 2 eggs a day."[180] That allowance would have saved lives in Sham Shui Po.

Another difference relates to the incidence of diphtheria. In contrast to the experience at North Point and Sham Shui Po camps, there were only four mild cases at Argyle Street Camp. Antitoxin was available and the Japanese "investigated the outbreak, sprayed everyone with carbolic, issued orders about the wearing of face masks and isolated contacts and carriers. No complications nor deaths occurred."[181]

The conclusion is inescapable. One's lot was significantly improved if one had the good luck to be an officer.

Camp "N"

On 21 May 1944, all non-Indian officers were moved back to Sham Shui Po, though to a separately designated section, "Camp N." (Argyle Street Camp was next used by Indian POWs.) The officers moved in two groups, on 7 and 14 May 1944.[182] Three months later, a remarkable event took place, a bizarre and unexplained though welcome augmentation of the officers' diet: "on Monday we received as *rations* 22 brace of *pheasants*!! can you beat it after no meat for over 2 years!!"[183]

On 26 April 1945, Lt. White, who had been in Sham Shui Po with the men since they left North Point Camp, noted a major shift, as he was one of 50 officers moved "over the wire" from "Camp S" to "Camp N."[184] "The wire separating the two camps doesn't mean much. There are visits back and forth all the time. Just got to be careful to dodge the Sentry."[185] And on 7 May 1945 this tireless diarist observed that many of the officers did their share of the necessary physical work, though he gives no numbers or proportions. "We even have an English Lord who does some cobbling."[186]

The officers remained in Camp "N" until the war ended.

Ma Tau Chung

Several refugee camps had been built in Hong Kong to accommodate the huge numbers of Chinese civilians who were fleeing Japanese domination on the mainland. The Hong Kong census by March 1941 was 1,650,000; three years earlier the number had been only 997,982. Arrangements to handle the human tide were inadequate in 1938, but eventually refugee camps were established at King's Park, Ma Tau Chung, North Point, Morrison Hill, Tai Hang, and Ngau Tau Kok.[187]

Col. Penfold recorded in his diary on 25 January 1942 that four days before, all the Indian Officers were taken out of Sham Shui Po and shown the former refugee camp between Argyle St. and Ma Tau Kok, where they were to live. The camp was called Ma Tau Chung. The following day they moved there. The Volunteers who had ended up at North Point after the capitulation came to Sham Shui Po and joined the bulk of the HKVDC already there. The Indians from Argyle Street joined the others at Ma Tau Chung, while the non-Indians at Argyle Street, mostly Volunteers, went to Sham Shui Po. Finally, the Navy marched out to North Point. The colonel considered all three— Indians, Canadians, and Navy—as having been in a way discordant elements in camp. Precisely why, he does not say. At Sham Shui Po it was decided to move all officers into the Jubilee Buildings.[188] Thus, with these various moves, the Japanese scheme of organization and segregation was fully revealed.

Ma Tau Chung Camp was located 300 metres from the Argyle Street Camp, on the opposite side of Argyle St. and set back from it. Late in January 1942 the Indian regulars were taken there from Sham Shui Po. The Indian members of the HKVDC were first taken to Argyle Street Camp, but then, after a day or two, they were taken on to Ma Tau Chung.[189] More than two years later, the Indians were moved from Ma Tau Chung to Argyle Street after the officers returned to Sham Shui Po.[190]

Indians from many units occupied Ma Tau Chung. These included the Rajputs and Punjabis, Indians of the Mule Corps, the Royal Army Service Corps, the Hong Kong and Singapore Royal Artillery, the Indian Medical Service, the Indian Hospital Corps, the Indian warders from Stanley Gaol, and some Indian Police reservists.

Bertram commented on the lot of the Indian POWs, whose fate has been little recorded, at least in English. He believed that conditions in Ma Tau Chung were much worse than those experienced by the British and Canadians. The Japanese were applying pressure on the Indians, hoping to force them to join Chandra Bose's Indian National Army (INA) and to fight against the British. But despite the rising tide of anti-British nationalism within India, the majority of the POWs held out with great fortitude. "The death roll among Indian troops was higher than for any other prisoners in Hong Kong—it was a demonstration of loyalty that I felt British rule had done little to deserve," was Bertram's comment.[191]

In May 1944 a POW on a working party near Ma Tau Chung saw some of the Indian POWs. There were over 200 of them still in the camp. Those he saw seemed to be in fairly good shape, but the camp was very dirty and looked "buggy."[192]

Endacott paints a more positive picture of the Indians' captivity. Those who had families in Hong Kong received parcels on a generous scale, even two or three times a week. Conversation with family members was forbidden, but sometimes a kindly Japanese interpreter or guard would ignore these encounters. Red Cross supplies from India provided flour for chapattis, and ghee. "So," he concluded, "on the whole, the Indian prisoners did not fare so badly. There was some beriberi and pellagra, caused mainly by switching to a rice diet to which most Indians were unaccustomed."[193] Despite this essentially positive description, the Japanese devoted much effort to propaganda and intimidation. The Punjabi and Hong Kong and Singapore Royal Artillery POWs were brought to Gun Club Hill Barracks for this purpose. However, almost all refused to collaborate, so they were sent back to Ma Tau Chung and closely confined, on subsistence rations.[194]

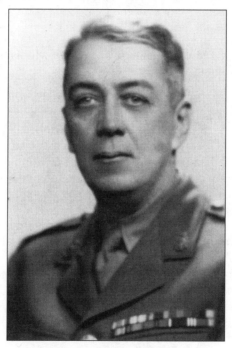

Figure 3.11. Maj. (Acting) Leopold W. Ashton-Rose, IMS (1896-1957). (Courtesy of Marjorie Ashton-Rose.)

Capt. Woodward was involved in the move of the Indian hospital on 17 April 1942. After wholesale discharge of the well and nearly well patients, the hospital was moved to a series of huts further down Argyle St., outside both Argyle Street Camp and Ma Tau Chung. The patients were chiefly Indians. Nursing staff was either RAMC or Indian Hospital Corps; the MOs were Maj. (A) Ashton-Rose, Capts. Woodward, Strahan, Evans, and Sundaram, all IMS, and about eight officers of the Indian Medical Department.[195] At Ma Tau Chung Camp, several patients suffering from dysentery or appendicitis died for lack of treatment, though separated from medical care by only a narrow lane and two wire fences. "The Japs just would not give permission for them to be brought to Hospital."[196]

On 16 June 1942, as usual without warning, the British, both patients and staff, were all removed from this hospital, which thereafter functioned as a purely Indian hospital. It was run by Jemadar Chetan Dev, IMD, described by a colleague as

> [O]ne of the best types of old style VCO. He carried on his duties under the most trying conditions with great patience, integrity and resolution and was completely aloof from the hurly-burly of plot and counter-plot resulting from the disaffection and scheming caused by the Japs' persistent efforts to get recruits for the INA. He held the respect of both Indians and Japs and is a man I am proud to call my friend...on those occasions of our operating at the Lower Camp Hospital he was not afraid to greet me with a friendliness and respect which must have jeopardised his position with the Japs.[197]

Dislocating the Indians from contact with the British was effected by the simple expedient of keeping physical separation complete. As part of the scheme to suborn the Indians, in October 1942 British POWs were made to do seemingly unnecessary manual labour just outside Ma Tau Chung Camp, presumably in order to humiliate them before the Indians.[198] However, propaganda seems to have been largely ineffective in turning Indians. Far more serious was the brutal intimidation practised on Indian officers and men, almost always because they resisted persuasion to join the Indian National Army. The most well-documented and surely the most vicious of these attacks involved Capt. Matreen Ahmed Ansari.

This man became known to Martin Banfill soon after the capitulation. Mixed in with the British wounded Banfill was looking after at Sham Shui Po immediately after the surrender were many Indians from the Rajputs and the Punjabis. A young Indian officer came along and asked Banfill to look at his men. Banfill tried to excuse himself, exhausted after caring for his own casualties, but the officer was adamant, so Banfill went with him. This man was Captain Ansari,

> a Muslim, an Indian, who had gone to Sandhurst, had a British commission. He belonged to a princely family, he was some connection of the Nizam of Hyderabad, and a gentleman, a really nice person. So I went with him and I stayed with him and he got me something to eat. He helped me and we bandaged up these Indians, and I slept with him that night on the floor. I remember sharing a blanket. The Japanese recruited a rebel Indian army under a man named Chandra Bose to attack the British, to prove that they were liberating India in their attack through Burma. They offered the command to Ansari, and Ansari said

he was a British soldier subject to the King, and he wouldn't. And they beheaded him.[199]

Some time in 1942 the British Army Aid Group (BAAG) contacted Ansari, and his escape probably could have been arranged. But duty compelled him to remain with his men—he volunteered to go to Ma Tau Chung Camp to stiffen the resistance of the Rajputs to Japanese propaganda.[200] Further details of Ansari's brutal treatment at the hands of the Japanese are described in the citation that accompanied his George Cross:

> ANSARI Matreen Ahmed, Capt., 7th Rajput Rifles, Indian Army....Captain Ansari became a prisoner of war of the Japanese when they invaded Hong Kong in December 1941...as he was closely related to a ruler of a great Indian State his captors tried to persuade him to renounce his allegiance to the British....When they found these approaches were useless he was thrown into Stanley Jail in May 1942, where he suffered starvation and brutal ill-treatment. On being returned to the prisoner of war camp he still proclaimed his loyalty to the British and in May 1943 he was again thrown into Stanley Jail where he was starved and tortured for five months. He was finally sentenced to death with 30 other British, Indian and Chinese prisoners and executed in October 1943. Throughout his long ordeal Captain Ansari's loyalty, courage and endurance never wavered and his example helped many others to remain loyal.[201]

Captain Ansari had been recommended for the Victoria Cross for valour in the field before he was taken prisoner. After the war, Compton Mackenzie found Ansari's grave in the cemetery at Stanley. Alongside Ansari are buried 20 of those who shared his convictions.

Ansari was the most prominent of those who were determined to reaffirm their loyalty to the King-Emperor, but there were others. Sepoy Nobat Khan, 2/14th Punjabs, caught while trying to escape, was strung up to a beam and bayoneted several times. In addition he was subjected to the suffocating water torture.[202] Fortunately the bulk of the Indians did not receive such personal attention. But more general methods were tried: "the Japs asked the Indian troops to volunteer for service with them, and when they refused they starved them for a week till they finally gave in. Then 150 of them were put to guard an air field in the New Territories and one night they all disappeared."[203] Endacott confirms this mass escape, "a striking success by the BAAG whose agents, with help from the villagers of Lin Ma Hang, in March 1943 succeeded in liberating a large contingent of Indian troops to Free China."[204]

In the last half of 1944, at a time when many Indian POWs captured in Malaya and Singapore were released and sent back to their homes in occupied areas, all local Hong Kong Indians who promised to work with the Japanese were released to their homes. (Chinese members of the HKVDC had been released late in 1942.) At the end of the war only three Indian prisoners, all members of the HKVDC, remained in the Argyle Street Camp.[205]

Immediately after the war, the former POW camp for Indians, Ma Tau Chung, was used, with other institutions, to house those in transit through Hong Kong and "for those unable to pay the heavy 'tea money' for house room."[206] Thus life began to return to "normal" in the area.

For the men who remained in Hong Kong, life was more or less as described, though with infinite variations of details and dates. But for many hundreds of the British, Canadian, and HKVDC POWs, this existence was profoundly changed when they were selected to travel to Japan. Indian POWs, for political reasons, apparently were not sent to be labourers in Japan. Drafts occurred several times in 1942, 1943, and 1944. The voyages themselves, and the life the men led in Japan, are described in Chapters Seven and Eight.

Chapter 4

Prisoner-of-War Life

in Hong Kong

It is difficult to appreciate without having seen it the tremendous loss
of morale and pride of a beaten and captured army.[1]

*I*f any one aspect of prisoner-of-war life stands out in the memories
of the men it is the sameness. Their lives stretched off into an
unknown and therefore interminable future punctuated by a relatively small number of memorable moments. Some of these were unpleasant, such as a severe beating, a tedious or painful disease, or the bitter
discomfort of a Japanese winter; happily, some also were pleasant
events, such as the arrival of mail, a spirited amateur play or concert,
or some successful if minor sabotage effort against their captors.

Yet despite the seeming greyness of their days, most of the men
did get through each day, one at a time; there were events and routines
to be learned, and lived, and survived. In an attempt to make these
days understandable, I discuss POW activities within several general
headings. There are sections on work, entertainment, sports,
Christmas, sex, and escaping, among others. In broad scope, these
experiences were common to all the POWs. Inevitably, details vary,
sometimes widely, from person to person, from camp to camp, and
over time.

When asked to identify the aspect of POW life that was most distressing, many ex-POWs have identified two related factors. They
were deeply concerned that their families were unaware of their fate
after 8 December 1941; and they lamented the extreme slowness of
postal communications and the resulting infrequency of word from

home. The Japanese, given their general denunciation of surrender, and thus of POWs, could scarcely have been expected to devote much energy towards assuring this or any of the other amenities expected by Western prisoners. Their efforts do not seem to have been more than perfunctory. Again, a cultural difference exerted a substantial effect here; there is much evidence that most Japanese soldiers had few or no contacts with home once they left Japan proper.

In addition, a logistical problem worsened the slowness of communication. The number of translators capable of reading English was grossly deficient. Every letter or postcard leaving any camp, and every communication arriving there, had to be censored by the Japanese. One consequence was that mail piled up. Often the POWs, visiting Japanese offices for some reason, saw sacks of mail piled in a corner, often the same sacks month after month.

Another offshoot of the translation bottleneck may have been the use of pre-printed cards that permitted only the deletion of certain words by the individual prisoner. Thus a card might read: I am well...working hard...in hospital. The sender was to cross out incorrect or inappropriate responses. Obviously, use of such cards greatly simplified the work of the censors. No additional writing was permitted, so the cards were in essence pre-censored. But the information the men could send home was minuscule, which only exacerbated deeply felt resentments. The card did ease the task of those noble-minded POWs who deliberately chose the "I am well" message even when so ill in hospital that they had to ask an orderly to mark and address the card. This tenacious desire to reassure their loved ones is a tribute to the mens' spirit.

At Hong Kong, outgoing letters were first permitted on 26 May 1942, each man to be allowed to write home once a month.[2] Within a day or two, a long list of restrictions regarding the writing of letters had been posted on the bulletin board. This was not to be a mass mailing, with a letter or card written by each man. Only a certain percentage could have this privilege: in Sham Shui Po, each hut drew lots to see who would write home first. But in North Point Camp, the Canadians who won the draw were to find that the matter was not a simple one: "June 2nd, 42. The men who wrote home have had their letters returned to them and told they must rewrite them, shorten to 200 words and not ask for a single thing."[3] Nevertheless, some mail did leave the camps, and some of the letters eventually reached anxious families, though rarely sooner than a year later.

Other kinds of communication were arranged by the Japanese, notably radio broadcasting of messages, again by only a minority of the men. Early in June 1942, Tom Forsyth of the Winnipeg Grenadiers was one of 10 Canadians who were permitted to send messages home in this way. They rode by bus to the dock, travelled by ferry to

Kowloon, and rode another bus about four miles to Japanese HQ. "We each spoke a short message into a microphone and a recording will be broadcast, picked up and relayed till eventually they reach Canada. We left camp at 12.30. Did not get back till 5, missed dinner, all the Japs gave us at H.Q. was two cups of pale, weak green tea. No cream, no sugar."[4] Many of these ethereal messages did reach their intended audience, often transcribed and forwarded by dedicated amateur radio operators in Canada and the United States.

Work

A visitor to Hong Kong just before the war noted "the apparently airy manner in which an engineer will say 'Oh, we'll just take the top off the hill and fill in the valley here.' The newcomer is even more impressed when he sees it done."[5] Hordes of Chinese labourers with picks, shovels, and rickety wheelbarrows, aided by women and children with baskets, attack the hill; in due course, it is carried into the valley. This was possible because labour was so cheap. Of course, this was exactly the technique by which the Japanese used POWs and impressed Chinese to construct Kai Tak airport. For the Japanese, the labour was very cheap indeed.

For military prisoners of the Japanese, the general principle adhered to was that privates worked, NCOs supervised work, and officers did not have to work. Exceptions were made by the Japanese to all these regulations, perhaps the most notable and substantial taking place during the cruel so-called "Speedo" period on the Burma-Siam railway, when many officers were forced to do brutally heavy work over 14- and 16-hour days along with the men. Gardening, carried out ostensibly for the POWs themselves, was an activity frequently assigned to the officers.

Of course, the major exception to all exemptions from work by officers, expected by the POWs and usually permitted by the Japanese, was that medical officers worked. Similarly, though not always without argument and persuasion before the captors permitted it, the medical orderlies usually could pursue their vocation. They and the MOs had the enormous advantage of being able to keep busy doing what they were trained to do. In both groups, the opportunity to work was seen as a great boon. Albert Coates, an Australian MO captured in the South Pacific, pointed out that although the Japanese often ignored the Geneva Conventions, at least they did use captured surgeons "with some humanitarian intent."[6] One former POW believes that the memoirs that have been written have overlooked the contribution made to prisoners of war by the medically trained men. "This group deserves much recognition for their dedication to their fellow men."[7] For the medical orderlies there was an added bonus. Work in the hospitals offered legitimate exemption from more onerous and often dangerous physical labour.

In most cases, non-medical officers would have preferred to be able to work. They knew they needed real exercise, both physical and mental. Inevitably, the Other Ranks would gladly have not worked or at least have worked less hard. Early on, officers at Hong Kong supervised the working parties. But when the Japanese discovered that the Chinese underground had established contacts with these parties, they forbade officers to accompany the men. Occasionally, an officer would work in place of a private by exchanging identities. Lt. White was one of these officers; in October 1942 he took off his rank badges to join a work party at a godown (warehouse) on the wharf. There, he handled Red Cross supplies, individual parcels, and other material.[8] This was not a rare event, but it was the Other Ranks who sustained the real, debilitating burden of exhaustingly hard labour.

The Japanese demanded working parties from Sham Shui Po as early as 24 January 1942.[9] In the beginning men sought to join the work parties because they assumed there would be opportunities to smuggle goods back into camp, and they were lacking much. One British NCO wrote of the trouble he had trying to get on a Japanese fatigue party. The RSM (Regimental Sergeant-Major) told him he would have to disguise himself as a private.[10] Before long, however, men schemed and connived to avoid working parties.

Canadians from North Point laboured both on the Island and on the mainland during the first summer in captivity. They did all kinds of work. Groups alternated, Grenadiers one day, Rifles the next, in sending 200 men to work on the airport.[11] One man reported that he was in a party of 39 sent to Bowen Road Hospital to cut grass and bushes around the electrically wired fence, to prevent current from being grounded. Later, this task would cost one man his life.

Kai Tak airport became the chief destination for working parties, which often gives survivors a certain grim satisfaction as their aircraft land at Kai Tak. (From 1998 this quasi-poignant opportunity has disappeared, as the international airport is now located elsewhere.) The men were required to move a large hill by filling baskets with dirt and stones and carrying them away. The POWs would get up at 4 a.m., have breakfast of rice and greens, and work all day, with perhaps a bun at noon. They returned anywhere from about 6 p.m. to as late as 10 p.m. at night. They were "like zombies," going around in a daze.[12] The weather often was rainy, cold, and miserable. In the winter months, work parties had to go out in the dark and return in the dark.

Many men were not up to the work, largely because they were chronically poorly fed. Conditions at the various work sites often included brutal harassment. On one occasion at the airport, when a POW didn't work hard enough to suit the Japanese guard, he hit the prisoner across the head with a rifle butt and knocked him down. "The guy got up and took a swing at the Japanese and another Japanese came up behind and stuck a bayonet right through his stomach. That was it."[13] No other Canadian I have questioned recalls this incident; the details may be exaggerated or the memory may represent some other location.

When working parties were first established, a man might be chosen to go out only every third day. But soon, more men were required by the Japanese. Coincident with the demand for increased numbers of workers was an increase in the sickness rate. By September 1942, many men whom the medical officers considered to be dangerously ill were forced to work. "Work party calls for 500 men these days, have to use many sick men. Japs won't consider any less."[14] Selecting sick men who would be least damaged by hard work was a heartbreaking and difficult task but one that most medical officers had to face.[15]

Gradually the number who were able to play games or do sports was confined almost entirely to officers who did not go on work parties,[16] or to cookhouse staff. It was a fact of POW-camp life—often deeply resented—that cookhouse staff ate better than run-of-the-mill prisoners.

Entertainment

Fortunately, work did not totally occupy the POWs' existence, though often it seemed that it did. Many activities took place that fell into the broad category of "entertainment." Organizing such activities generally signalled the beginning of accommodation to POW life, a perhaps depressing but necessary mental adjustment.

The Hong Kong POWs discovered one minor but real benefit of fighting a short war in a limited geographical area. Although they were lacking many things when they moved into their camps, other items survived almost miraculously. Thus many of the Canadian bandsmen arrived in camp with their instruments, though they would soon have been happy to trade them for a few tins of bully beef. Members of the HKVDC were able to have instruments sent in to the camps from friends and relatives outside. Consequently, some fine bands and orchestras sprang up.

The first concert took place remarkably early in what was to be a long and painful captivity. At Sham Shui Po, on 6 January 1942, the Japanese presented a band concert to which, as one Winnipeg Grenadier put it, they were invited to attend or else. What was left of the Grenadiers' band, plus the remainder of the Royal Scots, combined talents and played a few selections.[17] A Royal Scots bandsman gives more details: "Japanese 'Victory' Band plays at crossroads and we are asked to play for them. Staggered through 'King Cotton,' 'Light

Cavalry,' & 'Rose Marie.' Loud applause from the throng. Ended up with National Anthem (unsung and possibly unrecognized by the Japs, thank goodness)."[18] Later, presumably once the Japanese ear was more finely tuned, the musicians found that the anthem had to be avoided, but that Elgar's "Land of Hope and Glory" was allowable.[19]

The diary of A.J. Alsey is a particularly useful source of information about music in the camps. He was a sergeant in the Royal Scots and a talented musician. As early as 3 January 1942 he made notes about a camp sing-song at which a Canadian swing band played, "sax & clarinet very good indeed—approved swing style from trumpet."[20] But Alsey had to struggle throughout captivity to get acceptable instruments. The Royal Scots had not been as lucky as the Canadians. Their band instruments were largely "blown sky high."[21] Alsey borrowed a saxophone from someone in the Middlesex Regiment. But his real love seems to have been the violin. He searched for a long time, pursuing the rumour of one having come in over the fence in mid-February. This led him to Dr. Solomon Bard, another important figure in connection with music in the camp. But it was not until May 1942 that he had any luck. Then he needed violin strings and was reduced to getting the padre to persuade the loathed Major "Cissy" Boon to have some sent in.[22]

Lt. Solomon Bard contributed piano solos in the concert of 26 June 1943, and on other occasions served as accompanist, conducted band concerts, and played violin solos. Eventually he formed his own small orchestra (decades later he was, for a time, director of the Hong Kong Chinese Symphony Orchestra).

In June, Alsey met the owner of the other violin, who said he could borrow it when he wished.[23] Just a week later he was in a state of profound happiness, playing a violin duet with another prisoner, Tucker, so successfully that he wrote in his diary, "Would like to share this beauty with all."[24] Alsey later was a survivor of the sinking of the *Lisbon Maru* en route to Japan. It is evident from his diary that playing his music helped his morale significantly; undoubtedly his music lifted the spirits of others too. Though not invariably: in August 1942 he reported repairing a saxophone "so that she blows." The neighbours, apparently not music lovers, protested loudly.[25]

In at least a few cases there were quite remarkable feats of improvisation. Harry White wrote, in September 1942, that Maj. Maurice A. Parker, RRC, had made a cello out of an oil drum, "and it plays too! It's nearly as big as he is—looks funny as hell to see him trying to play it. He's a comical duck anyway. Kravinchuk made a guitar, damn good job he did of it too."[26] Another invention was "a curious stringed instrument" created by James Murray and Tom Weir, Winnipeg Grenadiers. Critical response was guarded in this instance, an observer labeling the output "weird sounds."[27]

Another form of entertainment was free-for-all concerts on the parade square. "Canadian Sgt. does conductor—horrible row."[28] At one of these concerts, the grand prize went to a Royal Navy man whose specialty consisted of singing, in a variety of styles, "Show me the way to go home." A young Canadian signalman, Will Allister, first appeared at an open air concert on the square at North Point Camp; he became an accomplished mimic and was considered to be "really a scream in the 'Fred Allen Radio broadcast.'"[29]

By the end of 1942, concerts were a regular feature in Sham Shui Po. In December it was decided that concerts and shows should be played on Saturdays and Wednesdays in the hall, on Monday evenings in the British general hospital and on Tuesday afternoons in the Canadian hospital.[30] At this time the orchestra of the Winnipeg Grenadiers was an important part of the musical scene in the camp.[31]

In addition to somewhat formal concerts, less organized but equally appreciated musical events took place. Sir Albert Rodrigues remembers playing in a quintet; they would go from hut to hut, playing a few selections at each. The challenge was to play songs requested by the audience—responding as best they could extemporaneously.[32]

Arthur Gomes recalled, during an interview in 1996, that before the war there had been a band in Hong Kong called the Aloha Serenaders. Many members of the band ended up in Sham Shui Po in 1942 and the band was revived. There, they were rehearsed by Capt. Njall Bardal; the chief instruments were mandolin and guitar.

In January 1943, Sgt. Ebdon noted that the choir of Russians in the HKVDC had given a splendid concert.[33] Will Allister joined the choir—he knew no Russian but memorized the words—and found it a joy to be to make music in those grim surroundings. Often they toured the camp, singing in the huts and hospitals.[34]

Sometimes the musicians played for non-cultural events. Early in 1944, the Japanese ordered the POWs to do PT to music. "Our little band has to get out every morning and play while the rest of us go through our stuff. Not too bad at that—takes the monotony off forced PT."[35]

Paralleling an experience we have all had, one Grenadier found himself unable to concentrate during a lecture early in 1943: "we could hear strains of music and wild cries from a nearby hut where a square dance was in full swing."[36] By this time, some Red Cross food had reached the camp, and the dietary supplementation obviously had had a beneficial impact on the energy of the square-dancers. Six months earlier—and six months later—square dancing would have been unthinkable.

Fortunately, the recurring Japanese interdiction of concerts and shows as retaliation for escape attempts were invariably short-lived.

For many of the men, what few happy memories they have from these years centre on musical events.

The Japanese, a POW officer reported, had supported the idea of concerts and plays from the beginning, spurred by strong urgings by the POWs themselves. The theatre thrived on miraculous improvisations. Wigs sprang from strings drawn from rice sacks, mosquito nets metamorphosed into evening dresses, wooden frames covered with paper became wings, and the Japanese provided some chalk colouring. One volunteer recalled the genius of CSM Baptista, who could create an idyllic Hawaiian beach with palm trees silhouetted against a moonlit sky, by "a deft mixture of ashes, salvaged from the kitchen refuse bins and mixed with water in the right measure."[37]

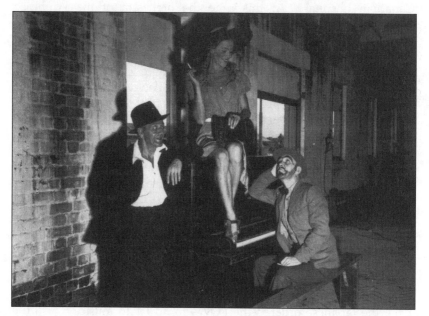

Figure 4.1. Sham Shui Po, theatre scene: l to r: Cpl. Richard Guy Falkner (WG), "Sonny" Castro (HKVDC), Maj. Maurice A. Parker (RRC). (Photo loaned by the late Dr. John Crawford.)

A memorable act involved that classic favourite, whether played for broad laughs or with subtlety—female impersonation. One of the best-remembered men in Sham Shui Po was "Sonny" Castro. He was a member of the Hong Kong Volunteer Defence Corps and spent the POW period in Sham Shui Po. His fame came from his activities in camp theatricals, where he specialized in the "female" singing and dancing roles. Carmen Miranda was the particular favourite; Castro frequently took on the persona of this performer, who at the time was a major box-office attraction in Hollywood movies.[38] The music she performed to was largely South American, particularly the samba.

One of the Portuguese lads 'Sonny' Castro, is a 'wow' of a girl....He's a good looking lad anyway, and his smile, the way he rolls his eyes, his hands, etc., he could pass as a girl anywhere. He used to make up a dancing team with his sister and that has helped him. Have to run the show 3 nights to get everyone—one night specially for the hospital. All the patients that can be moved are taken. It's wonderful for the morale of the whole camp.[39]

Sonny Castro was born (2 May 1919) Ferdinand Maria Castro, eldest of five children in a Portuguese Hong Kong family. After the war he was manager of Shun Hing Shipping Co., then manager and later social secretary to the Hong Kong General Chamber of Commerce.[40] He died suddenly 24 May 1985, unmarried.

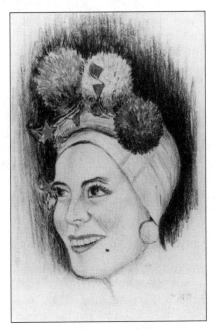

Figure 4.2. Colour drawing of "Sonny" Castro, HKVDC, wearing his famous "Carmen Miranda" costume and makeup. (IWM MS 85/42/1, Papers of CSM R.A. Edwards.)

Castro played the leading female role in the Portuguese show in February 1943, the minstrel show in April, *Boyadere* in June, *Here Comes Charlie* in July, *La Czigane* in October, and *Blue Rose* in November, all in the same year. He was a "true artist in every sense, remaining unspoiled throughout. Also designed and made majority of female costumes worn. No praise can be too great for work done."[41] This account was written under a caricature of Castro in black ink.[42]

Inevitably, perhaps, the question arises as to whether Castro might have been homosexual. Dr. Tony Coombes thought not. "Sonny was...damn good. He took up Carmen Miranda's line, with his 'Aye, Yi, Yi!' singing. I suppose people thought he was queer, but I never thought so. He was just slightly precious, perhaps. He used to call me 'Captain Tony.' A very good entertainer, first class chap, very nice fellow too."[43]

The Portuguese members of the HKVDC seem to have been a happy and homogeneous group of men. All 230 were Catholic. They lived in two adjacent huts in Sham Shui Po, "and the sound of laughter and singing to the accompaniment of stringed instruments and the strum of guitar could always be heard in the evenings."[44]

Two men must be singled out among the many performers, though not for any remarkable thespian talents. Cpl. John Harvey, RAMC, made frequent appearances as a vocalist; CSM Mark Tugby, WG, also performed in plays at Sham Shui Po. Under less savoury circumstances these men become central characters in Oeyama POW Camp in Japan, as described in Chapter Nine.

At the end of March 1943, a Kaufman and Hart play, *Once in a Lifetime*, was presented. Huck O'Neill was the producer; Lt. R. Simmons, RRC, Stage Manager; Cpl. S. Sheffer, WG, and Capt. Royal, WG, Properties. Of the 39 actors, at least 25 are identifiably Canadian. The document provides no explanation for this remarkably heavy Canadian participation. *Once in a Lifetime* was the last show to be held in "The Hippodrome."[45] By this time the camp population was much thinned by the drafts to Japan, and this presumably explains the decline of theatricals.

Much leisure-time activity centred on reading. George Porteous, Canadian representative for the YMCA, helped set up a library.

> Four titles come to mind as having more than literary significance for our situation. One was Maugham's *Of Human Bondage*, a sort of casebook for the physically and mentally lame POW. Then there was *Down the Garden Path*. Someone had crossed out the author's name and written in Mackenzie King. *Cheating Death* was certainly popular, but nothing had so much appeal as Seton's *Wild Animals I Have Known*.[46]

At Singapore, Russell Braddon found a new audience for a classic: he read *Winnie the Pooh* three times (to the initial disgust of his friends). At last they could stand his frequent bouts of laughter at the antics of Eeyore and the poems of Pooh no longer, and "they began furtively dipping into it themselves, and eventually it went round both tiers of our over-crowded and verminous hut. *Winnie the Pooh* is a book which all adults, particularly those whose lives have become difficult, should read."[47]

Only eight days after Hong Kong surrendered, the lure of sports had begun to be felt, at least by the victors. On 3 January 1942, a

Japanese soldier arrived at the YMCA opposite Argyle Street Camp, where the Sisters and nurses were quartered. He had tennis shoes and a tennis racquet and wanted a game. "In the end 3 Sisters and one soldier played tennis while a second soldier acted as ball boy! There is a tennis court in the YMCA compound."[48]

For the POWs, sports probably played a less important role in maintaining morale than did concerts and plays. As hunger became a serious problem the men gave up sports for lack of energy. By April 1942, a POW wondered where some of the men found the strength to play field hockey. He had none.[49] Recurrently, but temporarily, the food supply improved (for different reasons in different camps) and, often, men began to participate in sports again at these times. Officers had more energy and played sports more; this fact itself was often bad for morale among the Other Ranks. The sporting proclivities of Major Ashton-Rose are mentioned elsewhere. White, a prolific diarist, noted late in 1943 that a lawn-bowling green had been set up at Sham Shui Po, using a sand pitch that was tamped down with a roller borrowed from the Japanese.[50] Apparently this "lawn bowls without a lawn" was quite popular.[51]

Cricket, field hockey, and soccer were all played in the Hong Kong camps regularly until the summer or autumn of 1942. After that, such vigorous activities are mentioned less and less often. There were difficulties in addition to that of decreasing strength. Equipment was impossible to replace if broken or worn out. One reads of games abandoned, such as a cricket match after the only two balls, both old, burst.[52]

More sedentary pursuits continued to provide temporary escape. Card games were popular, including bridge. In April 1943, W.F. Nugent dedicated some ironic notes to "my dear friend, George Porteous, who wanted so much to be a publisher that a few notes have been dressed up as a book. May it, by improving his game, ease the strain on his many friendships, but not add still another to the already wide range on which he lectures." The slim book was alleged to have been typed, bound, and published in Sham Shui Po.[53]

The officers had much leisure time. One MO started a museum and participated in a chess tournament. "When I was in camp, sometimes, I used to play checkers all day long until it was time to go to bed....when I went in there I had never seen a checkerboard before. When I left there I *knew* how to play checkers."[54]

Trading

Whenever the Japanese permitted it, trading with civilians across the wire served an important function, increasing the food supply for at least a few of the men. On occasion, a guard actually helped the trading process. In January 1942, the guards at Sham Shui Po must still have been relatively sympathetic front line troops. Once, several Chinese traders were gathered at the barbed wire. One had four small loaves for which he was asking three Hong Kong dollars (about 60 cents). "Buck got busy and tried to get them for 2 dollars. A sentry standing near watched for awhile, came over, grunted at Buck, handed him his rifle and bayonet and proceeded to bargain for us. We got the loaves for 2 dollars alright."[55]

Sharp practices abounded on the part of the Chinese, and from these there was no remedy; they were outside the wire and indifferent to cries of outrage when a cheat was discovered. "Haunted the wire from 7 to 8 a.m. Got stung for $5.00 with rock salt & bag of sand for sugar. Loud laughter. Sat for hours breaking up salt."[56]

Cigarettes

Smoking was a problem from the start. In the beginning some men stopped, but most did not. Heavy smokers spent what time they had looking for butts, or trying to barter their few possessions. Later the POWs received variable issues, five, ten or at times more cigarettes a week, just enough to keep the craving up.[57]

One theme that pervades the literature about POW life in the 1940s, and that continues to punctuate the recollections of veterans half a century later, is the importance of the cigarette. We have a profoundly different view of cigarettes now, and they are no longer seen as either fashionable or healthy. However, in the 1940s, cigarettes were perhaps at their high point as a symbol of manliness and what came to be called "cool." This may be a result of the immense impact of motion pictures. In addition, smoking was something that essentially all soldiers did at the time.

Tobacco, one POW wrote, was the one thing for which the men never lost their craving.[58] The vast majority of soldiers smoked. If smoking cigarettes conveyed an aura of manliness, who needed that support more than men who had been defeated and captured by the enemy? But cigarettes acquired added importance in the prison camps. The ubiquity of the habit made cigarettes an accepted substitute for money, both within the camps and also cross-culturally, between POWs and guards or civilians in the surrounding population. The Americans found that the shortage of cigarettes was itself the cause of a significant morale problem on Bataan. To many of the troops, cigarettes were more essential than food.[59]

The prisoner-of-war camp can be seen as a microcosm of human social order. Forcibly confined together, a group of humans will—largely unconsciously—establish social institutions resembling those they know from normal times. For POWs, the most obvious difference from peacetime, aside from incarceration itself, was their unisex life. But that deficit aside, human social order imposed itself from the beginning.

In prisoner-of-war camps, goods were bought and sold, exchanged, sometimes stolen. POWs made things to be sold, hired themselves out to labour of many kinds,[60] negotiated loans, gambled, and struggled to find ways to survive. A POW's economic activity, exchanging goods and services, acted directly to enhance (or diminish) his material comfort. A POW in Europe pointed out that the spontaneity of this economic life was characteristic; "it came into existence not by conscious imitation but as a response to the immediate needs and circumstances."[61]

Trading was a universal activity. Most trading was for food, using cigarettes or other items in exchange, but the status of cigarettes soon changed from a normal commodity to that of currency. "Certain brands," Radford noted, "were more popular than others as smokes, but for currency purposes a cigarette was a cigarette."[62] Nevertheless, some of the cigarettes were offensive, such as a distasteful Japanese issue called "Ruby Queen" and some local "whiffs" that burned at an amazing speed.[63]

In a diary note on Camp Economics, a Canadian medical orderly at Hong Kong recorded some observations on the function of cigarettes. The main brands were Golden Dragon and United (both Chinese); before the war these sold for 9 cents Hong Kong for a package of 10 (about 2 cents Canadian); by March 1942, three months into captivity, the price had zoomed to $1 per pack (20 cents Canadian). At that time, one pack would buy a man a shirt or a pair of socks, a set of mess tins or a light sweater; two packs equalled a fountain pen, a suit of battledress, or three razor blades. Five packs might purchase a Ronson lighter or a silver cigarette case within the camp, while the Japanese guards might pay anywhere from 10 to 60 packs, depending on the make of the items and the relative bargaining skills of the principals.[64] Another Canadian observed, later in 1942, that cigarettes remained the principal means of barter or exchange in the camp: "One fag buys a bun, 2 or 3 a stew. Half of one a sweet sauce or an issue of black China tea."[65] At Hong Kong one POW, recalled only as "Newfie," was notorious for selling his food for cigarettes. "How he survived I don't know, but I would say that if he had three meals a week, he would be lucky."[66] But survive he did. Many did not.

Non-smokers had an advantage in the camp economic world because most men smoked and, during captivity, seemed to crave tobacco even more acutely. The fortunate non-smokers used their cigarette allotment as money to buy additional food, an extra piece of clothing when the weather worsened, or some favour for themselves. At a camp in Japan, an Australian medical officer gave up smoking and, with his ration of one cigarette a day, paid to have his sewing done (a mandatory labour in a shop run by the Japanese). He then was free to devote his time to reading surgery from books he had smuggled in from the hospital.[67] Few other POWs were able to find similar ways to better themselves in preparation for the longed-for time "after the war."

At North Point Camp in Hong Kong they put on concerts. One Canadian, Roy Robinson, wrote "The Rice-O" program, based on the then very popular Jell-O program starring Jack Benny. The incentive to write for the show was that for participating in the concerts, each man might be rewarded with a cigarette or two. And cigarettes were hard currency.[68] They were accepted as payment for all kinds of services and goods: "Binnie saves my life with 2 cigarettes, rewards for cutting hair....Jack brings in 5 fags from Kai Tak & King gives me one, a real field day...gave a fag to R.S.M. and one to Hale (my optician!)."[69]

At Stanley Internment Camp, a Crown Solicitor in Hong Kong was reported to have swapped a gold tooth for two packs of cigarettes.[70] In this camp a woman saw former gracious hostesses, who in their homes on The Peak had served the most elaborate of meals, fighting grimly for possession of a discarded cigarette butt.[71]

Entrepreneurs existed in every camp, again reflecting systems that paralleled those in the outside world. Some of these individuals retailed bizarre merchandise. At Hong Kong: "A Yorkshireman whose breasts swelled up with beriberi sent a note round the wards announcing that a genuine pair of knockers could be inspected at any time on payment of one cigarette to Lulu Wetherdale."[72] True, the quotation is from a novel.

Cigarettes could bring not only a simulation of the female body, but also, on occasion, the real thing. In Japan, for example, immediately after the war ended, suddenly ex-POWs set out to test the world of freedom and victory. Supplies had been parachuted into the camps, including vast numbers of western cigarettes. A dozen of the ex-POWs ended up in downtown Niigata in a hotel. For four days, if they ran out of "money" they sent someone back to camp for more American cigarettes. They never left their hotel room. "The Japanese girls bathed us, and fed us, and what have you. The thoughts we had initially were that we might have problems but we had no problems, we just went into the hotel. We initially paid with yen but we ended up paying with blankets and cigarettes."[73]

Aside from their purchasing power, cigarettes were made to be smoked. The ecstasy of one man, suddenly rich in cigarettes after liberation, is palpable. Ralph Sanderson, in Niihama, wrote: "What a day! As I write this it's 12 pm, I've smoked Lucky Strike, Phillip Morris, Camel, Chesterfield and Rawleigh [*sic*] cigs. Tonight, eaten all the chocolate possible and had fruit salad for tea and NO RICE for the first time in 3 years and 8 months."[74]

Non-smokers often find this addiction difficult to understand, but in all camps, and indeed in all occupied countries throughout the world, cigarettes became an item of currency for which people would exchange precious possessions. A cigarette would temporarily reduce the pangs of hunger.[75]

A novelist has caught convincingly the almost mystical aura that some men cultivated through smoking. The scene was set in a camp in Hong Kong:

> He lit one of the cigarettes which he had bought at the Japanese canteen out of his August allowance of military yen. It was a *Golden Dragon*, locally made, and burned with a musty reluctance. As he drew on it, distastefully but greedily, he decided that after the war he would acquire some reputation as a connoisseur of tobaccos. He would study the geographical distribution of the plant and the different methods of culture and cure; he would sample every brand of cigarette, cigar, and pipe tobacco on the market, and experiment with mixtures of his own devising, making careful assessments of such factors of enjoyment as appearance, feel, aroma unlit and lit, flavour, coolness, satisfaction of craving. He would invent a Matheson Rating [character's name was Matheson], which would be widely accepted as a standard of comparison for tobacco products, and would create for himself an aura of mystery by refusing to turn his talents to commercial purposes....He blew smoke, watching his resolve swirl into fantasy.[76]

Ray Squires, a medical sergeant at Hong Kong, believed that as many as 40 percent of the men would trade a slice of bread or half a rice ration for a cigarette. Squires goes on to express his chagrin at seeing Canadian soldiers bumming cigarettes and scrambling for butts discarded—often as deliberate enticements to humiliation—by the Japanese guards, "but such is the case."[77]

Perhaps half the cigarettes smoked were shared by several men, despite urgent warnings from the medical officers against this mouth-to-mouth sharing because of the likelihood of spreading dysentery and diphtheria. Sharing may have been unhygienic but it had survival value and morale value. Buddy groups or pairs were a fundamental and vital technique for coping. Everything the group had was shared carefully and fairly. "This sharing of your last fag is something real....The fag is cut in half, and cut in half evenly with a razor blade as I have often seen it done. Perhaps you may roll the half into a thinner one, but still you have a smoke each."[78]

Occasionally, some guards were comradely. As has been noted in all theatres of war and in many eras, the cigarette provided a social focus that permitted true, if brief, human contact between enemies. A New Zealander captured at Hong Kong recalled, years later, his extraordinary feeling of release when he was able to drive in a speeding army truck over the wooded hills of the New Territories. They had good Japanese guards in those first days, mostly combat troops who had fought in Hong Kong. "Often they would unstrap the helmets slung on their backs and share out the cigarettes they all carried in the lining. With the cigarettes came photographs of girls and war souvenirs."[79] So Japanese guards and interpreters did give the POWs cigarettes, at least occasionally: "The word 'presento' was very useful: it could mean 'That was a present to me,' or 'May I have that?' or 'Will you give me that?' The cheap Japanese cigarettes were referred to by the troops as 'Tojo presentos.'"[80]

In the camps, incoming supplies were watched with intense concentration, increasingly so as the tobacco inventory shrank. Thus on 8 March 1942, one attentive Hong Kong POW "[s]aw the cigarettes arrive and be deposited in the NAAFI. Roll Call at 6:15. Issue of 1 Pkt 'Golden Dragon' after Roll Call. It loosens everyone into humans again." A few days later, he noted with pain that tobacco was $70.00 a tin ($14 Canadian). Soon after came the inevitable moralistic intervention. The Church of England padre sermonized about people who sold their souls for cigarettes.[81] In this instance the moralists were prescient, as will be seen in later chapters.

POWs in the Far East were generally much worse off and much worse treated than their counterparts in Europe. One reason for this was the reluctance of the Japanese to permit substantial shipments of relief supplies, supplies that reached Western POWs in Europe relatively easily and in large quantities throughout most of the war. The difficulty in providing tobacco to Far Eastern POWs can be epitomized in the efforts (and failures) of a Canadian organization called the Over-Seas League (Canada) Tobacco and Hamper Fund. In a report issued in 1943 the representatives of the Fund indicated that they had shipped to Europe more than 103 million cigarettes, but none to Hong Kong. They had directed one million cigarettes and a thousand pounds of tobacco to the Far East some months before. These supplies were supposed to go on the second trip of the neutral Swedish ship, *Gripsholm*, but that trip was aborted by the Japanese. The cigarettes and tobacco were returned to Montreal.[82]

Yet despite this bad luck in getting cigarettes through official channels, some did arrive from home. For example, in February 1945 Donald Geraghty, RRC, in Sham Shui Po, had a bonanza. On the 23rd he received a Red Cross individual parcel containing Old Gold cigarettes, and four days later he received a parcel from his aunt and uncle that included 300 Buckingham cigarettes.[83]

The International Committee for the Red Cross (ICRC) attempted to respond to the need for tobacco by Allied POWs in the Far East, but they also were hindered by Japanese recalcitrance. Nevertheless, significant sums were expended. Because so few individual parcels could be delivered from Allied or neutral Red Cross societies, local purchase of foodstuffs, cigarettes, medical supplies, and other items became vital. One report shows a total expenditure of 663,000 Swiss francs for tobacco and cigarettes, of which 486,000 francs came from governments or Red Cross societies and 177,000 from local funds.[84]

Trading with One's Captors

It is important to understand the clear differentiation made by most POWs. One did not steal from one's comrades, but the captors were fair game. And one traded with the enemy with a ruthlessness and a level of chicanery that generally were not permissible when dealing with fellow POWs. But for some Other Ranks, their own officers seemed fair game. One enterprising American serviceman managed to get a number of packages of cigarettes and sold them to a Lieutenant-Colonel for a one-hundred-dollar check a pack.[85]

Trading cigarettes for food was forbidden in certain circumstances amongst POWs but always permissible with the guards and civilians. In Singapore a diarist recorded his benign trading activities. He spent some hours teaching a sentry English in return for a few cigarettes. Then he taught a wounded Japanese soldier to play the Chinese flute, for which he was paid with iced water.[86]

Less benignly, in the Philippines it was reported that medical corpsmen were trading sulfa drugs to Japanese soldiers for packs of cigarettes. The prisoners were making these tablets out of corn starch—totally lacking in sulfa or any other drug—and trading them to the Japanese for cigarettes. The Japanese thought they would cure their venereal disease.[87] Most POWs blithely ignored the potential ethical issue here.

Getting cigarettes was only the first step in the smoking process. If they were not to be traded, then of course they were smoked. To smoke a cigarette, one must light it. Methods of getting a light were numerous, matches being a rare and expensive commodity. One elaborate and ingenious solution appeared at Hong Kong:

> Smokers had a Heath-Robertson[88] sort of cigarette lighter. A small Marmite jar was fitted with a cork or wooden bung and about half-filled with salt solution; two tin-plate electrodes were separated by about $1/4''$, one to the mains and the other to a fixed carbon from an electric torch battery; another carbon was connected to the other side of the mains. To light a fag the smoker hooked in and an arc was thus struck between the carbons, the salt solution supplying the resistance. Nobody was electrocuted; how or why I don't know, but the buildings were like a fireworks display after lights out.[89]

In Malaya as in other locations, matches had vanished, and the everlasting search for a light had become a dominating factor in smokers' lives. A hut that boasted a piece of slow-burning rope was the object of "a steady pilgrimage of smokers from all over the camp."[90]

One man borrowed a pair of eyeglasses and used them, successfully, to magnify the sun's rays and light up a homemade cigar.[91]

A major reason for creating such elaborate and capricious devices was the cost of matches. Though one doesn't customarily think of matches as being a financial burden, in POW camp the cost became highly relevant. By October 1944, one man at Sham Shui Po had to pay the equivalent of one English pound, or about $5, for a "penny" box of matches at the canteen.[92]

A few Canadians at Hong Kong became notorious for a method by which they stole a few puffs from a gullible mark. The racket depended on the shortage of matches, so that one lit a cigarette by holding one end to a lighted cigarette and inhaling through the unlit cigarette so that the burning tobacco kindled the other. A Canadian would ask for a light from someone he saw already enjoying a cigarette. But the cigarette which the Canadian used was a hollow facsimile through which he could draw in several good puffs of the other man's smoke—"until most of us got wise."[93] This same technique apparently was discovered independently elsewhere, since the trick is described by POWs from Singapore as well.[94]

Smokers had many complexities in their lives. When several butts were obtainable, or loose tobacco, there arose yet another logistical hurdle: cigarette paper. The real stuff was rarely available. One critic noted that smokes were rather "throaty" when rolled with air-mail note paper.[95] Probably every conceivable variety of paper and leaf was tried by determined and often desperate smokers.

The acme of substitutes was unquestionably one that presented at least a few of the men with a moral dilemma. Was it acceptable to use pages from a Bible or a hymn book for rolling cigarettes? Most POWs found little to debate here, especially because the sanctified paper made excellent fags. Most chaplains seem to have accepted the inevitable and only urged plaintively that the men read the pages before smoking them. There was debate about where to begin dismantling the Bible. From the beginning, or selectively? As a contemporary historian has written: "An English chaplain said Revelations, which no one understood anyway. The Dutch Jesuit said the Old Testament, then the Acts of the Apostles because they were only practicalities, then the Gospels; leave the Sermon on the Mount for last, and learn it before smoking it."[96]

Other books also served this purpose. Any book would do for a desperate smoker with some scraps of tobacco. Since the pages in some books are made up of quite thick paper, the splitting of these pages became an art in itself.[97]

Need for Tobacco vs Drugs and Alcohol

One POW knew of two hard drug addicts in North Point Camp at Hong Kong; they had no problems in adapting to abstinence. But that was not the case with the heavy smokers.[98] And in Europe a padre, Hon.-Capt. John Foote, VC, saw men in the camps who, if they weren't alcoholics, certainly were heavy users. Most of them smoked, but Foote never heard anyone talk about liquor or complain that they missed it at all. They just stopped. "But the smokes were the things they *really* missed."[99]

Harrison wrote that women and beer rarely were mentioned. Next to food, the great need was seen to be tobacco, and many men found its hold almost terrifying:

> From start to finish the medium and heavy smokers were slaves to the habit and would take incredible risks to buy the weed, or to steal it from the Japanese. When they couldn't get it they smoked tea leaves, rope, dried hibiscus leaves—anything that faintly resembled tobacco. Clothes, presentation watches, and the most precious souvenirs of home, were all sold or swapped for it. Even in the depths of a Japanese winter, emaciated prisoners were still swapping their rice for tobacco.[100]

Many other substitutes for tobacco were used. Most were unsatisfactory, some disgusting. Dried pine needles, used tea leaves, used hops, eucalyptus leaves, and sweet potato leaves, all were experimented with in one camp in Hong Kong.[101]

Though in general POWs wouldn't steal from their fellows, inevitably there were exceptions. In Hamowa POW Camp, Japan, the prisoners' rations were separate from those of the guards, though cooked in the same galley. Two officers, successively, supervised the distribution. They tried to ensure a fair distribution, but the men stole from the food supply, both to eat themselves and to sell for tobacco.[102]

Almost invariably, the POWs kept such problems internal to the camp. Punishment was meted out by an aggrieved victim personally, or by vigilantes, or according to the decision of some form of judicial process. For example, in 1945 a British sapper in the Royal Engineers was beaten up by his roommates for stealing cigarettes and soap. This was seen by the camp hierarchy as punishment enough, and the War Diary stated that no official action was taken.[103]

Since cigarettes were both valued currency and a coveted gratification, they entered into efforts to discipline the prisoners. This was true of both the Japanese and the internal governance of the camp by the prisoners. In Niigata Camp 5B, Japan, the issue of cigarettes was only suspended, as punishment, when a prisoner did something seriously wrong. And usually the cigarettes would be given to the culprit by the camp leaders anyway, in some roundabout way.[104]

Two Canadians were court-martialled by the Japanese in Tokyo for disposing of various items of government-issued attire for cigarettes. After the war a Canadian war crimes investigator sent a copy of the documentation of their trial, thinking the men might enjoy it as a souvenir. "West [Sgt, Canadian Dental Corps], Soroka [Pte, Winnipeg Grenadiers]. Sentenced to eight and ten months, respectively, on 1 October 1943."[105] They served the sentence and were then returned to their POW camp.

Punishments by the Japanese usually took place immediately without any need for legal niceties. A cigarette might be the instrument of punishment: "P.W. were made to smoke a cigarette until the last ashes had been consumed, resulting in burned lips. This punishment was awarded for smoking elsewhere than in quarters."[106] In Burma, one ex-POW remembered vividly "Liver-lips," a Korean guard on the railway: "We couldn't smoke and maybe he'd come along and he'd give you a cigarette and then take a pole and beat the tar out of you because you were smoking."[107] An American POW was discovered by the Japanese smoking in the latrine, a forbidden activity. The Japanese NCO in charge forced him to kneel on sharp bamboo sticks, producing pain so severe the prisoner drew blood by biting his lips. After long minutes a friendly guard let him return to bed—which he needed help to do. He never smoked at night again.[108]

Within the camps, the use of cigarettes as currency grew, by logical extension, to include the payment of "fines" for offences against discipline or ordinary morality. In January 1945, in one of the camps in the Fukuoka area, some NCOs and Warrant Officers failed to accept the responsibilities that went with their rank. The POW officers believed that stoppage of Red Cross and other amenities including IJA cigarette issues was the only way to bring the men to realize "their duties to the Army and their fellow men."[109] For many offences the punishment would be the forfeiture of Japanese cigarette issues. "In cases where immediate effect is desired, it is our only means of punishment and as no offence can be punished twice no additional action under the Army Act is possible."[110]

The Hazards, Sometimes Lethal

"I will gladly pay you Tuesday for a hamburger today!"
J. Wellington Wimpy[111]

During World War Two, particularly in the Far East, food trading sometimes became a serious problem. Some instances have been cited already. Men might follow Wimpy's path, offering some of next week's food for an extra ration today. This was a slippery slope that led to serious difficulties. In Omuta Camp, in Japan, the call was: "Rice now, for rice and soup tomorrow." One of the survivors, an Australian, blamed the problem on the Americans who, he said, brought the system from the Philippines. In his previous camps it had been the custom for a man too sick too eat to give his ration to a friend. But in Omuta food was never given away, only sold. Some men "practically lived on the hunger and stupidity of others."[112]

Many men traded away part of their meagre ration for cigarettes. In several locations, formal action by the internal camp administration attempted to prevent these men from further undermining their already chronically poor physical state. Many men are believed to have starved themselves to death—or, one might say, smoked themselves to death—by trading more food for cigarettes than their bodies would allow. There seems no reason to doubt that physiological nicotine addiction and psychological addiction combined to create this extreme behaviour.

An Australian medical officer observed that some men, even though they were starving and could not stand on parade without fainting or falling over, would trade their bowl of rice for a cigarette. "I think," he wrote just after the war, "the reason was, they could take a few whiffs of the cigarette and this would ease their hunger, and some time later they would light up again and take another couple of whiffs."[113]

Cigarette trading for food became a problem at Bowen Road Hospital also. Col. Bowie's staff worried because some patients exchanged food, issued for treatment purposes, for cigarettes. "We took a strong line on this and the practice soon ended."[114] One soldier received a large number of cigarettes from home, though Bowie was puzzled as to how this could even have happened. When the soldier started to sell these at extortionate rates until the enterprise became scandalous, Bowie confiscated the cigarettes and distributed them, free, to all non-officers in the hospital. He was pleased and surprised that his action met with approval, rather than with disapproval of the high handed action, "which in fact it was."[115]

A Canadian POW in Hong Kong and in Japan took a strictly utilitarian view of the moral issue. Or, rather, he claimed to find no moral issue:

> Some men sold their rice rations for cigarettes; some people might think that the man who bought his rice for cigarettes was a bad apple, but you have to look at it in two lights, and I'm looking at it from a personal standpoint. At times I had sold my rice for cigarettes and other times I bought rice for cigarettes. A cigarette to me might, at that time, be more valuable than a bowl of rice. In Japan, we received 3½ American Red Cross parcels in our camp, and in those were 10 packages of American cigarettes, sometimes a mixture of Chesterfields and Camels, a pound of powdered milk, a can of butter, a bar of chocolate, cheese, sugar, a number of things. The first parcel we got I traded my can of powdered milk for 10 packs of cigarettes. I traded everything off. Being mercenary, a month later I could buy a can of powdered milk for one pack of cigarettes. That's a case, which way do you want to look at it—profiteering, or not? It was survival, you looked after number one first.[116]

This same man, however, took a different stance when a personal friend was the one trying to sell his food for cigarettes. One such,

George, "was always over to sell his rice for cigarettes and I never bought his rice. He did my laundry for a cigarette. You had to look at things that way. I knew if George sold his rice for cigarettes, if he was doing it all the time, he wasn't eating any rice."[117]

In addition to the fundamental hazard of starvation, there were specific medical problems associated with smoking. A Dutch physician reported on a disease that he labelled tropical nutritional amblyopia, or "camp eyes." This condition apparently was unknown in Europe. It was essentially a disease of adult males with blue eyes and fair or red hair. The specifics of the disease are unimportant here, but this physician believed that it was caused by a combination of gross deficiency of B vitamins, plus poisoning, perhaps by nicotine.[118]

This connection was only conjectural. Other diseases were less equivocal. In February 1944, 90 percent of the inmates of one camp had some degree of optic neuritis, a disorder of the nerve responsible for sight. The medical officer had seen cases go from 20/20 vision to difficulty in counting fingers in 10 days.[119] Efforts were made to eliminate tobacco as it was felt that smoking would further damage the inflamed optic nerve. "However, despite our warnings of total blindness, we could not stop the men from smoking."[120]

Another medical officer brooded over the likelihood that the sudden massive oversupply of goods to the POWs immediately after the war, the rain of chocolate bars, cigarettes, and butter, had put their feet "firmly on the road to the diseases of an affluent Western society."[121]

US President Clinton announced on 23 August 1996 that the FDA had labelled nicotine officially addictive. But the addictive capacity of nicotine has long been recognized, even if admitted by the tobacco companies only recently. Revelations show that, at least by 1972, this property was undeniable: according to Claude Teague, on the research staff of the R.J. Reynolds Tobacco Company, "Nicotine is known to be a habit-forming alkaloid, hence the confirmed user of tobacco products is primarily seeking the physiological 'satisfaction' derived from nicotine—and perhaps other active compounds....Thus, a tobacco product is, in essence, a vehicle for delivery of nicotine, designed to deliver the nicotine in a generally acceptable and attractive form."[122]

Tobacco literally was addictive to some men, and this addiction was life-threatening. The toss-up between food and smoking was too often decided in favour of smoking, so that an already significantly reduced diet was pared beyond the bone. Men died of starvation, clutching one last cigarette between nicotine-stained fingers.

Medical officers were aware of the risks and, in many camps, vigorous efforts were made to control those who could not control themselves. Early on, the medical officers tried to influence the men by persuasion. A POW in Java remembered informal talks in which their doctor told them what to buy with their meagre earnings, stressing particularly the need for bananas and eggs. If a man had some money and spent it on tobacco instead of fruit or eggs, then he must be responsible for the consequences. The doctors could only explain the situation, leaving the rest to the individuals.[123] Later, more active measures had to be taken.

The problem of cigarettes being traded for food became acute for a relatively small number of men, especially in the camps in Japan. The sometimes lethal implications of their addiction are well documented. The theoretical amount of food any individual's ration actually contained—derived by dividing the gross daily food intake in camp by the number of men, after deducting food that arrived spoiled—might not represent what any specific man in fact ate. For this difference two main factors were responsible. First was the almost universal craving for tobacco. "Depending on the cigarette shortage a bowl of rice would be valued from one to five cigarettes, and no amount of warning nor exhortation could suppress the practice." The second factor was gambling with the contents of Red Cross parcels, a popular pastime resulting often in a most unbalanced distribution of food. One or both of these habits, Robinson found, seemed to be universal amongst the American troops in particular.[124]

Gambling for food and bartering rations for cigarettes was a violation of Japanese camp rules in every camp. These activities nevertheless occurred and even provided potential mitigation for suspected Japanese war crimes if the events were recalled and if the offending parties could be identified.[125]

At Niigata there was "a living skeleton" who had to be forced to eat by threats of cutting him off tobacco and water.[126] This heavy-handed approach was all that could save some of these men. Even then, many did not survive. At Niigata some cigarettes always were available. The men got cigarettes outside the camp, occasionally, and a few men became cigarette barons. This was a major problem. Men who didn't smoke could trade a cigarette for a meal at times when rations were inadequate. They got fat and addicted smokers got thin.

> We tried all sorts of things to stop this swapping of cigarettes for meals, but of course, it was carried out at night, clandestinely, behind the latrine areas, or somewhere. We had more than one chap die simply from starvation. I think we selected about 20 persons who were in danger, serious danger, from swapping meals for a cigarette. We made them feed in the hospital, at least one meal a day, under supervision, and they had to eat it whether they liked it or not.

Officers made the men break their bargains with their cigarette baron. When word of this tactic got around, trading meals for cigarettes pretty well stopped.[127] The speaker was the British medical officer. One might wonder if this forced feeding differs significantly from forcible blood transfusion to a Jehovah's Witness. But it saved lives.

At Oeyama POW Camp, in Japan, as hunger increased the men became more difficult to handle. They would steal from each other—one of the most heinous crimes to a POW—and from the Japanese. These latter thefts often led to severe punishment.[128] In 1944, Oeyama Camp came to be run by four NCOs, one Canadian and three British, who worked with the Japanese, lived separately from the rest of the men, and had extra rations and privileges. On orders from the Japanese they would beat the men, justifying their actions on the grounds that they would not hit as hard as the Japanese. Rackets thrived in the camp, many of them involving food.

When a group of Allied POW officers was transferred to Oeyama late in the war they began to take control away from the NCOs. One of them wrote:

> We found that many men owed food to a gang of racketeers. A hungry man would obtain an extra half-ration of rice in return for a promise to repay a three-quarter portion at the end of the week. Believe it or not, some men, despite their hunger, would even buy cigarettes with a promise to repay in food. Several men were deeply in debt. Our senior officers (we had an Australian Major and an American Major) ordered that all debts were canceled, and arranged for all debtors to eat their rations together under supervision to protect them from the racketeers.[129]

A somewhat similar set of circumstances was recorded at Narumi POW Camp near Nagoya. Playing deadly games with their rations cost several men their lives, as will be described in Chapter Eight.

Conclusions

1. The cigarette was so generally desired that it became a unit of currency in many situations during World War Two, particularly in places of incarceration such as internment and prisoner-of-war camps.
2. Smoking cigarettes was a constituent in a social process that was important to most of the inhabitants of these camps.
3. As in any human situation, currency—including cigarettes—can be and was put to base uses.
4. For some men cigarette smoking was an uncontrollable addiction the demands of which caused their deaths from starvation. The principle inherent in Wimpy's desire for a hamburger now for a promise of two later strikes at the heart of the POW's situation: present gratification is real, while later inconveniences can be rationalized away. Let he who has resisted temptation cast the first stone.

Perhaps long-dead King James I deserves the last word. He described smoking as: "A custome lothsome to the eye, hatefull to the Nose, harmefull to the braine, dangerous to the Lungs, and in the blacke stinking fumes thereof, neerest resembling the horrible Stigian smoke of the pit that is bottomelesse."[130]

Sex

Severe dietary deprivation presumably reduces and eventually eliminates libido. And there is ample evidence that POWs in the camps in Hong Kong were significantly underfed. Nevertheless, at Kai Tak airport there were many Chinese women working on the construction of bays to protect aircraft against bombing attacks. They were, Lewis Bush noted, the usual working type; they wore jackets and trousers made of a material that looks like oilskin. Some of the men were on decidedly friendly terms with them, and would slip away to spend a few sweaty moments with them in the bomb bays out of sight of prying eyes. "Yes, sex had reared its ugly head, even among the prisoners. A British sergeant commenting on the amorous activities of some of the men said to me: 'I don't know how they do it on this food, sir.'"[131]

Understandably, the men were alarmed to think that the long-term malnutrition might produce permanent damage to their sexual capacities. Although some were able to provide definite reassurance immediately after the war—and a very few during their POW life—for most the answer had to wait longer. One study of Winnipeg Grenadiers in 1948 summed up this concern: "Some degree of impotence was universal on return to Canada but this has gradually improved so that now, it is a rare complaint."[132]

But for many men the test had to be made as quickly as possible. At Sham Shui Po, shaky POW control replaced the by then equally shaky Japanese on 18 August 1945. One of the first orders was that the men were to stay in camp; no Allied troops had yet arrived and the Japanese, though defeated, continued to exercise police functions. Inevitably, the order to remain in camp was ignored. At least by 25 August, some of the men brought a Chinese woman into camp. They had her in one of the empty huts, and apparently there was a substantial lineup. The fact was discovered because two of the men went to the medical officer for treatment. He had nothing to give them.[133] Nevertheless, there were some prophylactics in the camp, at least as Arthur Gomes remembered; he recalled a small table being set up in camp in late August, piled high with condoms. The Canadians were the first to get to the condoms and, presumably, the women. "They beat us!" Gomes recalled.

In the Philippines, on 30 November 1943, an American medical officer observed that his men were regaining their libidos. They had recently received some Red Cross food supplies. Several POWs told their MO that they had awakened with erections and had had wet dreams. "I told them I could take care of that. I'd see that the chow ration was cut down, for I didn't want them overfed and underfucked."[134] At Singapore, the situation was much as it was in Hong Kong and in Japan:

The semi-starvation, vitamin-lacking diet meted out by the Japanese kept most POWs so debilitated that sex, in deed and in thought, failed to exist. I had always considered myself the normal male and it was with a sense of shock that, during the latter months of Pudu and our stay at Changi, I found in myself certain homosexual tendencies. There was no desire...of a physical nature, but there was the urge for the companion-ship of one of my fellow men and the desire to be of service and to share all things with him. These thoughts and feelings were kept very care-fully to myself and I was gratified and relieved to find that this tempo-rary aberration vanished completely once we resumed the normal, hard POW work life some weeks later. Indeed, in all my POW days, I knew of only one man whom one could reasonably suspect of being homosexu-al and the Japanese recipe of poor food and hard work certainly elimi-nated what could have been a considerable problem to some 50,000 womanless young men.[135]

Homosexuality was inevitably both a concern and a fact—un-doubtedly more common than it was thought to be by the man just quoted. Fifty years ago this form of sexual expression was much less talked about and far more secret than it is at the beginning of the twenty-first century.

At Omori Camp in Japan, Bush noted an uncongenial phenome-non: "There was a nasty little American from New Mexico, who looked after the Japanese chickens. He seemed able to do more or less as he pleased, was always well fed and spent most of his time in the camp headquarters. He was rosy-cheeked, and had breasts like a woman."[136] Bush's suspicions of homosexual conduct are obvious if not explicit. In December 1944 a British naval POW commented cyni-cally on a Japanese order that, until extra blankets were issued, two men might sleep together. "The Nips have done at last what Nelson and sailors have been doing for ages!"[137] In Kobe House, a POW camp in Japan, a British soldier commented on this subject in his diary in July 1944:

> On the other point of Captain Boyce's talk, the homo-sexuality, some men professed to have believed that it did not happen in "Kobe House." However one sergeant said that he had heard of one case being found amongst the British; that the culprits were tried at a court-martial by Warrant Officers, found guilty, and there and then had their punish-ments administered, each of the men in turn were mounted on the back of one WO, whilst another gave them the number of strokes decided upon with his Sam Brown belt, buckle end. Another chap reported that there had been quite some cases of it, with one of the older Indian sea-men acting as a procurer. Sickening.[138]

Will Allister encountered invitations to homosexuality at camps in Japan. One invitee was a handsome British POW who offered him-self for three rations of rice: "a high-class whore."[139] The food supply must have been improving towards the end of the war, as masturbation was "a flourishing industry."[140] But it was the Japanese who harassed Allister on at least two occasions. A hancho, or work boss, a repulsively ugly man nicknamed Harpo, made constant overtures to him till, happily for Allister he was moved elsewhere.[141] At another camp a guard attempted to become both amorous and violent, but someone intervened and nothing further happened.[142]

Escaping

Western soldiers saw attempting to escape as both desirable and militarily correct. In Europe, escapes were numerous. At Hong Kong, attempts began soon after the capitulation on Christmas Day 1941. However, successful escapes presented hazardous risks. While the "military code" may have promoted escape attempts, most men simply ignored the whole idea and set themselves the task of surviving as POWs. Moreover, the officers quickly became officially opposed to escape attempts. The chief reasons were that such attempts were likely to fail, and that even if successful, retaliation would increase the misery and the risk for the vast majority who remained behind.

Among potential escapees, the likelihood of success depended on several factors. Aside from the ineffable and uncontrollable effects of luck, the most important of these was local contacts. Those who escaped most easily were those who had lived long in Hong Kong: in general, these were members of the HKVDC. They knew the city intimately and had families and friends who could help them; the process could be as simple as slipping under the wire while guards were diverted, and walking home. The Chinese found escape simple, but so did many of the Hong Kong Portuguese; being short and quite dark-skinned, their appearance favoured them. So did their detailed knowledge of the city and the crucial fact that they had relatives and friends to supply money and clothing and provide shelter. And they knew the local languages.

By the first week in February, before the Japanese had an accurate accounting, one English POW had heard that more than 100 had already escaped from Sham Shui Po. As he realized, "it was a simple matter for them to adopt 'coolie' dress of singlet & shorts and get thro the fence & they were 'home.'"[143]

Perhaps next in order of potential ease of escape were the Indians. Both the Rajputs and the Punjabis had been in Hong Kong for many years, and the city had a substantial Indian population.[144] These persons could be expected to assist at least their co-religionists who wished to disappear into the teeming city. There is evidence that some Indian POWs did effect escapes, including a mass escape late in the war.

For British POWs, escaping was more hazardous than for the non-European members of the HKVDC or the Indians. Marked indelibly by skin colour, appearance, and height, simply melting into the Hong Kong population was impossible. Those Britishers who escaped successfully, and there were a few, did so by leaving the Hong Kong area and reaching friendly Chinese forces on the mainland. To do this one needed trustworthy contacts and money. Many British members of the HKVDC were long-time, even lifelong, residents of Hong Kong; and the British regiments had been stationed in the colony for years, so such contacts often existed in abundance.

At the distant end of the spectrum from the HKVDC were the Canadians. They had been in Hong Kong only a few weeks. When I interviewed the late Dr. John Crawford in 1983, I asked him about attempts to escape at Hong Kong. Quickly he stood up and said, "Look at me!" Dr. Crawford was about 6'5" tall. Obviously, it was impossible for him—and by extension for even less lofty western POWs—to escape in Asia. Not only did they stand out like redwoods in a bonsai park, but the Canadians in particular had no reliable local contacts, having been in the colony only three weeks before war began. The chances of success were essentially zero. Nevertheless, one quartet of men from Crawford's regiment, the Winnipeg Grenadiers, did make the attempt. The results were tragic, as will be described.

Dr. Solomon Bard remembers the escape of a fellow HKVDC colleague, Dr. Lindsay Ride. He had been head of the Field Ambulance, but he was a physiologist and had never practised medicine. Therefore, Ride reasoned, he would be little help medically in the camp. He decided to escape. He also wanted to escape because he believed that things were going to be "dreadful" in the camps and he wanted to let people know. But, Bard remembers, he told his medical colleagues that they would be useful and needed. "I'm not going to tell you not to escape but I can tell you one thing—that you will be sorely needed as far as I can see here, looking after your people. I leave it to your own conscience."[145] Then he escaped successfully. This undoubtedly was a productive escape, since Ride then founded the British Army Aid Group (BAAG), which performed important Intelligence work throughout the war, as well as smuggling medical and other materials into the Hong Kong camps.[146] Ride left Sham Shui Po on 9 January 1942 and reached safety eight days later.

Until they had detailed records of who actually was in the camps, the Japanese could not know who or how many were leaving, so on 5 February they conducted a prolonged and painstaking roll call at Sham Shui Po, "with Japs ticking off each name in a particular book, lasts until 5:30. Everyone sleeps, or lounges, and of course cursed quietly. Even the cooks can't get away."[147]

The Japanese made some efforts to improve conditions in the camps, perhaps at least partially to remove one of the reasons for escaping. A British officer in Sham Shui Po noted in his diary in early February 1942: "The GOC, asked by Japs why so many men had escaped, replied that conditions, especially food, was the cause." The Japanese then did send in vegetables such as sweet potatoes, turnips, soya beans, and dried Indian peas. This allowed the men to have a passable soup once a day. The Japanese also let them have some Chinese tea but no sugar or milk.[148]

By the end of February, the Japanese had prepared (and read aloud to the prisoners in each camp) regulations about non-escaping that included a blunt statement of the fate that awaited a recaptured POW.[149] Nevertheless, escapes were so frequent by the spring of 1942 that the Japanese were forced to take more definitive action. Already there had been preliminary planning for a massive break from Sham Shui Po and Argyle Street Camp as a coordinated action. The Japanese discovered this, presumably because the patriotic Chinese outside, who were crucial to the plot, were betrayed by the Loa Kikan, a traitorous organization of Chinese criminals. The multitude of escapes led the Japanese to separate officers and men, officers going to Argyle Street Camp.

The shift of officers and men between Argyle and Sham Shui Po camps came just a few days after the latest escape, on 10 April 1942, of three officers—John Pearce, RA; Douglas Clague, RA; and Lynton White—and a sergeant, David Bosanquet, a 27-year-old Volunteer. They received no support whatever from the senior officers:

> We've been forbidden to go ahead with our plan. The CO has just told me that the disused hut is in the area which Maltby has designated as a hospital. We would be breaking the Hague Convention [sic] if we were to escape from it. Reprisals would be certain. And, what is more, if we go on with the scheme, the General says steps will be taken to see that we are unable to complete the tunnel.

They escaped nonetheless, departing Sham Shui Po through a storm culvert.[150]

These escapes galvanized the Japanese. They mustered all POWs on the parade ground for hours while searching every square inch of the camp. The next reaction by the IJA was to strengthen the barbed wire that encircled the camp. This was done by working parties of Indian POWs under Japanese command.[151]

Retaliation was swift. Bertram reported that the early discovery of the activities of a tunnelling party was disastrous to the camp as a whole. The cover they had used to conceal their meetings while planning the escape had been a Spanish class. Thereafter, all classes were cancelled, and a strict ban was imposed preventing any gathering of more than four prisoners. The sole exceptions were concerts (each of which required individual approval) and religious services.[152]

By the second week of May, the Japanese implemented the next stage in escape prevention. This was the contentious demand that each POW sign a statement promising not to escape. Obviously, making such a warranty conflicted directly with the instructions understood by Allied troops that they *should* attempt to escape, in hopes both of resuming military service and of harassing the enemy. In Europe, where the Germans and Italians accepted the validity of the Geneva Convention with respect to Western nationals held prisoner (but not to Soviet POWs), escape attempts during the war ran into thousands. But the Japanese held diametrically opposed views on prisonerhood and had not ratified that Geneva Convention. They insisted that the men promise not to escape, with death the declared penalty for breaking the promise.

Initially, the Japanese presented their demand to the prisoners but did not attempt to force immediate submission. The matter was being discussed on 12 May, but 10 days later, a senior officer was still touring the various units to learn their feelings on the question. The Royal Scots, at least, seem to have been unhappy about the issue, for a diarist recorded that "great noisy yelps" greeted Col. Ford when he raised the matter on parade. Meanwhile, the POW NCOs had been lectured about the need to mount pickets to discourage escape. The Japanese guards and officers had, apparently, been punished for previous escapes, so they were understandably testy on the subject. "The Japs *all* lost seniority when 4 officers got away."[153]

On 23 May 1942, discussion ended abruptly. The Japanese paraded everyone in Sham Shui Po camp to hear an address by Col. Tokunaga, the officer in charge of Hong Kong POW camps. He demanded that they all sign the declaration. Immediately after his harangue, officers and men were required to sign the "Escape Me Not" paper.

After much discussion, the officers recommended that all men sign. Because the undertaking was made under duress it would not be considered binding under any circumstance, the parade-ground lawyers claimed. Moreover, it was evident that failure to sign would bring severe repercussions individually and collectively. All but about 90 POWs did sign at that time. The 90 were taken away and threatened, after which all but 16 signed and were returned to camp. The final 16 were trucked to Stanley Prison, where they were "kept under insanitary conditions in a solitary cell on a diet of plain rice and water."[154] Ultimately, all signed.

Similarly, at North Point Camp, Lt. White noted on 24 May 1942, "We must all sign on oath that we shall not try to escape."[155] But attempts continued. In June and July 1942, Sham Shui Po Camp was under punishment because the four officers had escaped. Neither bread nor canteen was permitted. The daily caloric value of the diet at this time was about 1,400,[156] half of the minimal requirement to maintain health.

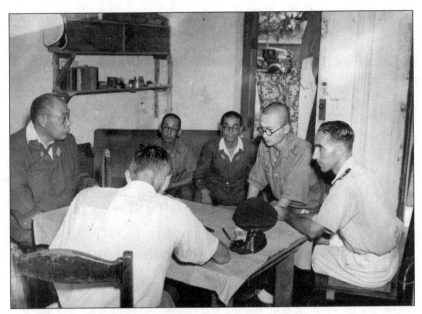

Figure 4.3. Col. Tokunaga Isao (far left) being interrogated by Lt.-Col. S.E.H. White, Royal Scots (back to camera), senior officer at Sham Shui Po, September 1945 (Imperial War Museum, A 30521.)

Two months later the Japanese found another escape tunnel at Sham Shui Po. A group of former dockyard policemen who were POWs had been digging it for weeks. The suspicion in camp was that informers were to blame.[157] As an immediate consequence, Japanese sentries were authorized to shoot anybody moving about after lights out. This event heralded a return to the nightly shooting that had gone on early in the camp's existence. "Bullets whistle all around & over the camp and it is almost suicide to go outside after lights out."[158] The date was 20 August.

Events were building to a tragic conclusion. That night, the camp was awakened by rifle shots. Everyone spent a miserable two hours on parade in the dark and the pouring rain, many with bare feet. The reason was that two Royal Engineers escaped through a typhoon nullah, or drainage ditch, outside the hospital for patients with skin diseases.[159]

The Japanese victors used grim and brutal object lessons to show how seriously they took their interdiction of escape attempts. One day after the Sham Shui Po escape, four POWs succeeded in getting away from North Point Camp. Sgt. John O. Payne, L/Cpl. George Berzenski (a medical orderly), Pte. John H. Adams, and Pte. Percy J. Ellis, all members of the Winnipeg Grenadiers, left the camp the night of 21 August 1942. One fellow prisoner recalled being in hospital at North Point in August 1942:

> One morning, the Japanese discovered that there had been an escape....One of the orderlies was a Lance-Corporal Berzenski of the Grenadiers and he was not there....The [Japanese] then came back to the hospital and started questioning the patients asking us if we had heard any noise or had seen anyone trying to escape. We said no. As a matter of fact, during the night I and most of the other patients had heard persons walking on the roof of the hospital and actually figured an escape was taking place because it was in this section of the camp that an escape had the best chance of success. This was because there were buildings close by which could be used for concealment, also there were guards posted only on the corners of the end of the Camp who used to do a beat back and forth and that end of the Camp was closest to the town and some Chinese lived in houses almost next to the Camp.160

Another Canadian, L/Sgt. William A. Hall, was also a patient in the North Point hospital that fateful night. His recollection was even more precise:

> I believe it was the 21st of August, 1942, when this escape took place. During the evening of the escape, I saw these four soldiers getting ready in the Orderly Room of the Hospital. My bed was at the end of the ward, closest to the Orderly Room and I had a good view of what they were doing. They each had a small pack, in which they placed food of all kinds. They were all dressed warmly and each one of them had a complete battle dress, which I believe they wore leaving the camp. I am not absolutely certain of the time I saw them in the Orderly Room but it was between 10:00 and 11:00 o'clock and it took them nearly an hour to complete their preparations.
>
> About 11:15 p.m. I saw the four of them leave the Orderly Room in the Hospital and about ten or fifteen minutes later I heard a clattering sound from the slate roof of the hospital and it was very evident that the sound which I heard was caused by persons clambering over the roof. The clattering sounded very loud in the ward and when the noise on the roof stopped it was very quiet and I heard no shouting or shooting at any time throughout that night....Immediately after I heard this noise on the roof stop one of the hospital Orderlies...came up to me and started to rub my feet to ease the pain, as I was suffering from beri beri of the feet and dysentery. This medical orderly remarked to me: "Well, they've finally got away."161

The four men were recaptured. Their execution was ordered by Maj.-Gen. Arisue, 23rd Army, Hong Kong.162 The lethal implications of the non-escape agreement were revealed. "The Japanese Commandant told us he knew we were supposed to escape, but he was giving us a direct order not to. Therefore, if we tried to escape we would be executed—not for escaping but for disobeying a Japanese order."[163]

Inevitably, despite the Geneva Convention on Prisoners of War, to which Japan did not subscribe anyway,[164] and the Hague Convention of 1906, to which it did, there were mass reprisals. On 29 August 1942 one POW wrote in his diary: "Everything has been in a turmoil all week—parades, searches, etc. Concerts are cut out, no sports, no canteen stuff to come in."[165]

Despite fears to the contrary, there were no reprisals directed specifically against the hospital or patients after this event. This is itself surprising since one of the escapees had worked there and it was the starting point for the escape.

The Japanese, a medical officer, Woodward, observed, always took a righteously shocked view of attempted escapes, since every escapee had signed an undertaking not to do so. "The agreement was given to me to sign when I was working as surgeon in the Lower Camp Hospital and was phrased that I should not escape 'while engaged in medical care of Prisoners of War.' As I should myself have been very displeased at anyone's escaping from the Hospital, with the inevitable repercussions on food, drugs and treatment I had no hesitation in signing this agreement."[166]

However, this same medical officer did not hesitate to steal parts for a hidden radio, discovery of which would unquestionably have had major repercussions for the hospital and its patients. "During the night, with the help of Jemadar Chatn Dev I got into the Jap store and acquired four radio valves from a set a Jap sergeant had stored there, and got them into the Camp next morning where I gave them to the OC Signals in General Maltby's presence. With only these valves a radio was eventually (six months later) improvised in the Camp chiefly by Naval Officers most of the work being done by Lt. Dixon RNVR. This radio got BBC direct and also the US advance airfield at Wai Chow 60 miles away. It was easily adjustable to transmitting and no doubt could have played a part in Colonel L.A. Newnham's scheme of escape."[167] This is a reference to a mass escape that was planned but betrayed, costing the life of, among others, Col. Newnham.

The status of medical officer carried with it heavy burdens. One that arose was an ethical and moral concern connected with making use of hospitals and patients for non-medical purposes such as escape work or the forbidden pursuit of communication with the outside world. Here, most medical officers would have agreed, the best interests of the patient had to come first. Coates described one situation he encountered at Nakom Patan POW hospital in 1945: "It had been suggested by some that a [radio] set should be operated under the bed of a very sick dysentery patient since the guards would be less likely to search there. I had to take the stand that I would not jeopardise the life of a sick man, even for the purpose of obtaining news."[168]

There were times, also—not many but memorable when they occurred, a welcome contrast to the grim details of executions and retaliation—when a certain aura of foolishness took over. One of the most bizarre happened at Kinkaseki Camp in Formosa (Taiwan). Because it may shed some light on Japanese attitudes towards managing prisoners it deserves mention here. When the POWs at Kinkaseki came back from the mine one evening, they saw an astonishing sight. One of the Camp Commandant's ducks, which he kept in small bamboo pens, was fastened on the parade square. "The poor bird was quacking away, its wings tied to two large stones! Before we could be dismissed after the usual roll-call...we were told the duck was being punished for breaking Camp Regulations!" In stilted English, the interpreter explained that the duck had "escaped" from his compound and was being punished "according to regulations," presumably as a warning to them all.[169] Japanese applied psychology? One has to doubt the efficacy of the warning, but the episode must have given the POWs at least a few moments of light relief (carefully concealed).

At Hong Kong as elsewhere, however, the atmosphere was as a rule devoid of amusement. Several books have been published describing some of the escapes made from camps in Hong Kong. Europeans who were successful almost invariably were men who had been resident in Hong Kong for many years.[170] But the fundamental fact is that for the vast majority of POWs at Hong Kong—and, indeed, in all Japanese camps—escape was never a viable option or possibility. They were doomed to remain prisoners until the war ended, whenever that might be, or until they died. A distressingly large number were fated to die.

Conclusions

While these events took place in the various POW camps, hundreds of thousands of Chinese, Portuguese, Indians, and others struggled to survive in Hong Kong. The process was little helped, it would seem, by the Japanese themselves. Though they had every logical reason to wish the city to function effectively, it did not. One Chinese observer noted some of the reasons: "I have only given a sketch of the complex Japanese administration machinery in Hong Kong. It could not work because of the almost impossible and cumbersome red tape; and besides, there was a great deal of quarreling and personal sabotage among the Japanese officers over private plunder and jockeying for promotion or lush appointments."[171]

POWs in the Far East suffered much during their years of imprisonment. That life went on as normally as possible is natural and expected, though the sometimes remarkable adaptations to horrendous conditions may border on the incredible. But human beings, especially those in their 20s and 30s, have enormous resiliency, a fact we may forget during less deprived times.

We have yet to examine one of the major hurdles that the survivors had to clear before suddenly finding a brighter future in the white hot devastation of Hiroshima and Nagasaki. This hurdle was the fact of disease joined with starvation to challenge their bodies to the utmost. And essentially every POW learned much about starvation and disease while in the Japanese camps in Hong Kong and Singapore, the Philippines and Borneo, Burma and Java.

In the next chapter, the scanty and often dwindling supply of food, and the resultant effects on health and survival, will be described.

Chapter 5

Trying to Cope

with Too Little Food

It's not much, God, when dinner comes
To find it's just chrysanthemums.[1]

*N*o subject surpasses food as the cardinal topic of recollections
and writings about POW life and of conversations with survivors. Among Far Eastern POWs the subject became an obsession.
Evening conversations usually gravitated quickly to food—when
they didn't start with that subject. Men remembered special meals of
the past, tried to conjure up the menus from favourite restaurants,
wrote down recipes, or invented combinations that sounded as if they
ought to be tasty. And they did this regularly. Daily. For hours at a
time. Here is one homely recollection from among hundreds: "I talked
to Benny Neufeld for awhile. He lived near Morden. Twelve in his
family, father came from Nebraska. They used to kill four pigs and an
ox every fall to see them thru the winter. His mother had a famous
recipe for baked beans. It makes us all the hungrier to talk about these
things but we can't help it."[2] Of course, hungry persons behave like
this in or out of POW camps. George Orwell described the process
when he was literally starving in Paris between the wars:

> Two bad days followed. We had only sixty centimes left, and we spent it
> on half a pound of bread, with a piece of garlic to rub it with. The point
> of rubbing garlic on bread is that the taste lingers and gives one the illu-
> sion of having fed recently…we wrote dinner menus on the backs of
> envelopes. We were too hungry even to try and think of anything except
> food. I remember the dinner Boris finally selected for himself. It was: a

dozen oysters, borscht soup (the red, sweet, beetroot soup with cream on top), crayfishes, a young chicken *en casserole*, beef with stewed plums, new potatoes, a salad, suet pudding and Roquefort cheese, with a litre of Burgundy and some old brandy."[3]

All this concern about food reflected the lack of it. The food in Japanese POW camps was usually bad. It was almost always unavailable in large enough quantities for western eaters, and was usually of inferior quality—far too often it was little but filthy rice. Here is the menu for Sham Shui Po Camp for Sunday 17 January 1943, a date selected at random from a Canadian POW's diary: Breakfast: rice, greens, tea; Lunch: rice, greens, tea, bully beef; Supper: rice, vegetable soup, tea.[4] And bully beef would have been small in amount and unusual.

Adjusting to this monotonous, rice-centred diet, so vastly different from what the men were used to eating, was difficult and, for an unfortunate few, impossible. Initially, the cooks didn't know how to prepare rice properly. They were not accustomed to cooking rice in large quantities, and lacked as well the necessary massive cooking vessels; in at least one instance a bathtub became the cooking pot.[5] Until the logistical difficulties were corrected, fuel was insufficient. In the beginning, cookhouses used available goods improperly.[6] Also, during the early months of imprisonment, the food tended to be overcooked deliberately because of fear of parasitic infections.

Some days, the only food was "rice bust," which meant there was nothing else but rice; nothing in it—no vegetables, no taro root (also known as "green horror"), nothing. The men were understandably unhappy over the way the food was prepared in the early days, and the word "mutiny" crept into one officer's diary on 14 July 1942:

> Some of the stews we made up for the men were pretty terrible to look at, stuff you'd hardly feed to the pigs back home. There was lots of grumbling and some refused to eat it. Had what nearly amounted to mutiny in 'D' Coy. Had about a dozen on orders and they were stripped of rank and told they'd be turned over to the Japs if there was any more of it. I really don't blame the men but what can we do.[7]

Initially, the POWs brought some supplies, including food, into the camps. Put under the charge of an officer, they were used to supplement the Japanese rice diet. However, after a few weeks these supplies were removed by the Japanese; the POWs were issued items now and then over a period of three months. "At the end of that time they ceased to give us any more of our own supplies and we lived entirely on the Japanese diet."[8]

Less than three weeks after the surrender, one British POW wrote of the need to guard precious supplies: "Taylor brings in 3 wee bits of meat & some fat, 4 Pn [pans?] Rice, meat & bean gravy. Jack digs up extra rice & 1 tomato and I do the 'steaks' in the outhouse—a risky job in front of prying hungry eyes. Oh Boy! but what a lovely treat."[9]

In Sham Shui Po, early on, there were actually extras on occasion. After everyone had been fed, a second line-up was allowed, the "buck-shee" line, and any extra food was doled out as far as it went. One reason for the existence of extra rations was illness: "Due to numbers in Hospital there is over half a boiler of rice buckshee." Inevitably, major inequities in food distribution were found, or at least suspected. A member of the Royal Scots complained: "All the cookhouses dish out meat except ours. The Middx [Middlesex battalion] go by with huge hunks of steak."[10]

The POWs could do virtually nothing to improve their dietary lot. Nor could the Japanese, or so they said:

A Japanese Supply Officer inspected the camp on 15 Mar 44, and after a list of those short of blankets and shoes had been taken, he made a speech in which he stressed the difficulty, in fact almost impossibility, of obtaining replacements, and also the great difficulty of obtaining food supplies. In fact, he virtually told P.Ws that he realised they were very short but he could do nothing about it.[11]

Earlier, assistance was obtained intermittently from the IJA captors. Dr. Selwyn-Clarke, who was permitted to continue his work as principal health officer for Hong Kong until 1943, did not find all the Japanese obstructive. He was careful, in his post-war autobiography, to identify "good" captors whenever he encountered them:

One of my first encounters with helpfulness from a Japanese officer concerned the reserve of four-gallon tins of biscuits, made of soya bean and wheaten flour with the addition of thiamine hydrochloride powder (against beri-beri), which I had had baked in the leading department-store of Lane Crawford against the anticipated siege. By good fortune the Japanese had put Lane Crawford in charge of a certain Lieut. Tanaka, who allowed me to remove all the tins for distribution to the POW and civilian camps and to those Chinese hospitals which had not been closed by the Japanese forces. Lieut. Tanaka subsequently disappeared, and rumour had it that he had been removed to Canton and there executed for displaying excessive concern for the Hong Kong prisoners.[12]

Other health-related preparations had been made before the war. For example, in the vaults of the Hong Kong and Shanghai Bank were six one-kilogram bottles of thiamine hydrochloride. The bank had been taken over as the Japanese military headquarters. But two courageous European members of the bank staff volunteered to open the vaults. With their help "the life-giving vitamin supply was carried out, past the Japanese guard, to my waiting ambulance. I was able to divide it between the Stanley internment camp, Bowen Road Military

Hospital, the two main Chinese hospitals and the POW camps at Shamshuipo, Argyle Street and North Point, in all of which the signs of beri-beri were already apparent."[13]

The key to many of the POWs' medical problems was, of course, the lack of vitamins in their food. There was little scurvy, so vitamin C must have been available, but the relative absence of the vitamin-B complex created major problems.

Rice was the staple food, as it is throughout the Far East. A medical officer described "the 'high grade' (highly polished) rice with which the British had stocked Hong Kong in preparation for a long siege and which was captured and supplied to us by the Japs."[14] Because this rice was polished it was markedly less nutritious than the unpolished grain. Much of the vitamin content is contained in the "polishings" that were discarded or used for fodder. Unpolished rice, ironically, is less expensive; but the Japanese were not buying rice for their captives, they were giving them captured supplies and these consisted of polished rice. The inevitable result was vitamin deficiency diseases, the main topic of this chapter.

A remarkable frequency of urination was associated with the predominantly rice diet. A medical officer noticed that "the ceaseless tramp of wooden clogs throughout the entire night" vanished soon after their return to customary western food, when relief supplies were dropped by American planes at the end of August 1945. He found it "one of the most dramatic of my medical experiences as a POW."[15]

In 1942 the diet was thought to have provided about 2,000 calories daily and contained little animal protein and few fats.[16] Working men need twice that amount. Consequently, by that first autumn, most of the POWs looked seriously emaciated, and deficiency syndromes were common, mainly due to insufficient vitamin B complex and, to a lesser extent, vitamin A.[17]

Throughout North Point Camp's nine-month existence, rations were desperately thin. A POW kept a detailed log of food received daily there. His cryptic notations give no quantitative measure but the message is unequivocal. Here is one day's entry: "B[reakfast]. Had rice, dates one Bun, tea & B[?]. D[inner]. Had two buns and B. tea. S[upper]. Had rice, fish one bun tea & B."[18] The Canadians at North Point were perhaps worse off for food than the British at Sham Shui Po. Certainly one Britisher believed that to be true, noting in September 1942 that the Canadians he saw working at Kai Tak airport seemed "much worse off" than he and his mates in this regard.[19]

A pragmatic solution to shortened rations was to find a way to work near the food, which meant either the kitchen or the storehouses. One prisoner contrived a job for himself with the camp ration party. Every month they spent time at the warehouses loading 200-pound bags of Hong Kong government rice. There was opportunity to steal food here. But there was also another benefit: "It was hard graft, but it broke us in as godown coolies [warehouse labourers], and was to prove very useful experience for Japan."[20]

Of course, the most prized jobs were in the kitchen. A prisoner in Sham Shui Po was understandably elated when a friend found an assignment in the kitchen: "Dev is going into cookhouse as Ration NCO. Starts well with a can of vegetable gravy."[21] So the benefits were direct and immediate.

Many camps suffered morale problems because of this preferred position of the kitchen staff, who always looked better fed than the bulk of the POWs. That they had a little extra food for themselves seemed to be accepted as inevitable, if enviable. But when rumours circulated about cooks trading food to the Japanese, or using food to buy better living conditions or other favours, then rancour grew. On occasion, resentfulness was expressed in physical violence. Morale fell even further when officers failed to punish those caught cheating their comrades. For example, in April 1942 a Sgt. Barker was "caught at 3 a.m. pinching a whole duff and Ford refuses to deal with the case."[22]

At Shinagawa Camp in Japan it was an open secret that the cooks, mainly British Other Ranks, both sold and traded food. They became the favourites of the Japanese, so that "they could and did defy the orders and requests of their own Officers in regard to matters of food and we could do nothing about it as they invoked the Japs....One could always tell a cook or a friend of a cook by his size and shape."[23]

Men developed various strategies for coping with the severe dietary restrictions. Many stole food compulsively, usually from the enemy but sometimes, unfortunately, from their comrades. Others developed defence mechanisms. For example, at Fukuoka 7 POW Camp one of the camp institutions was the Dutchman who ate continuously for 10 hours each day. He was carried on the rolls as a permanently sick man, relieved of all duties. He ate his three bowls of rice per day, one grain at a time. "All day, every day, from breakfast to 'lights out,' he munched away, timing each meal to finish just as the next was being issued."[24]

An Australian medical officer was convinced that it was the formulated policy of the Japanese "to keep us in a state of semi-starvation and disease to prevent escapes and other troubles as in the early stages when much looted tinned food was available and we had money we were never allowed to spend it and the contractor was forbidden to bring the food in."[25] There is no documented proof of this assertion, which many of the prisoners shared. The relatively good food supplies in Changi Camp at Singapore seemed to refute the claim of a policy of starvation to rule. There, the camp was huge and breakout perhaps especially to be feared, yet the men ate well enough for the camp to earn the sobriquet of "Changi Hilton."

Bland and tasteless as it was prepared in the camps, the rice needed flavouring badly. A clove of garlic was a treasured thing. Sliced with a razor blade and mixed in the rice, it made an enormous difference.

Food sometimes differed considerably between an ordinary camp and, for example, Bowen Road Hospital. It could be argued that patients should be able to eat especially nutritious food. Yet, despite recurring rumours to the contrary, food at Bowen Road Hospital was not always sustaining or even pleasant. Tom Forsyth noted, on 5 March 1942: "My morning egg was rotten....A very skimpy supper, two wafer thin slices of bread and half ounce of cheese."[26] Still, he did have a morning egg.

Only 11 days later, another Canadian found a markedly different situation. While he was in North Point Camp, L/Cpl. Martyn became ill and was transferred to Bowen Road. He was keeping a daily diary of food and he not only continued this in the hospital, but apparently also had a friend make notes for him of the North Point Camp food. Thus we have a direct comparison. For example, on Monday 16 March 1942, in Bowen Road Hospital, Martyn was served: Breakfast: tea, milk, two slices white bread, peach jam; Lunch: rice, turnips, a slice of corned mutton, salt issue; Dinner: tea, milk, sugar, two slices white bread, a hard-boiled duck egg, and butter. In North Point Camp he would have received: Breakfast: rice, sugar sauce, tea; Lunch: rice, sauce, tea, vegetable soup, bread; Dinner: rice, squid sauce, bread, tea.[27] So at Bowen Road he had both meat and an egg, but would have received neither at North Point. No wonder men often welcomed the thought of going to hospital.

But why was there such a difference? Was Forsyth on a diet because of whatever illness had taken him to Bowen Road? Had the military hospital received augmented food supplies between March 5th and 16th? Both statements come from contemporary diaries, so memory deficit should not be the explanation.

What is certain is that when a hospital was inside a camp, rather than being a separate institution such as Bowen Road, no differences existed between rations for the sick and the well except those of quantity imposed by the Japanese. One of the problems that POW medical officers struggled with in all camps was the Japanese regulation that the sick, because they were not working, deserved and should receive less food than the healthy workers. This was not simply a perversity practised upon defenceless prisoners; the principle of rations proportionate to work level was laid down in the Japanese Army ration standards, which allowed only 2,400 calories daily for a man lying in bed all day (in the IJA this could only mean a very sick man), 3,400–3,500 calories daily during training, and 3,600–4,000 calories daily for a man in action.[28] And on average, a Japanese soldier was much smaller than his Canadian or American counterpart. Prisoners rarely if ever saw such generous absolute amounts, but the proportional difference was insisted upon by the Japanese.

At Changi Camp in Singapore the same principle was followed. The issue of rice to British POWs was graded according to the type of work done: heavy workers received 300 grams, light workers 250 grams, and non-workers—including the sick—200 grams. Thus men who, due to illness, required a full or even a special ration to restore them to the category of worker were not considered at all. However, a reserve of food was created "through the use of the camp messing funds, from which the messing officers bought useful items through the local Japanese commander."[29]

Amputees make an interesting comparison with the ordinary population of the Hong Kong camps. These men did not go on work parties, nor could they participate in sports, but they received the same diet as everyone else. They did not suffer from nutritional disturbance until late in their internment, nor did they suffer as severely as their fellow POWs.[30] Thus amputees had an unexpected and unappreciated advantage in POW camp. Two Canadian medical officers pointed out the most important reasons: no work requirement and regular food rations. What they do not emphasize is the fortuitous enhanced impact of the "normal" diet: amputees were feeding less body on the ration than were men who had all four limbs, because the amputees *had* less body. Thus the nourishment they received benefitted them relatively more.

Theft of food infuriated the Japanese. At Niigata Camp 5B, in Japan, the men returned from work late in 1943 to find their beds and kit strewn around the huts. Some rations had been stolen. The men who ultimately were found to have stolen the rations were thrown in the guardroom, except for two who were tied to a post outside, overnight.[31] In December, in Niigata, this was essentially an execution.

Caloric Value of Rations

There was an excess of medical officers at Argyle Street POW Camp, at least 15 for about 600 POW officers whose health was reasonably good. One consequence was that studies were made of such things as the dietary constituents, research there was little or no time to do in the other camps. Table 1 outlines the rations available at Argyle Street Camp and their caloric value:

The steady decrease in caloric intake is obvious and ominous.[32] And this occurred in a camp supposed, by the men, to be much better off for food than was Sham Shui Po. They may have been correct; the table shows Japanese issue rations, but in addition, officers had money to buy supplementary food. The men had little or no money for such purposes.

At Sham Shui Po, Canadian medical officers arrived at more optimistic estimates for late 1942. An abrupt increase in calories to 2,700–3,000 daily followed the receipt of Red Cross food supplies in October 1942.[33] But even Red Cross parcels could cause medical problems, as Dr. Coombes observed. One man became extremely ill, and Coombes found him vomiting and suffering from diarrhea, just after they had received a Red Cross parcel. "I looked at him and asked a few questions, and it transpired that he'd eaten or drunk a whole tin of butter. The Red Cross sent in butter in a tin, but it had been out in the sun and heat, and it was completely liquid. But he got the top off and he drank the lot just like that."[34] The shortage of dietary fat was felt keenly. The POWs suffered with the cold much more than usual. Fat was rare in the ration since there is almost none in rice.

Table 5.1
Report on Rations, December 1943

| | 1942 | | | | 1943 | | | |
| | October | | November | | October | | November | |
	Gm	Cal	Gm	Cal	Gm	Cal	Gm	Cal
Rice	437.3	1560	435	1553	384	1371	384	1371
Flour	123.2	453	123	453	100	368	65	239
Fish	43.6	23	43.5	23	55.6	30	59	32
Peanut Oil	15	118	18.5	142	14.4	113	13	103
Sugar	7.2	29	6	25	4	16	4.5	18
Grn Vegs	260	60	240	55	274	63	387	89
Beans	2.9	9	1	4	63	54	20	17
Swt. Potat	100	86	163	140	20	17	—	—
Cal/man/day		2,338		2,395		2,032		1,869

Source: PRO, WO 224, File 188, *Interrogation Report of Lt. R.B Goodwin*, 8.

Inevitably, men lost bulk rapidly, sometimes halving their prewar weight. CSM R.A. Edwards, HKVDC, kept a list of his weights at various times during captivity. The figures ranged from 168 lb (76 kg) on Christmas Day 1941, through 134 (61 kg) at the end of 1942, 121 (55 kg) at the end of 1943, to his low point of 115 lb (52 kg) on 13 June 1945.[35] Ray Squires noted wryly in December 1944 that he was "Weighed today by the Nips. We all showed a 40 lb increase over last month. I jumped from 134 to 180 but still weigh 134 on hosp. scales."[36] So the miracle was short lived and spurious. Colin Standish went into POW camp weighing 175 pounds. When his war ended in Japan in 1945 his weight was 71 pounds.[37] Every man had a similar story. Moreover, weight loss could spell accelerated dietary catastrophe in a camp. Coates, at a camp on the Burma-Siam railway, noted that scales were used regularly by the Japanese authorities. "This provided the commissariat with a ready means of estimating the caloric requirements. The lower the total weight, the less food need be supplied!"[38]

Table 5.2
Weight Loss among POWs at Oeyama Camp, Japan*

Rank	Normal Wt(kg)	Aug. 1944	Sept. 1944	Oct. 1944	Nov. 1944	Dec. 1944	Jan. 1945	Feb. 1945	Mar. 1945	Apr. 1945	May 1945	June 1945	July 1945	Aug. 1945
ORs	74.99	56.94	55.75	57.26	55.89	55.44	55.65	56.14	55.15	55.61	55.50	55.33	54.88	54.88
NCOs	76.48	61.23	60.09	61.02	59.71	58.34	58.07	57.48	57.23	57.98	57.55	57.86	57.96	60.09

Source: *Journal of the History of Medicine and Allied Sciences* 46 (1991): 65-85.
   *Mean weight changes (kg) in Japanese POWs at Oeyama during the period August 1944 to August 1945. Weight changes are demonstrated by rank for ORs (Other Ranks) and NCOs (Non-Commissioned officers).[39]

No matter how inadequate the food was on a day-to-day basis, every effort was made at Christmas-time to provide, if not that utter impossibility, a typical "home" holiday meal, at least one distinctively different from the monotonous, scanty, tasteless, daily fare. For example, the hand-coloured printed menu for 25 December 1942 at the Isolation Hospital, Sham Shui Po, begins with the words "No Rice" underlined firmly. "Breakfast, 8:30 am, porridge, stewed pears, eggs; Tiffin 1 pm, bully beef, fried tomatoes, roast yams, fried vegetables and tea; Tea, 3 pm, tea, cake, biscuits; Dinner 6 pm, M & V [meat and vegetables] (Fried fish), boiled fruit pudding, tea, jam sauce."[40] Yet in the memory of one Canadian POW, Christmas was just like any other day; "we knew it was Christmas Day, but that was it."[41]

Unusual Foods

In Sham Shui Po, every blade of grass in the camp disappeared. Pet dogs and regimental mascots that had followed the men into camp were eaten. The POWs snared wild birds for food and snakes were considered a delicacy.[42] The Chinese inhabitants of Hong Kong were hungry too. Each evening the wire around Sham Shui Po was electrified, and there would be a dead dog or cat in the wire every second or third morning. The current would be shut off, and hungry Chinese waited for the animal to be taken off the wire and thrown out, when they would pounce on it. One man came across the body of a large black cat lying on the rails in Niigata, cut in two by a train. "We immediately exclaimed 'Here's something for the soup.' If you didn't know what it was you might have thought it was rabbit." A week later, the Japanese foreman dragged into camp the body of a police dog; a POW skinned it and cut it up, at which the foreman took both hind quarters and walked off with them; inevitably, the Japanese guards ended up with all the best meat.[43] Late in the war, the men in this camp were given a collection of old horse heads and other bones to make soup. They found that it made very good soup. "We make soup with them twice then send them on to another camp. We also got 50 or 60 large snakes for soup. I detest the darn things. One time we got wheat, barley, rye and some millet and now only rice."[44]

In the Philippines, Dr. Calvin Jackson recorded a series of poignant entries in his diary as he hand-fed his pet chicken, Cordelia, on one occasion splinting her broken leg. When ultimately he was forced to eat her, eight months later, he preserved the bone with the healed fracture. It is uncertain whether this represented affection for the chicken, pride in his veterinarian skill, or both.[45]

Ft/Lt. R.D. Millar, who spent his captivity in Java and Sumatra, noted that in at least one camp, a form of food supplementation was carried out that many, less starved, might consider disgusting. Some men caught maggots in the latrines, washed them, fattened them on rice, and ate them to get the extra protein. "Believe it or not, IT IS A FACT"[46] (emphasis in original).

Internees developed the same capacity as the POWs to eat nearly anything; those who failed to do so often failed to survive. Fastidiousness about food disappeared. "Prisoners pushed flowers, grass, weeds, dogs, cats, rats, snakes, grasshoppers, and snails down their gullets, where desperation plus the force of gravity carried it to their stomachs, the stomachs hurried it on to intestines, which hurried it on to the next place. The following day, we, as gardeners, passed it back to the potato beds. Somewhere along the yards of irritated mucous membrane we received the impression that we had had a meal."[47]

The impact of long-continued hunger was profound. George Orwell saw its ravages amongst starving tramps between the wars: "Hunger reduces one to an utterly spineless, brainless condition, more like the after-effects of influenza than anything else. It is as though one had been turned into a jellyfish, or as though all one's blood had been pumped out and lukewarm water substituted."[48]

A Canadian medical orderly, thinking about the departure on a draft of many of his comrades, summed up the general position in the camp and in himself:

> Another draft left today, which leaves only a thousand in camp....Food here is getting worse. $3/4$ oz bully per man. Hot feet are getting bad again, mine kept me awake until 2 a.m. yesterday. Can only read with one eye; this is very common due to vitamin deficiency. The men's spirits are remarkably good.[49]

Particularly in the two decades before World War Two, diseases caused by poor nutrition had been studied in various parts of the world. Many of the studies were in the Far East where, among the poorest inhabitants of China, India, and other countries, diseases such as beriberi and pellagra were endemic. What many of the investigators concluded was that whereas each individual disease could be shown to have a specific cause—for example, insufficient thiamine in the diet causes beriberi—the overall cause of these diseases was poverty.[50]

In a very real sense, this generalization applies to the prisoner-of-war cosmos as well. Within this world the prisoners were in general desperately poor. But there were exceptions. The well-to-do, relatively speaking, included the officers, cookhouse personnel, non-smokers, men with special skills needed in camp, and men who had local contacts to supply supplements of food and materiel.

The economy of the camps was artificial. The fundamental necessity, food, was rigidly controlled by the Japanese. But in terms of effect, this circumstance might be likened to a major drought striking an area with consequent hunger and onset of nutritional disorders among the poorest, first, while those better off lived on stored surpluses or were able to purchase food. In the POW camps of the Far East, the drought was general and lasted three and a half years.

The POW medical officers clearly anticipated problems with vitamin deficiencies. Long before these attained their full epidemic proportions, yeast-containing substances were being concocted at Sham Shui Po and given to the prisoners regularly. According to A.J. Alsey, this seems to have been a weekly event: 21 April 42: "Medical Officer's Inspection. Yeast Parade at 12." Then, 28 April 42: "M.O. Insp. at 11:15 followed by yeast Parade. The yeast is certainly stronger now....Our rice thieves get a public smacking from the Japs."[51] Yeast contains thiamine and other B-complex vitamins in varying amounts.

The whole question of separating one type of deficiency disease from another was, and remains, most difficult. One investigator, himself an ex-POW, has written about "unnecessary preoccupation with the task of forcing all tropical illnesses presumably due to vitamin B deficiencies into the category of either beriberi or pellagra, in this way beclouding the issue."[52] And a medical officer who was in camps in the Philippines and Japan confirms this opinion: "In my experience, there was no deficiency which presented itself as a pure entity."[53] Despite these warnings we must try to separate them for consideration here, since throughout their captivity in the Far East, both medical officers and patients referred, sometimes confidently, sometimes with uncertainty, to each disease by name.

Moreover, the records that have survived must be examined with caution. For reasons that remain conjectural, the Japanese forbade POW medical officers to make certain diagnoses. Thus, at Bowen Road Hospital, Col. Bowie was told that he could cite a diagnosis of avitaminosis, but such diseases as pellagra, beriberi, or other vitamin deficiency diseases could not be shown. Thus all cases under these more specific headings had to be categorized as avitaminosis, further less-ening the accuracy of those records that survived.[54]

Beriberi

> Now polished rice is extremely nice
> At a high suburban tea
> But Arbuthnot Lane remarks with pain
> That it lacks all Vitamin B,
> And beri-beri is very very
> Hard on the nerves, says he,
> "Oh take your Vitamin B, my dears!"[55]

Medical officers captured in the Far East were often handicapped in caring for their patients by their own ignorance—not culpable igno-rance but simply reflecting the reality that the majority had little train-ing in tropical diseases and hadn't been in their garrison posts long enough to have acquired experience. Notable exceptions were medical officers in the Netherlands East Indies forces and those civilian doctors in Hong Kong and of Singapore who had practised in the region and had a working background in these diseases; some British medical officers had been stationed in Far Eastern posts long enough to have sufficient knowledge. Most did not.

An irony is that some of the Canadians could have known about beriberi. The Royal Rifles of Canada had been on garrison duty in Newfoundland and Labrador for 11 months immediately prior to trav-elling to Hong Kong, November 1940 to early October 1941. During this time, and for decades before, Newfoundland and Labrador had been suffering under endemic beriberi. Indeed, studies carried out there in the 1930s were significant signposts on the road to finding a way to combat the disease.

Beriberi in Newfoundland was a disease of the outports and other remote settlements that needed to stockpile food each autumn because they could not be supplied over the winter. By late spring the poorest inhabitants of these settlements were essentially out of food; beriberi was a common consequence. The replacement of whole meal grains with refined white flour contributed to the problem.[56] The situation was analogous to that in the Far East where polished rice replaced unpol-ished as the dietary staple—the pernicious impact of "civilization."

The chief investigator of the disease in Newfoundland stated unequivocally that beriberi was a disease of economics, easily pre-vented by improving the diet.[57] The same was true for the POWs; those who found ways to supplement their diet consistently had little beriberi. Those who could not do so and who were forced to rely on the Japanese-provided rations suffered from this and other deficiency diseases.

Clinical work with these victims in Newfoundland would not, however, have been possible for the medical officers of the Royal Rifles, both because of the remote nature of affected outposts and because, if the victims did get medical aid it would have been civilian, not military. Thus, despite spending almost a year in an area where beriberi was common, the Royals had to wait till they were in North Point and Sham Shui Po to learn the cruel nature of beriberi—and how little they could do about it.

Beriberi first appeared at Hong Kong in 1889, or at least was first diagnosed in that year.[58] The disease was studied scientifically for only about 70 years before World War Two began. In the last third of the nineteenth century, when this research began, the medical world was enjoying enormous success identifying bacterial causes for diseases such as tuberculosis, diphtheria, dysentery, septicemia, and many others. Inevitably, then, researchers expected to find bacteria causing most diseases, many of which actually had other causes. Beriberi was one of these.

Those studying the disease fell largely into two camps: those who believed that some as yet undiscovered germ caused beriberi, and those who believed that some equally undiscovered poison or toxin was to blame.[59] It was, however, generally conceded that rice was a crucial element in the etiology of beriberi. The questions were, how was rice at fault, or what kind of rice was at fault, and why? One researcher, Braddon, who thought a toxin or poison was the cause, had nevertheless, by 1907, shown convincingly that milled rice or white rice was implicated, whereas neither cured (or parboiled) rice, nor home-pounded rice, nor red rice, were. He worked in Malaya, and studied beriberi in conjunction with the rice-eating habits in the four major population groups in the country. The Malays used home-pounded rice and suffered from beriberi rarely; the Tamils used cured (parboiled) rice and never had beriberi; the Chinese ate by preference imported white rice and had a very high incidence of beriberi; and the Europeans, who ate little rice, did not have the disease.[60] Though he failed to demonstrate the reason for this difference, Braddon was absolutely correct about the relationship between polished rice and beriberi.

About the same time as Braddon's research, Eijkman, on Java, had shown by experiments that chickens, if fed exclusively on white rice, acquired a disease that closely resembled beriberi. Other investigators found that confined populations such as those in prisons or insane asylums could be made more (or less) likely to suffer from beriberi depending upon the proportion of white rice in their diet.

The problem was that this research brought scientists closer to understanding the disease, but one mental hurdle still needed to be leapt. Attention had been directed towards finding some entity that caused the disease: toxins or bacteria were the two commonest proposals. What was required was realization that the absence of some entity also can cause disease. This new concept proved difficult to comprehend.

Hopkins suggested that there were substances in addition to carbohydrates, fats, and proteins—perhaps present in tiny amounts—that were needed by the human body for adequate nutrition. Finally, early in 1910, researchers in the Philippines stated unequivocally that beriberi was a disease of metabolism and that white rice was deficient "in respect of some substance or substances essential for the normal metabolism of nerve tissues."[61] Thus from 1910 on, the bad effects of a diet largely or totally based on white or milled rice have been recognized.

Early in the twentieth century some Japanese physicians advised their patients that barley combined with rice was a healthier staple than the polished white rice that the Japanese preferred to eat. One of these knowledgeable practitioners, Takaki Kenkan, became famous because he was the Imperial Japanese Navy surgeon who eliminated beriberi through diet.[62] So the Japanese medical profession knew about beriberi and its causes and effects, just as did western physicians.

There is some evidence of the apparent ubiquity of beriberi in Japan as recently as the late 1930s. Tanizaki Jun'ichiro's novel based in this period. *The Makioka Sisters* describes a well-to-do though declining Japanese family in Osaka. Tanizaki makes many references to beriberi, suggesting that the disease and its cure were common then: "Beri-beri was in the air of this Kobe-Osaka district, and every year from summer into autumn the whole family—Sachiko and her husband and sisters and Etsuko, who had just started school—came down with it. The vitamin injection had become a family institution. They no longer went to a doctor, but instead kept a supply of concentrated vitamins on hand and ministered to each other with complete unconcern. A suggestion of sluggishness was immediately attributed to a shortage of Vitamin B, and, although they had forgotten who coined the expression, 'short on "B"' never had to be explained."[63]

So common was the process that it became part of a child's play: "One day he saw Etsuko at play....Taking a worn-out hypodermic needle, Etsuko gave her straw-stuffed Occidental doll a shot in the arm. What a morbid little game, Teinosuke [Etsuko's father] thought. That too was the result of a dangerous preoccupation with hygiene."[64] And there are many other references to beriberi in the novel.

Beriberi remained a problem in Japan until during the Second World War, when mandatory limits were placed on the proportion of bran that could be removed during milling. But the death rate in 1940 was almost identical to that in 1900, about 15 deaths per 100,000 population, so that 7,000 to 8,000 Japanese died each year from the disease.[65] Whatever reasons explain the high rate of beriberi among their prisoners, ignorance of cause and cure cannot be argued on behalf of the Japanese.

Padi, or red rice (unmilled rice, which may in fact have a variety of colours) retains intact the full outer cover of the grain (pericarp) containing the essential vitamin. Home-pounded rice is red rice pounded by the home owner to remove the husk and pericarp; the methods used are inefficient enough so that the pericarp is never fully removed, sufficient remaining to protect against beriberi. Cured or parboiled rice, used largely by East Indians, leaves much of the pericarp firmly adherent to the rice, so the protection remains. But milled rice or white rice has so much of the pericarp removed that the vitamin content is insufficient to preserve health. Thus the explanation of Braddon's findings: what caused beriberi wasn't a toxin but rather the absence of a vital factor—what came to be called a vitamin.

Therefore the direct cause of beriberi is a prolonged deficiency in the diet of thiamine or vitamin B^1. The disease occurs in two forms: so-called wet beriberi is less painful but more hazardous to life. The danger stems from the swelling produced by the body's retention of large amounts of fluids (a state called edema), which begins in the feet and progressively affects more and more of the body as the disease worsens. If enough fluid collects so that the chest becomes involved the victim often dies of heart failure; the pressure of fluid compresses the heart until it cannot function effectively.

Most Europeans were unfamiliar with acute severe beriberi, though they may have known its visible symptoms among Chinese labourers and factory workers. When the disease is in its acute form,

> the whole body swells like a drum and the wretched patient, unable to sit and unable to lie down, tries to prop himself in a position where the fluid will not enter his lungs. Once our doctors had the thiamine, a few injections did the trick, and we collapsed from Michelin advertisements into rather gaunt but otherwise normal-looking individuals.[66]

In the dry form of beriberi, on the other hand, there was no edema, and the men remained extremely thin. Often the patients had pain but it was confined largely to the feet, legs, and hands.[67] In both forms of the disease, the men became dull and apathetic.[68] It may be more accurate to consider three forms of the disease, the two already cited plus a group of patients with serious heart problems. "Amongst a large number of cases of beriberi every possible blend of these three sets of symptoms will be encountered."[69]

Some, at least, of the manifestations of malnutrition that have been labelled beriberi in diaries and in post-war memoirs probably were not. This point is evidenced by examining the characteristic symptom associated with wet beriberi, edema, which produces swelling of the legs. Denny-Brown, a widely experienced British neurologist, observed that swelling of the ankles or legs below the knees, without loss of ankle-jerk reflexes and without muscle wasting or weakness, occurred frequently in POWs. "It is essential not to confuse this common condition with beriberi, which it has often been called by medical officers and by the patients themselves."[70]

Thus, many of the cases diagnosed in the Far East during World War Two as beriberi may have been instances of edema due to low levels of protein in the blood. Once protein was increased in the diet, the edema disappeared quickly.[71] Since the vitamin deficiencies were general, resulting from lack of many dietary elements, diagnosis of specific diseases was extremely difficult and often, in retrospect, impossible.[72]

According to a Royal Navy POW at Sham Shui Po, a Japanese sentry apparently died there of beriberi during 1942. Most of the sentries, he claimed, suffered from wet beriberi.[73] Yet as has been discussed, the Japanese knew as much about beriberi as did other nations. Beriberi was a major problem in the Imperial Japanese armed forces late in the nineteenth and early in the twentieth centuries. Takaki managed to persuade first the navy, then the army, to change the diet of the men. One of the steps taken by the IJA was to decrease the amount of rice and replace that portion with barley; a generation later, Allied POWs noted that their beriberi improved when the same dietary change was introduced. But this change had been made in behalf of imprisoned Japanese on their own land as early as 1875.[74]

As will become evident, beriberi was a significant problem for many—perhaps most—Allied POWs held in the Far East between 1941 and 1945. At Hong Kong the incidence was high. Many of the men who were sent to Japan welcomed the opportunity through a naive belief that they would be better fed there. In a few camps the men received reasonably adequate rations, but the vast majority did not.

When Maj. Alfred Weinstein was transferred to Mitsushima POW Camp in October 1944, he found beriberi a daunting problem. Of 200 men, 180 had "extensive clinical evidence" of beriberi. The situation was so bad that Weinstein persuaded the commandant, Lt. Kubo, to permit him to select a group of 30 of the sickest of the 180 patients, to be excused from heavy manual labour. Weinstein described Kubo as "one of the few good Japanese commanders I have met."[75]

The chosen patients continued to work—in Japan one worked or one starved—but the allotted tasks were easier. The men made straw footwear and raincoats. In June 1945, a Japanese sergeant assembled these men, who all wore a red ribbon to indicate that they were severe cardiac cases. "They were to climb into the mountains into a forest which had been lumbered and carry back heavy logs weighing from 50 to 120 pounds on their shoulders. This area was approximately two miles up and down the mountainside (two miles each way) from the camp."[76] Despite vigorous protests these severely sick men were forced to do the work, though the sergeant relented to the extent of permitting the five most seriously ill to return to their light work. One of the unfortunate remainder, an American private, "collapsed while carrying back a log and was brought back to the hospital, where he died three hours later. I feel that Sergeant Arai is as directly responsible for his death as if he had shot him through the head."[77] When the POW was dying, the MOs sent for Arai and showed him what had happened. "He appeared abashed and silent. He never sent the detail out again."[78]

Electric Feet

> This scourge struck about half the men in gaol...but made up the balance by striking them with a pain twice as severe as anything any of us had ever seen before.[79]

"Electric feet" was probably the most painful disease caused by malnutrition that afflicted prisoners in the Far East. First the toes became numb, they began to twitch, then shooting pains started. Often the pain continued day and night, though usually worse at night. The condition was first seen roughly three to five months after the Japanese established their large prison camps. The number of cases increased rapidly over 1942, but in general had decreased substantially by the end of that year.[80]

Hibbs has written perhaps the most evocative description by a physician of this unusual syndrome. He wrote of what he had seen personally in the Philippines:

> The first symptoms of a peripheral neuritis were stiffness, heaviness, or a tired feeling in the arches of the feet. Soon there was aching in the arch and soles of the feet. This progressed to a dull, throbbing, deep bone ache in the whole foot. Soon sharp, shooting pain appeared, radiating from the arch to the tip of the toes. Burning pain, especially on the soles of the feet, paresthesia, and extreme tenderness next developed. These symptoms increased in severity until the patient was "half crazy." There was no relief. He would rub his feet or just look at them and cry. A common practice was for patients to sleep side by side, with heads in opposite directions, so that each could rub the other's feet. Soaking in water was a frequent, but not too successful remedy. Some unfortunate victims were unable to sleep, and their nights were spent in crying, moaning, and begging for relief. The pain soon spread up the legs to the knees, occasionally to the hips and a few even had pains and paresthesia across the abdomen, chest and scalp. After the feet were severely involved, pain developed in the fingers. Rarely did the symptoms advance beyond the elbows. In severe cases of long duration, the patient complained that the extremities were going to sleep or were dead. This anesthesia afforded some relief.[81]

"Electric feet," "hot feet," "happy feet," or "burning feet," as the disorder was wryly referred to by the men who suffered from it, was usually thought of as being a symptom of the acute disorder affecting the peripheral nerves known as dry beriberi. But the exact causation remains uncertain. The debate is medical, not historical, and the precise cause or causes make no difference to this narrative of the POW lives of Allied troops in Hong Kong or in Japan. That "electric feet" was related somehow to malnutrition cannot be questioned.

Many observers, medical and non-medical, took it as a given that the disorder was a manifestation of beriberi. Most of the patients did suffer from beriberi, though difference of opinion exists as to whether beriberi and "electric feet" occurred simultaneously or successively. Bush stated that this disorder was experienced only at Sham Shui Po Camp in Hong Kong,[82] but this suggestion of exclusivity certainly was wrong. At North Point the first four cases occurred in April 1942.[83] Tom Forsyth wrote in his diary in August 1942 that many men at North Point had "so called electric feet," and that one of his company sergeants was delirious with the pain.[84] Nor is there any reason to suppose that the Indian POWs at Ma Tau Chung were not affected.

Medical officers found that the painful burning of the feet sometimes required injections of morphine. The disorder was usually unaffected by therapy. The suffering was genuine and often severe. One Canadian, Donald Geraghty, developed this condition in the autumn of 1942. Late in October he recorded having gone without sleep three nights running, and, six weeks later, on 3 December, he noted that he had stopped soaking his feet and they felt and looked better. "But I can't sleep very good. Today I got 2 hrs deep sleep, first in a week."[85] On 13 May 1943 he was still in hospital, his stay then exceeding seven months.

Two Canadian POWs visited one of their comrades in the Sham Shui Po Camp hospital on New Year's Day 1943. They found Rfn. Adams in the "agony" ward. He looked extremely ill, being blind, deaf, and "light in the head all due to Malnutrition also Electric feet."[86] A few days later one of them commented that many of the men were ill with weak hearts, supposedly due to "electric feet" and pellagra.[87]

"Electric feet" progressed in stages. Nights made sleepless by pain produced, in turn, exhaustion. The agony gradually drove some men mad. They could neither eat nor sleep. A few, fortunately a minority, wasted away and died:

> A hut was set aside for the advanced stages, again dubbed Agony Ward. Their gaunt figures bent double on the floor, weaving and bobbing and rocking back and forth in pain, like penitents at the Wailing Wall, rubbing their tortured toes and weeping, made a haunting sight. I had never seen grown men cry. It roused pity, disgust, horror, fear—fear that this was awaiting me.[88]

Nor did this problem cease when the men arrived in Japan. There, prisoners still sat up at night wrapped in blankets, their painful feet submerged in buckets filled with icy water that froze over at night. "the sufferer would break the ice to shove his feet into the water for relief while he shivered under his blankets."[89]

A former POW medical officer at Hong Kong remembered vividly that sufferers used to stamp up and down all night on a concrete floor, thumping their feet vigorously as a sort of counterirritant to the pain. Some used the electric fence around the camp, lying down with both feet on the wire, which at this time had only low voltage, like a cattle barrier. The electrified wire gave temporary relief. A British medical officer remembered giving morphine, using the old British army issue of tubes of tablets that had to be dissolved. He had many men with severe cases of electric feet; they could have an injection only every third night during periods of severe pain. "They used to beg for it. And you'd say, 'Sorry, your turn tomorrow,' and they stuck it out. I remember so well that not a single one became addicted in any way."[90] Fortunately they were well supplied with morphine.

For those with less severe discomfort there was little effective therapy. One man claimed that the feet were literally so hot that when they were put in cold water, steam would rise from the water after a short time. This may be an exaggerated memory, but more significant, perhaps, is that in 1987 he still had very little feeling in his legs below the knees.[91]

One prisoner claimed that he could think of no worse torture to subject anyone to than to give them electric feet. The only similar experience he could suggest was when you had your ears frozen as a youngster and they started to thaw out, with stinging prickling pain. That was similar. "But it's day and night. It did drive a lot of guys mad. Some guys died from it. They soaked their feet too long. You know, you'd try anything. They put them all in one ward, the agony ward."[92]

Despite allegations or suspicions of superior rations, officers were not exempt from "electric feet." At any rate, the officers who remained in Sham Shui Po with the men suffered. Lt. Harry White, WG, first mentioned the topic in his diary on 23 December 1942. The painful-feet epidemic was worsening, and all that the medical officers were sure of was that malnutrition was an important factor. "Go into a hut and see man after man on his bed, holding his feet, rubbing them, many of them crying like babies, and they can't help it—it gradually breaks down their nerves."[93]

Less than two months later, he was himself being treated for this miserable syndrome. He started on a 20-injection series of treatments with nicotinic acid. Maj. (A) Ashton-Rose, IMS, had been able to get the drug through the black market. Officers who needed the treatment paid 5 yen. By levying this charge, Ashton-Rose could obtain more drugs for the men, though they couldn't get nearly enough. "After the needle you flush all over—quite a sensation."[94] Nor is there any doubt that White's attack of "electric feet" was a severe one. His feet were still bad at the end of February and he could get no sleep. For 10 days and nights he claimed not to have had a half-hour's sleep.[95]

Col. Bowie discussed the deficiency diseases in his detailed monograph on Bowen Road Military Hospital. When he referred to the phenomenon of burning feet,[96] he failed to mention that he himself suffered from this disorder. But his clerk, Cpl. Norman Leath, remembers a time when Bowie was "under the weather" with "electric feet."[97] If the commanding officer of the major military hospital was so ill-fed as to develop this syndrome, one can infer how inadequately casualties were supplied, men who should have had extra food to promote wound healing.

As the disease progressed, the pain in the feet subsided. From too great sensitivity the symptom became too little sensitivity and, ultimately, anesthesia.[98] When effective dietary therapy was possible, the patients then experienced these states in the reverse order, going from anesthesia to hyposensitivity, to hypersensitivity, finally and usually arriving back at more or less normality.

Some idea of the nutritional state in Stanley internment camp on Hong Kong Island comes from the diary of a nurse who ended the war there. Reminiscing about travelling to Hong Kong on shipboard, when she made friends with two nurses, she realized that they would have been incredulous at what the future would bring. They couldn't have known that a time would come, in Stanley Camp, when one of them, lucky enough to obtain a pinch of curry powder, would invite the other two to help celebrate her birthday on curried banana skins. She had found the skins in a refuse bin.[99]

Dean Smith, a scientist, was an internee in Hong Kong, Michael Woodruff a POW medical officer at Changi, Singapore. In 1951 they published a scientific report based on studies done in their respective camps and incorporating the research and observations of a number of others as well. One reads this article hoping for answers to some of the questions that are obvious throughout the preceding pages of this book. However, the conclusions which emerge "are disappointingly meagre in comparison with the mass of observations collected."[100]

Smith believed that several circumstances combined to reduce the normal and beneficial bacterial synthesis of vitamins to a minimum. These included the sudden change from a European to a poor Asiatic type of diet, the common occurrence of diarrhea and dysentery, and the marked deficiency of dietary protein needed for the nutrition of the beneficial bacteria of the intestine. For these reasons the dietary vitamin B^1 requirement for inmates of the camp probably was higher than it would have been under circumstances of more normal intestinal function.[101]

Smith and his colleagues gave their patients various dosages of vitamin B^1 orally, hypodermically, intramuscularly, intravenously, and even intrathecally—into the spinal canal. Of the 270 patients who received the vitamin for three months or more, only 17 percent were sufficiently relieved to stop the injections and the condition of 55 percent was unchanged.[102] Nicotinic acid, or niacin, given intravenously or on an empty stomach, sometimes resulted in marked flushing and temporary relief. But it had no permanent effect. Smith concluded that the temporary effect was simply due to transient enlargement of veins in the feet.[103]

Thus Smith concluded, with respect to the "burning feet" syndrome, that there was no doubt that this was the same condition as that associated with beriberi and also with ariboflavinosis in many parts of the world. In the Hong Kong cases, one-third had anesthesia and one-third had diminished or absent reflexes. Symptoms improved after adding beans, rice-polishings, and yeast to the diet; "it seemed to us that the condition must be caused by lack of some B complex factor or combination of factors, other than B^1 or nicotinic acid, and closely related to riboflavine."[104]

Hibbs observed beriberi over a period of 34 months in approximately 8,000 fellow American POWs in the Philippines. Every man had some form of beriberi at one time or another, and more than three-quarters of the men had painful neuritic feet.[105] A few of the patients—less than 100—received reasonably adequate treatment for about five months. This occurred because a Japanese medical officer decided to do a "scientific" assessment. Scientific it was not, but the selected severely ill men did get vitamin supplements of various kinds during the study period. There were eight groups, of which only one had complete treatment. All improvements were temporary, the patients regressing as soon as they were back on the routinely insufficient dietary regime that they shared, again, with the rest of the camp.[106]

The chief conclusions of the study were that in patients with beriberi, appetite, nervous manifestations, and heart disorders such as a rapid heart rate improved when they took thiamine. The peripheral neuritis that they assumed was caused by beriberi responded sooner to vitamin B complex as a whole than to thiamine alone. There may be nutritional causes of polyneuritis other than lack of thiamine. Generalized red rashes on the palms of the hands and the soles of the feet were seen consistently in dry beriberi. There may be few or no motor manifestations in beriberi peripheral neuritis; that is, the muscles continue to work properly. Irreversible destruction of the optic nerve may occur in patients who have severe beriberi, resulting in blindness.[107] Their most practical observation was perhaps that more vitamins can be bought in a grocery store than in a drug store.

In Japan, few new cases appeared among prisoners transported there from the South Pacific, though many old cases recurred or became aggravated during the first winter.[108] Despite the evidence that the incidence of "electric feet" decreased significantly in Japan, a Welsh POW has provided a powerful image clearly showing that the disorder did not disappear. He was sent from Hong Kong to Oeyama, where the POWs worked in a nickel mine owned by Oeyama Nickel Company: "On the journey back to camp, sitting on benches fixed across the trucks, the noise of our stamping 'electric' feet almost drowned that of the engine."[109]

Surg/Lt. Stening was at Fukuoka 2 Camp, where he had many opportunities to study patients with "electric feet." Loss of sleep was less during winter because most of the men had partly frozen feet and the anesthesia reached almost to the knees. They could not avoid freezing their feet: the men had to go out to work, often without socks and wearing worn-out boots. Many were supplied with Japanese canvas and rubber boots that soaked through quickly and were impossible to dry. The men worked in appalling conditions, exposed to winter winds. Eventually rubber wellingtons were provided, but by then many of the men were too weak to lift their feet in them, so they had to go back to wearing their smaller, soggy, canvas boots.[110]

The Japanese claimed to have seen, in Japan, some bad consequences from this disorder. A report referred to an affliction of the nerves giving severe pain in the legs and especially in the soles. In one case they were obliged to amputate one leg because of the gangrene that developed after the painful leg was exposed to coldness to ease the pain. They also found that while vitamin B[1] had some effect, it was powerless in serious or advanced cases.[111]

Pre-War Observations

The disorder did not arise *de novo* during World War Two, but was little known to western physicians because it was confined to non-Europeans who were either very poor or were in prison.

The first neuropathies were seen during the British Burmese War of 1823–1826. Native Indian troops were heavily affected by a disorder called, by the British medical officer who studied it, "a burning in the soles of the feet."[112] So many men had it that a medical board in Madras offered a substantial monetary prize to the author of the best publication on the subject.[113] J.G. Malcolmson won the prize in 1835. His account contained no references to Europeans with the syndrome, showing that this is certainly not a disease limited to Europeans, as some twentieth-century writers have claimed. Malcolmson made a definite connection between "burning feet" and poor nutrition.[114]

Between 1888 and 1897, Strachan reported 510 cases of a neuropathy that had many characteristics in common with POW neuropathies. After admitting such a patient to hospital and observing further progress, he noted that at night the patient often would be awake for hours, rubbing his feet and legs and moaning with pain."[115]

Sharples studied a similar phenomenon in the decade before World War Two began. Burning feet were seen in Hindu women labourers working in British Guiana. He thought the disorder was the result of eating poorly cooked rice as a staple. The condition occurred only in Hindu women workers between 17 and 40 years of age, who experienced intense burning of the soles of the feet when walking, "as if they were walking on fire."[116] Some of the patients had difficulty keeping themselves from falling when they stood with eyes closed.[117] Most of the rice was milled, thus removing much of the vitamin content. The Hindus prepared their rice with too much water, which was discarded and which contained much of the remaining vitamins. On a full diet including eggs, fruit, beef or chicken soup, and milk, the patients improved quickly.

Post-War Follow-Up

The disorder did not disappear completely after liberation and the resumption of normal diet. "Electric feet" continued to affect a very large number of the Hong Kong POWs. One study in 1947 examined 300 former members of the Winnipeg Grenadiers who had been imprisoned both in Hong Kong and in Japan. This is a remarkably large sample; of 916 Grenadiers who went to Hong Kong in 1941, 263 died in the Far East and 653 were repatriated home in 1945. Thus this scientific study encompassed 46 percent of the survivors; and of this large proportion of the battalion, 83 percent had abnormal sensations in their feet and legs, affecting both sides symmetrically. The sensations were variously described as "tingling," "burning," "aching," "numbness," "sharp shocking pains," and "cramps."[118]

Many still complained of paresthesias, and about half had minor neurologic signs. These were improving and did not interfere with normal activities. Two Canadian doctors became convinced "that moderately severe peripheral damage can be present even though our relatively crude methods of investigation are unable to prove it."[119]

John Crawford reported an extensive analysis of many of the Canadians who returned from Hong Kong. Medical files were examined for the first 400 (alphabetically) of 1400 HK veterans for the presence of various symptoms, changes in their incidence since 1945, and their distribution in the various military districts of Canada.

Eight complaints were studied—fatiguability, sweating, paresthesias, optic atrophy, edema, cardiovascular complaints, gastrointestinal complaints, and nervousness—in 1945 and again in 1949. Crawford cites one case history of a man who had had some paresthesias, died suddenly from another cause, and was found at autopsy to have major neurological changes: "One should therefore guard against the assumption that the complaint of paresthesia is entirely or even mainly psychogenic in origin."[120] In 1949 it was apparent that rehabilitation of these ex-POWs had not proceeded as well as had been hoped or expected.

A clinical analysis of 482 ex-POWs from the Winnipeg Grenadiers who had been in Hong Kong compared their findings in 1956 to those in 1947. The symptoms and signs fell into three groups, probably corresponding to different lesions. The most relevant to the present topic were neurological changes due to spinal cord and optic atrophy. The severity of pain and paresthesias bore little relationship to signs. There had been much improvement in all symptoms since 1946, but less change in neurological signs and in optic atrophy. The vast majority were then fully employed.[121]

Gopalan seems to have been the first to suggest a connection between electric feet and deficiency or absence of pantothenic acid in the diet. He claimed that therapy with pantothenic acid produced rapid alleviation of symptoms, and he also showed that marmite (a multivitamin food supplement) improved the symptoms, that pantothenic acid did so more rapidly, and that thiamine, nicotinic acid, and riboflavin all failed to help. Most of his 53 patients were poor malnourished Indians; signs suggesting deficiency of riboflavin were almost invariably present. The Tamil expression for "burning feet" is Kal erichal, and that is what the patients call the disorder, which usually involved only the soles of the feet but, occasionally, the palms also; sometimes the sensation spread up to the top of the foot. There was almost nothing abnormal to be seen when examining the feet except for marked perspiration. There was no loss of sensation: "touch, temperature and pain sensations, the vibration sense, the sense of position and passive movement are all retained even in advanced cases."[122] When these patients ingested marmite, symptoms subsided in four weeks; with calcium pantothenate improvement came in three weeks.

One type of behaviour that indicates uncertainty in medicine is a profusion of names for what appears to be the same disorder. Clearly this uncertainty exists in connection with electric feet. Glusman, himself an American POW medical officer, wrote about the syndrome after the war, coining the name "nutritional melalgia." "Melalgia" derives from the Greek and means limb pain.[123] He studied this condition in the Philippines and in Japan. The striking observation was that burning feet could occur as a distinct disorder by itself. "Electric feet" were being complained of almost simultaneously in widely separated areas such as Hong Kong, Singapore, Java, and the Philippines, in all locations by July 1942.[124]

"Electric feet" probably was a syndrome of avitaminosis due to vitamin B deficiency generally, not to lack of a single component of the complex. Vernon, himself a POW medical officer in the Philippines and Japan, wrote about this disorder in 1950. He followed Glusman's lead in calling it "nutritional melalgia." And he believed that it was not beriberi. But the principal stimulus to writing his account was "to disseminate information for the benefit of a misunderstood group of patients." These patients were ex-POWs who were having much difficulty convincing civilian physicians that such conditions as "electric feet" were real.[125]

Recently the US government recognized a pensionable link between edema experienced while a POW and post-war ischemic heart disease, though admitting that no connection has been proven.[126] Though this pronouncement provides pensions benefits to some US veterans, such decisions do nothing to clarify the medical problems.

The experiences of those thousands of Allied POWs who suffered with this strange disorder seem not to have had much impact on subsequent medical research or practice. For example, writing in 1984, one expert on neurological diseases in the tropics wrote:

> BURNING FEET SYNDROME. This is a painful, chronic sensory neuropathy of unknown etiology found in the tropics. The pain is of a burning causalgic type in the feet and lower legs and is associated with excessive sweating and with minimal objective sensory, motor, and reflex signs. The pain is often worse at night and is exacerbated by heat; analgesics are required. Pantothenic acid or B complex vitamins sometimes give improvement. Diabetes, isoniazid, or chronic alcoholism may produce a similar syndrome.[127]

Surely the numerous published papers derived from experience with POWs and other subjects must have contributed something to knowledge of the cause. The author cites 14 references published between 1955 and 1980, but none seems (by title or author) a POW-based article.

Pellagra

Pellagra is the disease of three D's: dermatitis, diarrhea, and dementia. It affects skin, gut, and brain. Yet it can exist in the absence of these three symptoms, a fact that seriously complicates diagnosis. Characteristically, the skin lesions affect the backs of the hands, forearms, face, and upper surfaces of the feet, and are described as "fish-scale" skin. Other symptoms include failing vision, painful feet, and polyuria—frequent bladder emptyings.[128] But perhaps the most serious feature of pellagra was its propensity to cause mental disturbances in its victims. Dementia is a late sign, often preceded by a fourth D, depression.

Though pellagra once was thought to be caused by eating spoiled corn or maize, by the 1920s it was widely recognized that long-term dietary deficiency of niacin or nicotinic acid (vitamin B[3]) produced the disease.[129]

The problem in POW camps was that "pure" vitamin deficiencies were unlikely. The diet was so uniformly poor that limitations rapidly occurred, not only of niacin but also thiamine, riboflavin, and the other B vitamins. When several vitamins are missing from the diet, symptoms of several disorders can co-exist, to the detriment of the patient and the confusion of the medical officer: "every conceivable permutation and combination of the lesions of pellagra with those of deficiency of riboflavin and probably of other factors as well, was seen in the camps."[130] Pellagra differed from camp to camp, at least according to two investigators who found that in Hong Kong (where one of them was imprisoned) pellagra was mostly oral, whereas in Singapore (where the other author spent his war) it was mostly seen as skin lesions.[131]

Crawford and Reid described a "typical" POW in the spring of 1943. There is intermingling of signs and symptoms from beriberi and pellagra, as well as other diseases. But the signs of pellagra in their depiction are obvious:

> His skin is dry and rough, loose and inelastic, and subcutaneous fat is absent. There is an area of brownish pigmentation over his malar prominences [cheekbones], and the bridge of the nose and the elbows. He has had a "pellagrinous" dermatitis on the posterior aspect of the knees and the dorsum of the wrist, but this has now cleared up. There are cracks at the corner of the mouth. At the nasolabial folds there are patches of a seborrhea-like dermatitis. He has a deep ulcer on the calf of the left leg. His tongue is sore, smooth, and very red at the margins and tip.[132]

As was true with so many western medical officers, A.H. Coombes knew nothing about pellagra until he read textbook accounts in a book approved by the Japanese, so that they were allowed to retain it. "I saw pellagra for the first time, classic stuff, dermatitis with its special distribution around the neck, and the diarrhea you got with it, and dementia. I saw half a dozen cases perhaps of dementia, all died. Real dementia which we put down to pellagra."[133]

Loss of Sight

A common problem that, again, related directly to inadequate diet over long periods, was loss of sight. This was more often partial than total and more often temporary than permanent. But it was a major worry for POWs when it occurred and, for some, it is a lifelong burden. In May 1943, a medical orderly at Hong Kong estimated that 10 percent of the POWs couldn't recognize a person's face at 40 yards and, he supposed, would be permanently affected.[134] Walter Grey "had a cataract operation recently and the doctor told me he couldn't bring the sight back because the inner eye was too badly scarred from malnutrition."[135] One prisoner remembered getting vitamins in an unusual form: "A lot of people started losing their eyesight and they brought in these little caramel fish candies and if your eyesight was really bad you got one candy in the morning and one at night."[136] Presumably the "candies" contained or were thought to contain some sort of vitamin supplement. Frank Harding woke up one morning in Camp 3D, Kawasaki, Japan, and couldn't see more than four feet in front of him. His medical officer called it malnutrition blindness. "Somehow he got some vitamin shots for me. I wasn't the only one. Lots of people had eye trouble."[137]

Standard theory suggests that such lesions represent avitaminosis B, but the Hong Kong POWs sometimes acquired visual defects while in reasonably good shape, and the deficit often did not improve with intensive vitamin therapy; hypoproteinemia may play a role, and "there is considerable evidence that a toxin may exist in mouldy rice."[138] The original condition suggested the existence of nerve inflammation behind the eyeball, eventually causing the optic nerve—which mediates sight—to atrophy.[139]

One former medical officer at Hong Kong wrote, after the war, that ocular problems were usually associated with a general neuropathic syndrome. Extremely painful feet were usually prominent at some stage, along with profound loss of weight. Like others, Durran found the textbook accounts of beriberi, pellagra, and central neuritis "confuse my attempts to classify the condition under discussion, which does not appear susceptible of being neatly docketed under any of these labels."[140]

Visual examinations and detailed histories were done on 375 of a total of 560 surviving members of the Winnipeg Grenadiers in 1947. Of the 375, 95 had partial optic atrophy. One puzzle is why only some men had these lesions, which appeared most frequently in autumn 1942, when everyone was living in much the same state of starvation and avitaminosis. Crawford pointed out that although the response of vision to vitamins was poor, beriberi would respond somewhat.[141]

Conclusions

As is apparent, the deficient supply of food caused many problems for the Far Eastern POWs—some temporary, some permanent. The spectrum of symptoms, diseases, and syndromes is wide. Essentially all the men and many of their officers experienced genuine hunger of a type they had not known even during the Depression. A large percentage had beriberi and "electric feet"; many had to cope with pellagra and with diminution or loss of sight. And a host of conditions affected prisoners that could not be diagnosed accurately, nor usually treated, but that were almost certainly also the result of the poor nutrition that these men experienced for so many years.

That these were not the only medical conditions among the POWs will be spelled out in detail in the next chapter. It deals with all the other disorders, those not directly traceable to insufficient rations of inadequate food.

Chapter 6

In Sickness, Rarely in Health:

Life and Death in the Camps

and Hospitals

At one stage in Thailand I had had eighteen separate medical complaints at the one time and my range included ulcers, scabies, beriberi, malaria, dysentery, gingivitis, vitaminosis [sic], conjunctivitis, colic, debility, dermatitis, plus others which I cannot now recall. And of course there was always the raw tongue and the weeping scrotum.[1]

*T*his remarkable constellation of illnesses may have been more likely to occur under the extreme conditions of the Burma-Siam Railway, but POWs in sites such as Hong Kong ran the same basic risks. They lived fundamentally unhealthy lives, underfed, overworked, unable to keep clean, often living among swarming parasites, flies, rats, and snakes. No wonder disease rarely came singly, but rather as bizarre and sometimes undiagnosable combinations of several conditions. How did such a medical nightmare come about?

After the capitulation of Hong Kong on Christmas Day, the Japanese found themselves with about 8,000 prisoners of war. Canada had sent 1,975 troops to Hong Kong in October; one died during the voyage and 290 were killed in action (including those wounded who subsequently died of their wounds) or were murdered by their captors in the few frenzied days just before and during the surrender; 1,684 Canadians remained alive. The following five years were not kind to the Canadians—nor to the British, the Indians, or members of the HKVDC. A total of 128 Canadian POWs died of disease in Hong Kong, on the high seas, or in Japan, most of them in 1942 (including 54 dead of diphtheria alone; 4 more died of that disease later). And four Grenadiers were executed for attempting to escape. Thus, of 1,680 Canadians who were neither killed in action nor executed, 128, or 8 percent, died in Japanese captivity. Of the entire Canadian contingent of 1,975, 423 died during the war from all causes (21%).

Diphtheria was perhaps the most frightening threat to the POWs at Hong Kong. But the men suffered from diverse and complicated combinations of several diseases. Foods, their lack, and the resulting medical problems, were considered in the previous chapter. This chapter will consider other diseases of all kinds.

Figures have survived for hospital admissions of Canadians at Hong Kong in these early months of captivity. But admission to the so-called hospital at North Point Camp was reserved for the most seriously ill minority of men. Then and throughout the unremitting years of captivity, the actual incidence of illness was always far higher than figures for hospitalization suggest. Nevertheless, there are data for January 1942 (for most of this month the bulk of the Canadians were at Sham Shui Po), and for February through July, when all Canadians had been consolidated at North Point. In both locations, and at almost all times in Hong Kong, the Canadians maintained medical facilities separate from the other national groups in the camps. This was not the case in Japan, as will be described in a later chapter.

Table 6.1
Monthly Returns, 1942

Period To:	Remaining	Admitted	Discharged	Died	Transf'd	Remain
31 Jan	0	117	94	0	1	22
28 Feb	22	100	99	0	7	16
31 March	16	87	78	0	9	16
30 April	16	142	125	0	16	17
31 May	17	132	93	0	14	42
30 June	42	91	70	0	39	24
31 July	24	118	99	0	22	21

Source: MG30, E213, *John Crawford Papers*.

The data from 1942 are derived from files maintained by "C" Force personnel in the camps, particularly S/Sgt. Robert Boyd acting for the senior medical officer of "C" Force, Maj. John N.B. Crawford.[2] Maj. Crawford returned these files to Canada after the war. A summary chart for 1942 gives some indication of the amount of serious illness.

These figures tell us, for example, that in both April and May 1942, almost 10 percent of the surviving Canadians were sufficiently ill to be hospitalized. The actual amount of sickness can only be guessed at, but certainly several other men were unwell for every man who could be admitted into hospital.

The zero figures in the "Died" column should not be misunderstood. During these first seven months of captivity the Japanese allowed severely ill POWs to be sent from North Point Camp to Bowen Road Hospital, perhaps because both sites were on the Island itself. This movement wasn't always timely but it did occur. As indicated in the "Transf'd" column, 108 of the sickest men were sent to Bowen Road; a proportion of these men died there.

Unhappily, some men approved for transfer to Bowen Road didn't make it there. In the middle of June, Tom Forsyth noted in his diary that two men very sick with dysentery were finally granted permission by the Japanese to go to Bowen Road Hospital; loaded on the back of a truck, one died on the way, the other just after arriving.[3] Although the Japanese did permit transfers of sick men they often delayed implementing the move—sometimes, as in this instance, with apparently lethal results. Whether these delays represented sheer bureaucratic incompetence or malevolence cannot be decided with certainty. But evidence of ineptitude in the Japanese POW bureaucracy was widespread and pervasive.

Diphtheria

Diphtheria was a common disease among western POWs in the Far East. Diphtheria is a highly infectious disease, especially among young adults, and living in cramped, unsanitary conditions increases the risk. The disease is caused by bacteria and, in the western world, the usual form affects the tissues of the throat. Patients often develop a heavy membrane on the inside of the throat, sometimes so thick that it prevents breathing. As the bacteria grow inside the body they also produce a toxin or poison that interferes with the function of nerves, including those that permit swallowing, heart action, and movement of the arms or legs. The damage done by these toxins often results in muscular paralysis that occurs many weeks after the disease seems to have disappeared. Patients who die usually do so because of asphyxiation from the membrane in the throat or later, from heart failure, when the heart is affected by toxin.

In addition to the variety of diphtheria that attacked the throat, many cases of diphtheria in the Far East involved skin,[4] including some especially difficult and often fatal cases in which the organism invaded the already cracked and inflamed skin of the scrotum, damaged by vitamin deficiencies. Many men had skin lesions from other causes, particularly ulcers on the legs and feet, which provided an ideal breeding ground for the diphtheritic organism.[5]

Diphtheria occurred all over the Far East. At least as early as June 1942, cases were diagnosed among the American POWs in the Philippines. A few days later, in the camp where Calvin Jackson was a medical officer, there were 37 cases, yet there was only antitoxin enough for 10 patients.[6] In Changi Camp, Singapore, diphtheria was also diagnosed frequently. Here is one medical officer's recollections:

> Diphtheria became very prevalent during the third month of captivity. There was never any antitoxin....Two common lesions seen were diphtheritic balanitis [infection of the penis] and infection of a scrotal dermatitis. The latter cases presented a pitiful picture: the whole scrotum was involved in an extensive ulcer and no treatment was of any avail. They all died. Several cases definitely had the disease twice. It appeared that immunity to the disease was lost under the conditions of avitaminosis.[7]

Thus the protection that customarily arises from surviving an infection of the disease failed to occur in the starved men.[8]

Diphtheria came to be a significant medical problem affecting western POWs in Singapore, the Philippines, Java, and Hong Kong by late spring and early summer, 1942. Because these locations are many hundreds of miles apart, the epidemics must have begun spontaneously in the various camps, indicating the ubiquity of the causative bacteria throughout the Far East and the relatively poor state of immunity among American, Canadian, British, and other young men in the Allied forces.

Maj. H.G.G. Robertson, RAMC, kept a diary at Sham Shui Po. He first queried the possibility of a diagnosis of diphtheria on 28 June 1942, and by 3 July was seeing many cases of "sore throat." Some were suspicious, but no laboratory diagnosis of diphtheria could be made: there were no facilities for making one, nor for treating any of the cases.[9] By the end of July the diagnosis was certain. A month later, Japanese personnel were wearing face masks for anti-diphtheria reasons. The POWs were given Condy's gargle, the ubiquitous purple potassium permanganate.[10] According to the Japanese, the gargle would kill diphtheria germs. Ineffective as it was, it was all they had.

Cases of diphtheria first began to be seen at Bowen Road Hospital in July 1942. Most or all of these cases would have been contracted by men in hospital already for other reasons, or by Canadians from North Point Camp, since at this time the Japanese permitted transfer of seriously ill men from that camp but only rarely from Sham Shui Po or Argyle Street on the mainland. The first death from diphtheria, Sapper T.Y. McMasters, RE, was recorded on 27 June 1942. On that same date, Spr. F. Wilson died of the disease at St. Teresa's Hospital. Lt. White noted cases of diphtheria among the Canadians at North Point Camp as early as 16 August 1942,[11] though he was actually about a week behind the actuality. There were 18 diphtheria admissions to Bowen Road in August and 59 in September, an ominous portent.[12]

On 11 August 1942, the patients from St. Teresa's Hospital in Kowloon were transferred to Bowen Road Hospital. As Maj. Bowie noted at the time, these men "brought stories of an outbreak of diphtheria in Kowloon,"[13] and the Japanese required Bowie to isolate 10 of the 24 patients, thinking they might have diphtheria. It turned out that they did not. Nevertheless, diphtheria had occurred at St. Teresa's; a roll of deaths there shows a man dying of the disease on 27 June, six more diphtheria deaths in July, and one just three days before the transfer to Bowen Road.[14]

Sister D. Van Wart, a nurse who was at St. Teresa's, recalled the period vividly. A diphtheria epidemic started in the mens' camp; the patients arrived at St. Teresa's, but there was no serum to give them.

> I was put in charge of the ward, having had previous experience and had been immunised. The Japs were terrified and wouldn't come near us. The Matron pleaded for serum which they wouldn't give us. Then one evening the Jap doctor called the Matron to the gates and threw a package over saying: "Here is your precious serum you want so much, now stop bothering me about it."[15]

There was enough outdated serum for 8 men and more than 100 patients were dying. The medical officers and the matron had the heartbreaking task of deciding which patients should receive the serum. One VAD had a septic throat, was given one shot of serum, and recovered quickly. Miraculously no other staff caught diphtheria. An ex-POW thought that someone did bring serum to the camp gate, "but it was thrown on the ground in front of the POWs and smashed by one of the guards."[16] Where this happened is uncertain—most likely at Sham Shui Po, if the story is accurate.

Inevitably there were some especially distressing cases. The medical officers had to do tracheotomies on some suffocating men, who were black in the face when they arrived. Many did not survive. A doctor who came to St. Teresa's from the officers' camp at Argyle Street hid instruments for the operations in his socks. "Matron removed them surreptitiously while he was scrubbing up, while another doctor kept the Japs occupied outside."[17] Coombes did a number of tracheotomies, but it wasn't to save the man's life, "we couldn't have done that, it was just to ease their frightful restriction of breathing. And you could put a piece of hollow bamboo in, or pieces of rubber tubing boiled up and so on, and secured as makeshift intubation."[18] Dr. Anderson remembers doing tracheotomies on men desperately ill with diphtheria, and doing them without anesthesia.[19] Probably these men were so near death that they were beyond pain.

Most men with diphtheria admitted to Bowen Road from North Point were critically ill. Once the Canadians were transferred to Sham Shui Po, on 26 September 1942, no more patients with diphtheria arrived at Bowen Road.[20] Of the 77 patients admitted there with the disease before the end of September, 19 died (25%). The chief medical officer at Bowen Road noted that supplies of anti-diphtheritic serum were inadequate, a shortage that seems to have been general throughout the Far East. When the epidemic began, there were 31,000 units of serum at Bowen Road. In September they received 37,500 units from the Japanese, and in October, 50,000 units.[21] Since Bowen Road had no cases of diphtheria in October, it is apparent that they had access to 68,500 units for 77 patients, or an average of 890 units per patient. The customary dosage was 8,000 to 10,000 units per patient.

Two Canadian MOs, John Crawford and John Reid, wrote about their experiences with diphtheria. The first case diagnosed positively among the Canadians was seen 7 August 1942. The disease quickly became an epidemic. In the next six months, 459 cases developed among the Canadians, peaking in October: 12 cases in August; 67 in September; 248 in October; 106 in November; 20 in December; and 6 in January 1943. A few cases occurred in the spring of 1943. The severity of the epidemic owed much to the unfortunate timing of their transfer to the mainland on 26 September 1942, since their captors insisted that they take active cases of diphtheria with them. The Japanese refused to admit the disease was diphtheria and provided no antiserum. Of the early cases, 101 received no serum and of these 38 (37.6 percent) died; most would likely have survived under then-modern treatment.[22]

Immediately on arrival at Sham Shui Po, diphtheritic Canadians began to swell the ranks at sick parade. Dr. John Crawford had to take at least six men with frank diphtheria from North Point Camp to Sham Shui Po.[23] As well, the British were already wrestling with a major epidemic:

> The most elementary safeguards (if only to protect the Japanese guards and staff) should have included medical tests and the provision of anti-toxin. Yet for several months, in the summer of 1942, the epidemic was allowed to run its dreadful course, striking down inevitably the strongest and fittest men. Only when the death roll was already into three figures did the Japanese send in serum.[24]

The epidemic was so severe that at least some men contemplated suicide when they heard the diagnosis. One soldier remembered that when Capt. Reid told him he had diphtheria it was like a death sentence. "I looked at the electric wire fence and I considered putting an end to myself. I don't know why I didn't do it, but I didn't. That's the lowest I've ever been."[25]

At Sham Shui Po, anti-diphtheritic serum was in short supply. A certificate in the Hong Kong Public Records Office indicates total absence of serum between 21 August and 4 September 1942.[26] Significantly, on 5 September, 16 patients received serum, including men from all battalions and branches of the services, though no Canadians.[27] They were still at North Point at this stage, with diphtheria occurring but not yet epidemic. At Sham Shui Po there was certainly an epidemic. In July 1942 there were 40 cases with 10 deaths, in August 89 cases with 19 deaths, and in September 56 cases of whom 15 died.[28] Thus the mortality rate was 44 of 184, or 24 percent.

There was so much diphtheria among the British at Sham Shui Po that many men had to be removed from a Japan-bound convoy. The Japanese wouldn't risk introducing this epidemic into their homeland. One man described the ship as "a terrible old hulk," and he was pleased that one of his friends was unable to make the trip. He was taken off at the last moment as a suspected diphtheria carrier, and isolated in the hospital.[29] His potentially infectious state probably saved the man's life—the "old hulk" was the ill-fated *Lisbon Maru*, sunk on this trip with hundreds dead.

Capt. Anthony Coombes recorded amounts of diphtheria antitoxin used at Sham Shui Po. Dosages ranged from 2,500 to 10,000 units. Between 12 August and 30 November he administered antitoxin to 45 men. But there is a major gap between 14 August and 24 September, during which time no serum was given. Sgt. Britwell, RAMC, received two doses, 5,000 units on 16 November and 10,000 units on 30 November, by which dates the supply of serum was adequate. Otherwise all were single doses. Most significant is the gap between 12-13 August, when seven patients were treated, and 25 September when, apparently, antitoxin again became available. The Canadians arrived at that camp 26 September, and they had no antitoxin to give their diphtheritic patients until 5 October; but during this time, 14 patients in the British diphtheria ward were treated.[30] Since the list is entitled "Unofficial antitoxin," it was probably obtained *sub rosa* through Dr. Selwyn-Clarke or the black market.

A mystery surrounds the availability of serum. Coombes stated unequivocally: "No serum was available until September 5 1942, after which date *plentiful supplies* were on hand."[31] Perhaps the reference was intended to be 25 September, which would be consistent with the list cited in the previous paragraph showing a gap in serum use (and, presumably, availability) between 13 August and 25 September.

But if serum was "plentiful" at Sham Shui Po from 25 September, why were the Canadians (who arrived there on the 26th) without serum until 5 October? Did British medical officers withhold serum from Canadian medical officers, and therefore from Canadian patients? The former medical officers I have interviewed, in Canada,

Britain, and Hong Kong, all say that this would never have happened deliberately; medical cooperation was generally good even though the establishments were separate.

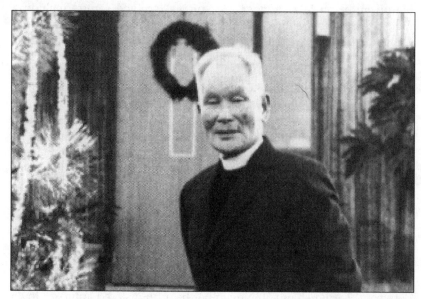

Figure 6.1. Former IJA interpreter, the Reverend Watanabe Kiyoshi, "Uncle Jon." (Frontispiece, Sir Selwyn Selwyn-Clarke, *Footprints: The Memoirs of Sir Selwyn Selwyn-Clarke, KBE, CMG, MC, C.St.J., MD, BS, FRCP, MRCS, DPH, DTM & H, Bar-at-Law, Former Governor and Commander-in-Chief, Seychelles* (Hong Kong: Sino-American Publishing Co., 1954)

Maj. Donald Bowie stated that in September 1942, Lt. Mackenzie, a Hong Kong resident, informed him that a stock of serum had been stored in the Dairy Farm Storage Godown, or warehouse. Bowie asked the Japanese to get the serum. "I never found out whether the supplies we were given came from that stock or not but Sergeant Seino told me that no serum had been found in the Dairy Farm cold store."[32]

Some serum was smuggled into the camps, and at least one of the smugglers was Japanese. Dr. Selwyn-Clarke was permitted by the conquerors to continue as chief civilian medical officer of Hong Kong for two years after the surrender. He made prodigious efforts to aid the POWs and internees. In his account he gave full credit to Watanabe Kiyoshi, a Christian minister who was an interpreter for the Japanese army and who was known by the informal code name of "Uncle Jon." As Selwyn-Clarke recorded, "[w]henever the purpose was particularly vital, for example in getting anti-diphtheritic serum to the Canadians, I would entrust the phials to Uncle Jon."[33] The question of the shortage of serum and Japanese unwillingness or inability to provide adequate amounts is a painful one still for the survivors, especially those who had medical responsibilities; and, of course, for the families of men who died of diphtheria but who might have been saved had anti-diphtheritic serum been available. There is circumstantial evidence to suggest that the dairy godown mentioned by Lt. Mackenzie may not, in fact, have contained serum by September 1942. By then, Japan was severely depleted in most medical supplies. Although the civilian allotment of diphtheria antitoxin in Japan itself for the years 1942-44 totalled 17,300 litres, actual production amounted to only 5,700 litres and the military took 1,700 liters of this, leaving for the civilian population only 4,000 litres or about 22 percent of the estimated required amount.[34] Thus domestic supplies were low, and it would not be surprising if captured serum was promptly shipped back to Japan to make up this deficit.

The POW medical officers had to fill out death certificates for Tokyo. When they wanted to cite diphtheria, the Japanese tried to insist that it couldn't be diphtheria, which is infectious. "I remember getting a slap, a wallop, for saying, 'Just put "heart stop."' And he said, 'No, no.' I thought it would be good Japanese for heart failure or something, just put 'heart stop.' Eventually they agreed to put diphtheria, and I think as a result of that we did get the antitoxin."[35]

Dr. Coombes remembered that the medical officers used to have meetings after they had received some antitoxin, because there wasn't enough to treat the disease thoroughly. They had case conferences about who should get one of these doses of serum. It was frequently life-saving for those who received treatment.

Some men acquired diphtheria from sharing cigarettes. Some had open sores on their legs and developed ulcers covered with a diphtheritic membrane. "I remember this so well. When you saw that you said, 'You're all right, you're going to recover, you won't get laryngeal diphtheria, you've been immunized by this. So we'll just keep you quiet and it will clear up.' And it did."[36]

One consequence of the shortage of serum was an experimental approach to therapy at Bowen Road Hospital. Faced with four patients with severe acute diphtheria, Maj. G.F. Harrison proposed to give transfusions of whole blood from patients who had recovered from the disease. The hope was that a transfer of immunity would occur. After anxious consultations among the medical staff, the transfusions were carried out. Two of the patients recovered.[37] Apparently the experiment was not repeated, though the medical approach had logic. In Sham Shui Po a similar trial was contemplated but, for lack of equipment, could not be attempted.[38]

Tom Forsyth, of the Winnipeg Grenadiers, kept a detailed diary that contains much information about the impact of diphtheria. On 14 August 1942, still at North Point, he heard that diphtheria raged in Sham Shui Po, with an average of one man dead every day. "Only one case here yet but we are warned to keep to our own areas, no mixing with the Rifles. No more soft ball games nor classes, nor bat. parades."[39]

For what seemed endless months to patients acutely ill with diphtheria and to their medical attendants, the disease raged essentially unchecked. Resistance obviously was low, and the germ had found susceptible victims. Dr. Solomon Bard for the first time thought he could really "see the terror in people's eyes."[40]

D.L.W. Welsh, a Canadian POW, can represent some dozens of his mates. He entered the hospital in Sham Shui Po on 29 September 1942, just three days after the Canadians moved there from North Point Camp. Up until that autumn he had kept a terse diary, largely limited to entries about the food. Welsh's final entry was 5 October, when he wrote: "B[reakfast]. Never eat anything all day (couldent, [*sic*] swollen)."[41] He died that evening.

At first the Japanese claimed that it wasn't diphtheria at all. Then they said they didn't have any serum. Weak doses of the small amount that was available were given to the orderlies who were looking after the diphtheritic patients. But there was none for the patients themselves. Thus:

> in 1942, in the twentieth century, we witnessed an untreated epidemic of diphtheria, which was something I never thought I would see when I studied it in my medical school. I never thought that I would see that, with the full blast of its complications, including paralysis of the diaphragm, vocal cord paralysis, quadriplegia, and death. Every day when there was a death in our hospital a black flag would be hung up, so that the Japanese headquarters outside the fence, outside the gate, would see it and make the preparations for coffins to be delivered, for burial.[42]

By September the Japanese finally began to take diphtheria seriously. About mid-month they ordered that masks be worn, "a Japanese custom and damn good, I'd say."[43] Moreover, they meant that the masks actually be worn. They beat up men they saw not wearing a mask, or going near the diphtheria hospital. "Used rifle butts on one man. Broke three ribs."[44]

Diphtheria among the Canadians

In the autumn of 1942, 74 Canadians developed diphtheria before any antitoxin became available; of these, 54 died. The Japanese ordered that all diphtheria patients and carriers with positive throat swabs must be isolated. On 24 October the patients and the Canadian MOs were sent to the Jubilee Buildings, thereby separating them by the width of the parade ground from the rest of the camp. The Canadians were given one end of this large building; part of the remainder was designated as the isolation hospital for the British. The Canadian section was portions of four floors, 40 small rooms used as wards for two to five patients, tightly packed, lying on the cement floor. No beds were available.[45]

The orderlies who worked in these wards "all should have been given medals because they knew damn well that there was no treatment."[46] Some of these men were especially singled out for praise by the men they nursed: "I want to take this opportunity of paying a tribute to Freddy Drover of Newfoundland. He was the finest medical orderly we ever had. The only orderly who never lost his patience or his temper. He never lost hope and always did his best to inspire it in others."[47] Ray Squires was praised by all for his selfless work, often among the most dangerously ill. The helpers in this isolation ward were all volunteers.[48] Most of the volunteer orderlies had had no medical background of any kind; a few, from both the Royal Rifles and the Winnipeg Grenadiers, were illiterate.[49]

A former member of the HKVDC recalled: "The small group of Canadian orderlies, led by Sergeant Reg Kerr, who in peacetime had been a Salvation Army member, were a motley crew, and easily the best of the Canadians I met in our camp. The group I was with in the hospital were all from the Winnipeg Grenadiers."[50]

Sgt. Lance Ross, Royal Rifles, developed diphtheria on 10 October 1942. His diary records something of the medical situation at that time. He had been placed in a makeshift ward in an old building without windows, along with 200 other patients. They were all lying on a cement floor. Some died every day. The suffering was terrible. "11th—Can hardly write so sick. Tonsils are as big as eggs; can hardly breathe. 12th—Three died last night."[51] The diphtheria patients were transferred to the Jubilee Buildings about 24 October. He found that location much preferable to the windowless huts. It was cold, however, and they were living five to a room, lying on the floor because there were no beds.[52]

During October 1942, Maj. John Crawford and his Canadian medical colleagues admitted 283 cases of diphtheria to the Canadian wards in Jubilee Hospital; 41 of these men died. Thus the mortality rate had improved impressively from 73 percent in September (54 deaths in 74 patients) to 15 percent (41 of 283). Much of the credit goes to the increasing availability of anti-diphtheritic serum. On 3 October, Crawford had been able to purchase some serum on the black market, and soon after, the Japanese issued a small batch. As well as the black market, there were other sources of drugs. "The work parties also served, unknowingly to most of us, as a contact with the Chinese guerrilla movement who were a source of medications denied to the camp by the Japanese."[53] These drugs were supplied by the British Army Aid Group (BAAG), perhaps via guerrillas.

BAAG also supplied news to the outside world of what was happening to the Hong Kong POWs. Thus, during 1942, the Canadian government learned about the diphtheria epidemic,[54] information that at least made Canadians begin to be aware of what was happening to their loved ones.

In Sham Shui Po, treatment with serum had to be rationed. Any patient who had a throat membrane 48 hours or more before serum became available did not receive treatment with antitoxin.[55] Their disease was too firmly established to be treatable with the still quite limited resources. Serum was given only to new cases, where a small quantity would do the greatest good. The maximum dosage was 2,000 units, the typical dosage was 1,000 units. In normal circumstances, 10 times that amount would have been used. But even this small quantity saved lives. By mid-October it was being administered routinely, and one victim wrote nonchalantly in his diary (13 October 1942): "Today or rather this morning I contracted the 'Dypth' [sic]. I had a needle this afternoon."[56]

Diphtheria killed many prisoners of war in Hong Kong; ironically, though, some believed that diphtheria also saved lives. As the supply of serum increased, reasonable therapeutic dosages were able to be given, thereby minimizing the danger of the disease. More importantly, patients with diphtheria and diphtheria carriers were isolated for long periods, saving them from exhausting and debilitating work parties.

CSM Colin Standish was a diphtheria carrier. He has described the strange existence these men led for many weeks or months. They did little because the Japanese didn't want them to transmit diphtheria to other POWs or the guards. On principle they wanted the carriers to work, but couldn't put them on regular work details. The carriers weren't ill; they just had to wait with little to occupy them. "I got some of the boys making wreaths for the ones that died because we were losing quite a few people every day. They had to be cremated so we sent [hibiscus] wreaths out with bodies. The morgue was in our section where our buildings were."[57] There was no work for them—there were enough recuperating patients to do the light work in the camp.

But the problem hung on for many discouraging weeks. On 11 November 1942, there were 301 Canadians in hospital, being cared for by the four medical officers and 40 medical orderlies (almost all untrained volunteers).[58] By Christmas 1942, fewer cases of diphtheria were being diagnosed, and eventually the Jubilee Buildings were closed as a hospital. By the end of the epidemic, 494 Canadians, almost one-third of those captured on 25 December 1941,[59] had suffered from the disease. Many more had spent long periods in isolation as diphtheria carriers. On the first Canadian draft sent to Japan, 296 of the 663 Canadians (45%) were identified as having had diphtheria; on the second Canadian draft, 119 of 336 (35%); on the third Canadian draft, 21 of 98 (21%); and on the fourth and last draft including Canadians, 11 of 47 (23%). Thus, of the 1,144 Canadian POWs shipped to Japan, 447, or 39 percent, had acquired a diphtheritic infection in Hong Kong, almost all during the final six months of 1942.[60]

There was a common theme that dismal autumn: "Pleased to see Neville is with us, then learn he's in isolation, Diphtheria carrier."[61] By early October, between 75 and 100 of the approximately 1,500 Canadians had been found to be carriers and were in isolation.[62] A Royal Navy POW noted:

I have not mentioned the diphtheria epidemic which was raging when I first came to Camp S. The whole S.W. quarter of the camp was wired off for dip. suspects and it was packed. How the Japs arrived at such a high proportion I don't know, but we were all swabbed frequently and carriers or suspects segregated. Inside the compound was the hospital for the confirmed cases.[63]

Capt. Woodward, IMS, sarcastically described the Japanese efforts to intervene in the diphtheria epidemic. Sometime in the autumn of 1942 "the Jap organisation excelled itself" and throat swabs were taken from everyone in Sham Shui Po with, the surgeon noted, "a fine disregard for aseptic technique." A box full of swabbed plates was dropped on the ground, most of them breaking, but repeat swabs were not taken to replace these. Woodward felt that the Japanese organization for epidemics was quite good; "if it were not staffed by Japs it would be effective instead of just amusing."[64]

The carrier state was serious. Carriers have the offending germ in their systems, can infect others, but do not get the disease and seem healthy. At Singapore it was decided that because the POW authorities could not deal with the carrier problem, they would not investigate it. "By a misunderstanding, the staff of one (non-diphtheria) ward were tested. Some 25 to 35 per cent were positive on culture, if my memory serves me."[65]

Remarkably, none of the Canadian medical officers and few orderlies contracted diphtheria despite their constant exposure. Dr. Banfill recalled that his younger brother had the disease when they were children; he must then have developed a sub-clinical infection and, thus, protective immunity.[66] One volunteer orderly who did develop diphtheria was Harry Atkinson. (Actually, Atkinson recalls clearly that he was less a volunteer than one who was "volunteered" by his CSM.[67]) Having his breakfast one morning, he noticed that it was difficult and painful to swallow.

My throat, while it wasn't swollen up on the outside, seemed to be constricted inside. I went down to Sergeant [Ray] Squires' room where the doctor was, and while he wasn't there Ray had a look at my throat and said, "Hell, you've got diphtheria!" And he said, "Freddy Drover will fix you up right now. Just drop your pants and bend over." And that was it. I was in the ward laying on the floor with four other fellows and in about 10 days I was back to work. Mine was a very mild case.[68]

Atkinson was lucky enough to get ill after supplies of serum had become plentiful.

Although the two Canadian regiments had not been immunized systematically by the army, some individuals may have had the protective injection before joining the service. And some would of course have acquired immunity from exposure, as Dr. Banfill possibly did. During the 1920s, the claims made for protection by diphtheria toxoid, a laboratory-treated suspension of the diphtheria bacterium that was non-infective but produced protection, encouraged authorities in Canada to introduce immunization campaigns. Although progress was slow initially, Canada became a world leader in antitoxin and, later, toxoid production at the Connaught Laboratories in Toronto. In 1926-27, Canadian investigators found that the incidence of diphtheria among 9,000 unimmunized controls was 11.44 per 1,000, whereas it was only 1.55 per 1,000 among those who had been immunized.[69]

Subsequent success obtained in Hamilton, Ontario, attracted worldwide attention. There the incidence and mortality from diphtheria had shown little change for many years up to 1925, when the immunization campaign began. Diphtheria deaths in Hamilton ceased after 1930, and no case of the disease was documented after 1933. There were almost no deaths from diphtheria in Toronto between 1934 and 1939, and none from 1940 on. In Canada as a whole, 1,300 persons died from diphtheria in 1921; approximately 300 per annum in the years 1943 to 1945 (the last three years of the war); and only six in 1958 (in an area where immunization had been neglected).[70]

The Winnipeg Grenadiers had trouble with diphtheria long before they arrived at Hong Kong. Early in 1940, while still in Winnipeg before shipping out to Jamaica, there was a small outbreak. The battalion War Diary notes on 19 January 1940: "All ranks were confined to Barracks with effect from 1200 hours this date, five cases of Diphtheria having been discovered. The Medical Officer began a Schick Test of all ranks."[71] Two days later, Sunday, church parades were cancelled as a precaution against spreading diphtheria. But on Monday, 22 January, the prescribed confinement to barracks was lifted. On 1 February 1940, then Capt. J.N.B. Crawford, RCAMC, a pediatrician who would have known diphtheria, which was relatively common among children in the recent past, was attached to the battalion for duty as medical officer.[72] The War Diary also records that in January 1941, in Jamaica, all men received TAB (anti-typhoid and paratyphoid A and B) inoculations.[73] Diphtheria immunization was not carried out.

In Sham Shui Po POW Camp, Capt. Saito, the Japanese medical officer, routinely carried with him a length of rubber enema tubing with which he beat any POW—officer, NCO, or Other Rank—who transgressed the rules of the camp. On one occasion he beat the senior medical officer, Maj. Crawford, about the face and head because he and his men had proven negligent in their medical duties—"proven" by the fact that so many of their charges were dying of dysentery and diphtheria.

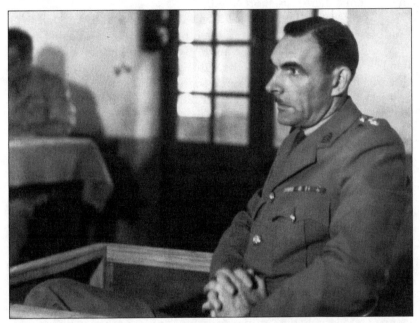

Figure 6.2. Lt.-Col J.N.B. Crawford, RCAMC (1906-1997), testifying during war crimes trials in Tokyo, 1946. (Photo courtesy of the late Dr. Crawford.)

Whether or not this was the medical officer referred to by Bush in the following anecdote is uncertain. Certainly Capt. Saito was never removed from his position.

During 1942 [the POWs in Sham Shui Po] had experienced a severe outbreak of diphtheria. A large number of men had died painful and unnecessary deaths. The Japanese medical officer at that time maintained that serum for diphtheria was not available in the Colony. At the height of the epidemic a senior Japanese medical officer arrived on a tour of inspection from Tokyo. When he saw the conditions which prevailed and heard the complaints concerning lack of serum he apparently became furious with the Japanese medical officer, and obtained it within an hour. This put an end to diphtheria and the Japanese medical officer was removed from the camp.[74]

This particular episode, ending in removal of the Japanese medical officer, I have not seen corroborated elsewhere. Possibly it is the Crawford story embellished during repeated retelling. But the Japanese finally did provide anti-diphtheritic serum.

In the officers' camp, whether at Argyle Street or later at Camp "N" connected with Sham Shui Po, diphtheria was only a real problem in July 1942, when they were feeling the hopelessness of a medical catastrophe: eight deaths out of 10 cases of diphtheria.[75] Fortunately, the epidemic there was short-lived.

No disease seems to have affected the officers at Argyle Street Camp as severely as the men in the other camps. At the beginning of November 1942, when Sham Shui Po was reeling under a major epidemic, dozens of men having died, there was one case at Argyle Street, three or four days old. "But more segregation for the hut concerned and restrictions about going to other huts, bridge etc—and we have to wear funny little mouth masks." A week later there had been no further cases of diphtheria. The hut concerned came out of quarantine. By the middle of the month another case cropped up. Precautions were resumed: huts in quarantine, masks, and gargling. "We have all had swabs taken this morning, which one hopes may produce some information." As a result of the swabs the Japanese found one diphtheria carrier. His hut was put in quarantine and all the restrictions were on again.[76] The MOs at Argyle Street Camp administered the Schick test for diphtheria, an injection in the skin of the arm. Men with positive tests were to have diphtheria inoculation.[77]

Capt. Warrack, RAMC, wrote about this small outbreak of diphtheria—perhaps four mild cases—in Argyle Street Camp. By this time the serious outbreaks of the disease at Sham Shui Po and North Point camps were largely over, and a supply of antitoxin was available.

At the post-war trial of Dr. Saito Shunkishi, the chief IJA medical officer in charge of POWs at Hong Kong, the question of serum and its availability was pursued at great length. Mr. Razee Nazarin testified as accountant of the Harry Wickin Co., which had a contract with the Hong Kong government to store quantities of serums, including anti-tetanus, diphtheria antitoxin, and anti-dysentery serum. In December 1941, "the stock we had, I believe, would ordinarily last 2 years."[78] Mr. Lewis Guy testified as a chemist with Watson & Co. that they also had a 6-month supply of various items such as diphtheria antitoxin, as well as sulfapyridine, nicotinic acid, and other related products. Asked if he knew what became of these stocks during the Japanese occupation, Mr. Guy replied: "No I do not exactly know what became of them, but in February [1942] the Japanese civilians took me from Stanley to go over the wholesale department. When they came there they found the Navy were in occupation and we were not allowed to go in. So I presume that the Navy had it."[79]

There is a diary entry for 13 January 1942 that supports this view: "Major Manners says that there are some millions of tons of goods in his warehouses at the Wharves. These are being put in Japanese ships as fast as possible. A convoy of 30 ships went out recently, all laden to the Plimsoll line, from the Kowloon Wharf."[80]

Throughout the war, a dog-in-the-manger attitude frequently characterized relationships between the Japanese army and navy, between the Kempei Tai and the rest of the army, and between all the armed services and civilians. That this was counterproductive in innumerable ways seems obvious.[81] In this instance it may well have cost POW lives, for it is entirely possible, and even likely, that the Japanese navy had confiscated these medical supplies for its own use, or to ship back to the main islands of Japan, and they would truly have been unavailable for use in the camps and, perhaps, by the Japanese army. Though the debate on this question cannot change the fatal end result, nevertheless, the Japanese camp officials may genuinely have had great difficulty in obtaining medical supplies—as they assured the POWs regularly—despite the POWs' belief that the supplies existed in profusion in Hong Kong.

The Court found Dr. Saito Shunkishi guilty of several charges, among which the alleged failure to provide serum weighed heavily. He was sentenced to death by hanging (sentence later commuted to imprisonment for 20 years).[82] The commutation apparently stemmed largely from the impact of a letter written by Dr. Selwyn-Clarke on 17 February 1947, seeking clemency for Saito. He wrote: "From my personal observations on Captain Saito, I am inclined to the opinion that he is not altogether normal mentally." He also cited instances where Saito permitted medical supplies into the camp at Ma Tau Chung when Selwyn-Clarke was imprisoned there. Selwyn-Clarke attached to his letter one from his deputy, Dr. Isaac Newton, who concluded: "Dr. Saito's relations with me were those of a fellow doctor working in very difficult circumstances and I hold the impression that shortcomings that existed were the result of his lack of authority in the Japanese Army and not of intentional cruelty on his behalf."[83] Why Selwyn-Clarke and Newton were not subpoenaed to appear at the trial (which was held in Hong Kong, where they both lived), and why this post-trial information should have weighed so heavily in the minds of the reviewing officers of the Judge Advocate General's office, is unknown.

By early 1943, worry about diphtheria ended. There were occasional cases but no further epidemics. Unhappily, there was no shortage of other diseases to torment the weak, hungry, harassed survivors and to vex and frustrate their medical attendants.

Dysentery

Dysentery was a constant, painful, and often lethal problem in Far Eastern POW camps. Bacillary dysentery and amoebic dysentery were the two varieties occurring among the POWs during their captivity.[84] These diseases must be distinguished from ordinary diarrhea, which at some time afflicted every POW and which had many causes including profound change in diet. Dysentery, on the other hand, was characterized by severe abdominal pain and frequent evacuation of stools containing blood and mucus. In many men, blood loss was considerable. Those unfortunate enough to have hemorrhoids simultaneously were particularly subject to bleeding, a common reason for doing hemorrhoidectomies in the camps.[85]

Although sulfa drugs combated bacterial dysentery effectively, as emetine[86] did amoebic dysentery, dysentery patients seldom received specific treatment because the drugs were rarely available. Often, men with dysentery received some combination of warm tea enemas, magnesium sulphate, charcoal, and a diet of rice gruel.

In the Philippines, American medical officers found plentiful supplies of emetine for treating amoebic dysentery; the drug had been sent from the United States to Japan in 1923 after a catastrophic earthquake: "We were in essence using our own medicine after a lapse of nineteen years."[87] In less fortunate camps patients with amoebic dysentery most often did without emetine. Occasionally, ingenuity overcame the shortage. A Dutch chemist named van Boxtel achieved local fame among some of the Burma-Siam Railway camps by finding a method for extracting emetine from its naturally occurring precursor, ipecacuanha. This achievement saved many lives.[88]

Warrack, a medical officer whose POW experiences encompassed both Hong Kong and Japan, gives a succinct description of the course of bacillary dysentery:

> The onset was sudden, consisting of a feeling of malaise accompanied by rigors and hyperpyrexia the temperature rising to over 103 F. Diarrhoea commenced about six hours later and was accompanied in many cases by severe [blank] and collapse....Mild cases were treated with 2-hourly doses of magnesium sulphate until the stools became clear of blood. This usually occurred by the third or fourth day, the patient being then discharged to make room for more serious cases....Severe cases were given from four to six grams of sulfapyridine. The effects of this drug were in most cases dramatic, the stools often becoming firm and clear of blood in 24 hours....By February, 1942, the supplies of sulfapyridine were exhausted and all cases were treated with sulfanilamide.[89]

Thus the most effective drugs against dysentery had been used up less than two months into what became a 44-month period of captivity. Supplies of drugs were rarely replenished. At Hong Kong, the painful clutch of dysentery had been felt almost immediately. Twelve days after the capitulation, Maj. H.G.G. Robertson, RAMC, noted that 120 cases of dysentery had arrived at Sham Shui Po from Argyle Street

Camp. Most of these patients were Indian troops. There were only 50 beds, all of which were already in use. Yet the patients were there, desperate for treatment; those well enough lined up at the latrines in nervous agitation, the rest soiled themselves, their belongings, and their neighbors. Naturally, the epidemic spread.

By mid-February the Indians had been transferred to Ma Tau Chung, but the situation remained chaotic. One medical officer reported the occurrence of a death outside Bowen Road Hospital: 48 hours after they had requested transportation, the patient was taken out of camp, but with the cold weather and the lack of drugs, "the poor chap had no chance. Except for the odd bottle of Mag. Sulp. [magnesium sulphate] which doesn't go far among 50 dysenteries, we have had no supplies for over a month in spite of our repeated demands."[90] One response by the Japanese was to remove this medical officer from his position, replacing him with Maj. (A) L.W. Ashton-Rose. The "principle" invoked was to become familiar: the duty of the medical officers and medical orderlies was to heal the sick; if the sick died, the medical personnel had failed in their duty and should be punished, or replaced, or both.

Other forms of treatment were used for dysentery, some of them undreamt of by the distinguished physicians who wrote textbooks on the subject. One Canadian with severe dysentery had been given tooth powder that proved to be useless for cleaning teeth. Driven by hunger, he ate the whole thing—and it cured his dysentery.[91] In camps along the Burma-Siam Railway, sulfa drugs were effective against bacillary dysentery but hard to get. Even the supply of magnesium sulphate ran out after some weeks, and castor oil and calomel (which contains mercury) were used.[92] Medical therapy was slipping back into methods used in the nineteenth century and even earlier. Treatment with magnesium sulphate was unpleasant and old-fashioned. It had been replaced by more modern agents that worked well—when they were available.

Early in 1942, Ray Squires had an experience with this antiquated and drastic therapy at North Point Camp, where the so-called hospital was overwhelmed. The ward was in a barn; manure was everywhere, flies swarmed. Squires had severe dysentery. There was no room in the ward and he lay out in the open the first night, nearly freezing to death. Hong Kong nights can be bitingly cold in January, especially to sick men. "About four in the morning I said, 'Can I come in and sit on the toilet?' They said, 'Yes. As soon as somebody goes you can have their hole.'" Later the doctor gave him 17 straight doses of magnesium sulphate. "On a torn up bowel that's very, very painful but it cured me, it did the job."[93] He was better in two weeks.

In those increasingly rare situations where sulfa drugs were available, most of the men who had bacillary dysentery did well. Dr. Crawford observed a remarkable feature of dysentery in the camps—the response of acutely ill patients to what he termed such "homeopathic" doses of sulfapyridine as half a gram every four hours for four doses; normal dosages would be several times this amount.[94]

The burden of disease affected all patients individually, but it also pressed heavily on the medical staff. There weren't enough medical officers or trained medical orderlies to care for these patients. Fortunately, volunteers took on the task of helping. Lewis Bush was one of these unsung heroes: "I paid my first visit to the dysentery ward to read to the patients as one of Philip Samuel's team. There were about fifty inmates, all of whom were in a serious condition. The stench was horrible."[95] Another POW, assigned to the hospital for dysentery ward fatigue, returned to his barracks after a stint on the wards. Asked by his Regimental Sergeant Major, "'What do you do?' I poke my [odorous] fingers under his nose."[96] The fundamental nature of orderly work in a dysentery ward was all too evident.

At Sham Shui Po in the middle of 1942, dysentery had become a major problem and, in combination with other illnesses, the strain began to tell. One night there were more than 150 dysentery patients in the hospital, over 40 admitted on one evening. The medical officers threatened a strike of some sort—"chucking in duty"—if they didn't get more help.[97] Given what we know about dealing with the Japanese, the threat must have been very muted indeed, and perhaps existed only in the minds of the officers. But the need cannot be questioned. Possibly the threat was intended to spur or shame more men to volunteer their aid.

At Bowen Road the SBMO, Maj. Donald Bowie, noted that on the night-duty hours for 23-24 September 1942, on the dysentery ward, patients' bowels moved 232 times. Two nursing orderlies were on duty.[98] The exertions required of these two men merit recognition and commendation, though awards seldom are given for expertise and perseverance in dealing with overflowing, stinking bedpans and desperately ill, excrement-coated patients. A similar calculation was made at St. Vincentius Hospital, a POW institution in Java. There, one orderly on night duty carried pairs of bedpans 243 times on one shift, walking an estimated 19,440 yards in nine hours.[99]

Will Allister was hospitalized at Bowen Road because he had dysentery. He recalled especially the so-called diet. "The cure was simple: starvation. No food, only tea, for four days. Then I was placed with the others on quarter-rations. The only catch was that the entire hospital was already on quarter-rations because of the uncertainty of the food supply, and we were allotted one-quarter of that quarter."[100]

The pandemic of dysentery, bad in 1942, was little better in 1944. A Royal Navy officer passed Ma Tau Chung Camp where the Indians were imprisoned. The Indian POWs that he saw were in a bad way.

"They all had dysentery and were sitting on the window sills of their huts crapping outside, being too weak to get to the toilets."[101]

Amoebic dysentery was much more a killer than was bacillary dysentery. Given the general shortage of emetine, the death rate predictably became much higher. In turn, emetine, as with so many other potentially life-saving measures, had to be rationed. It was the specific for amoebic dysentery, and it was necessary to preserve it for patients who seemed certain to die without it. More hardy patients had to be denied the drug, to cope with their infesting amoebae as best they could. "These discriminatory decisions had to be taken, just as in a battle, a shipwreck or a train disaster. Priorities had to be determined and the only criterion was a medical one."[102]

All POWs remember the infamous rod test, though not with affection. Some found it amusing, some humiliating and offensive, but all regarded it as bizarre, which it was, and useless, probably true also. The procedure is best described by one of the victims, in this case a Hong Kong POW at Formosa, en route to Japan:

A launch came alongside and up the accommodation ladder came half a dozen Japanese dressed in white coats, and two young women. I was called in to the saloon and Joe explained that each man would have a chopstick inserted up his rectum around the end of which would be wrapped a piece of cotton wool. Whilst this was taking place the man would hold in his hand a test tube into which the chopstick would be placed when the operation had been completed....We then organized the men in lines on each side of the deck. "On the word One," shouted White, "drop your trousers!" "On the word Two, touch your toes!" This all quite naturally encouraged a great deal of ribald laughter. None liked the idea of the young women being present but they seemed to be part of the team and made notes on cards as each man was attended to.[103]

Dr. Ben Wheeler recorded his opinion of this same undignified procedure, a unique and as far as he knew useless method of checking for dysentery carriers, because he had never heard of the Japanese culturing any organism, even from acute cases. Twice before leaving Singapore and twice in Formosa the POWs had to line up and, with hands on knees and trousers down, have an eight inch glass rod with a rather twisted knob forcibly inserted in the rectum, turned and withdrawn. The material on this rod supposedly was used to grow and identify disease-causing bacteria. "In one camp, where I had over one hundred undoubted cases of dysentery, we were forthwith pronounced dysentery free, and cases thereafter were called diarrhoea."[104]

This rectal probing was a routine Japanese practice, instances being recorded from all over the Pacific theatre of war. In at least one case, the procedure seemed to be part of a substantial research project. This was in the Philippines, from August until at least early October

1942. An American medical officer, Calvin Jackson, recorded two episodes: "Jap lab started working in dysentery area. They stuck small glass rods up rectum, then stroked rod across a Petri dish of plain agar....Japs were dressed in long white coats, gum boots, and face masks."[105] On 2 October 1942 he noted that the Japanese lab was still functioning. The technicians were again dressed in white coats, rubber boots, and face masks; they said they were on a research project.[106] No result was evident, or at least nothing was ever reported.

Malaria

> Sympathise with any wretch who tells you that he has malaria. A temperature of 105, a headache like the hammers of hell, cramps in the legs, and a tendency to vomit, terrific shakes, shivers, and sweats.[107]

Malaria seems to have been an inevitable risk in Hong Kong from the beginning of its colonial existence. During the initial British occupation of the Island in the 1840s a disease thought to have been malaria was described as being "severe and fatal."[108]

Malaria has afflicted human beings for thousands of years, though its parasitic cause was determined only a century ago. Long before that, a relationship was seen between marshy land and the disease; this was particularly true in central Italy, where the odours arising from swampy land were believed to cause disease. As a result, the disease came to be referred to in Italian as *mal aria*, or "bad air." The cause was not the stench but rather the parasite transmitted by the bite of the mosquitoes that bred in their millions in standing water. But this was not understood until relatively recently.

Three centuries earlier, however, a reasonably effective treatment had been found in South America: the cinchona tree has bark that, when ground to a powder and ingested, relieves the symptoms of malaria dramatically. It is not a cure, for the disease recurs, but it does allow victims to suffer less and to be ill for shorter periods. Almost 200 years ago, cinchona bark was found to contain several active substances, of which quinine was the most effective anti-malarial.

A century and a half ago, the cinchona tree began to die out in South America. Fortunately, seeds or seedlings were planted in India and in what is now Indonesia.[109] The latter became the main source of quinine and, because the Japanese conquered the Netherlands East Indies (Indonesia) during World War Two, quinine was available to Japan from that source. Some small portion of that may have reached POWs.

What does it feel like to have malaria? One victim compared it to dengue fever (referred to by the troops as "dingy"), which he had experienced while stationed in Jamaica. There are definite similarities in their symptoms. Thus when he became ill with chills and nausea in Hong Kong, he "thought it was dingy fever first off, and then I had the diarrhea with it too and then with the combination of the two, I can't really remember too much about it. I was pretty sick."[110]

A POW who had just escaped from Sham Shui Po, David Bosanquet, observed one of his fellow escapees in the throes of malaria: "We found Henry lying in a corner of a hut, wrapped up in a blanket, very ill. His whole body was shivering with malaria. He listened to Fong and through chattering teeth then told us that all necessary arrangements had been made for us to go."[111] So the successful escape into mainland China continued for the other men but not Henry, who was at least temporarily incapacitated.

Malaria is characterized by severe shaking chills, high fever, and extreme weakness. Those are only words; in reality, in a severe bout of malaria the victim shakes uncontrollably, perspires voluminously, has a raging fever, and often is capable of doing nothing but lying weakly in bed, hammock, or on the floor, while waiting out the attack—often hoping to die, though usually failing. The patient can be reasonably sure that he will be less ill the next day, though distressingly weak. He also becomes fatalistically sure that in two or three days (depending upon the variety of malaria that infests him) he will again experience the chills, fever, and weakness. And this cycle can go on for weeks or months in the absence of proper therapy.

Malaria is the result of infestation of human red blood cells by parasites. First observed in 1880, there are four species of Plasmodium parasites that can cause malaria: *Plasmodium falciparum* (the symptoms typically recurring every 24 hours), *Plasmodium vivax* and *Plasmodium ovale* (48 hours), and *Plasmodium malariae* (72-hour intervals).

For its transmission the parasite requires the active participation of the Anopheles mosquito. There are almost 400 species of these, but only 60 can transmit malaria. In all these species it is only the female mosquito that feeds on blood and that therefore can serve as the source of the disease.

When the parasites are injected into the bloodstream by a mosquito they travel to the liver. There they infect cells and reproduce until they burst the liver cells and invade the bloodstream. They enter red blood cells, reproducing again and feeding on the hemoglobin in the cells. The red cells burst and release asexual parasites into the bloodstream where they infect new red blood cells, the cycle repeating. Sexual forms develop in the red blood cells where they can be ingested into the body of the next Anopheles mosquito that bites the victim. It is the breakdown of the red blood cells by the immune system that produces a sudden flushing of red-cell and parasite proteins into the bloodstream. Reaction to these proteins causes the dramatic symptoms.

Mosquitoes in turn bite the now-malarial patient, thus ingesting large quantities of the parasite. The sexual parasites develop in the gut of the mosquito and are then ready to be injected into another victim in about 21 days, thus perpetuating the disease.

Controlling malaria in the long term means controlling the mosquitoes that carry the disease to humans. Mosquito control is a combined engineering and public health task. Before the war, Hong Kong officials had paid particular attention to the malarial menace within the cities of Kowloon and Victoria, and in many places on the Island in addition to Victoria. Unfortunately, the Japanese did not maintain these works after the colony became their responsibility.

An engineer's account of the work done to construct the heavy gun sites on the Stanley Peninsula, before World War Two began, noted that:

> The RAMC [Royal Army Medical Corps] interested themselves in the work at an early date and were extremely helpful. Since July, 1936, they have had a gang of coolies on the site carrying out anti-malarial work under a specially trained orderly. This squad themselves tackled all minor local troubles, and reported any new places that required the construction of permanent drains. The paddi and surrounding low-lying ground were dealt with by first constructing a system of French drains, and then filling over the whole with spoil from the various works. This area when turfed over will form the playing-fields for the new barracks.[112]

But these anti-malarial measures did not extend into the New Territories, where the war began. Malaria made substantial inroads upon the fighting strength of the Allied troops at Hong Kong during 1941. The Royal Scots were particularly seriously affected with this disease. During the malaria season just before the war, this battalion was heavily involved in work constructing defences along the so-called Gin-Drinkers Line, which was located in notoriously malarial country near the Chinese border.[113]

The Royal Scots had been in Hong Kong since 1938. By 1941 some men would have had recurring malaria. When they were assigned to defend the left sector of the defensive line north of Kowloon their medical fate was set. One historian says that only 180 members of the battalion had malaria severe enough to require treatment. That seems like a large proportion of a battalion of about 770 men. But this same writer claims the RAMC predicted that malarial casualties in that mosquito-ridden area might have been expected to reach 75 percent. He credits the smaller actual figure to "discipline and precaution."[114] Nevertheless, some companies were hard hit. "C" Company had only 35 men when they went into action on 10 December.[115]

Maj. Bowie, chief medical officer at Bowen Road Hospital, commented on this severe outbreak of malaria among the British troops.

He emphasized that many of those defending the mainland felt weak and shaky from the fever and anemias of their malaria. Nevertheless, they had to fight for their lives over hilly, tortuous country.[116] Many of the men were rushed out of hospital, or sick bay, or the malaria convalescent depot at Murray Barracks, and into distant company positions to fight the Japanese.

Nor was it only the British troops long stationed in Hong Kong who were affected. Malaria proffered an ugly welcome to the Canadians as well. For example, Lloyd Doull, RRC, was but one of many who had malaria at the time of capture at Hong Kong, only six weeks after arriving in the colony.[117] Numerous men fought despite their illness, but military efficiency suffered. Moreover, the Canadian medical officers were seeing tropical diseases for the first time. They were at least temporarily mystified at the exotic symptoms appearing among their patients. It would not have helped them to know that in Canada, a century earlier, their medical ancestors were well accustomed to coping with malaria, which ravaged most of the then settled parts of Ontario.[118] Nor, of course, were they alone in their ignorance. Most US medical officers arriving in the Southwest Pacific were also unfamiliar with the local diseases.[119]

Malaria flourished in Hong Kong between 1941 and 1945. Among the 1,500 Canadians imprisoned there, 41 percent had clinical malaria while they were prisoners.[120] Few had been exposed to the disease before so they were virgin soil. Nor were all possible measures taken to avoid the disease. One former prisoner has pointed out a surprising complication: in Sham Shui Po they were supplied with mosquito netting, "but we found out that [the nets] provided too convenient a shelter for bed bugs, and most of us preferred to run the risk of malaria rather than the certainty of being bitten by bed bugs."[121] Of 26 Canadian ex-POWs interviewed in 1987, 22 stated that they had suffered from malaria at Hong Kong. Only five of these men recall receiving quinine while they were ill as POWs.[122]

In April 1942, the OC Canadian troops, Col. J.L.R. Sutcliffe, died. A Winnipeg Grenadier lamented in his diary: "Heard this morning that Colonel Sutcliffe died last night at 7 o'clock of Malaria, dysentery and anemia. I think myself he died of a broken heart."[123]

When it struck in Hong Kong, malaria often dealt a heavy blow. Harry White testified in early 1943 that after being in hospital about a week with malaria he had lost 20 pounds.[124] A Canadian medical orderly noted in 1944 that a member of the Canadian Dental Corps had died that day of amoebic dysentery and malignant tertian malaria, "a tough combination."[125] Nor was much treatment available in these camps. Sometimes there was quinine, often not. As one ex-POW recalled, Maj. J.N.B. Crawford was sympathetic and would listen to the problem, but that was about all he could do: "I had malaria one time and I went and he said, 'Well, the only thing I can tell you is go and lie down. That's about all there is.'"[126]

Heroic treatments sometimes worked. A Dutch physician made up an injection to treat malaria. He obtained used battery acid to dissolve his quinine sulphate and gave injections of about 1 grain of quinine per case. He had a patient who had cerebral malaria—commonly a lethal form—who survived on this treatment.[127]

In December 1942, a British officer wrote of spending a week in bed with malaria. In his feverish stage he had temperatures up to 40.5°C.[128] Hundreds of other men, had they kept diaries, could have made similar entries. Another ex-POW recalled that malaria was the first disease that attacked him. "I got no medication whatsoever, and I know I was in a coma for about two days....The first thing I remember, everything tasted like rubber. The rice, whatever they fed us. I don't remember much about it. No quinine. Nothing at all. They had no quinine."[129]

Maj. Cecil "Cissy" Boon was a constant irritant to most of his fellow prisoners in his position as Japanese-designated senior POW officer. His general role was discussed in Chapter Three, but there is direct evidence of one event specifically harming his fellow-POWs suffering from malaria. An RAMC officer who had been sick in Bowen Road Hospital was sent to Sham Shui Po. He brought two pounds of quinine sulphate, needed urgently in Sham Shui Po where quinine was unobtainable and the incidence of malaria heavy. The officer mistakenly gave the quinine to one of Boon's NCOs.

> This creature was requested to give the quinine to Ashton-Rose but instead carried it to Boon who gave it to the Japs. The probable results were reprisals on the BMH [British Military Hospital] especially to the CO who had been forbidden to send drugs to Camps, and the closure of the same avenue for future drug supplies and the loss of two lbs. of life saving Quinine to dangerously ill patients. The only possible gain was in Boon's popularity with the Japs.[130]

Woodward heard of these events directly from Brown and Ashton-Rose, and they happened while he was in the camp.

In the cities of Kowloon and Victoria, malignant malaria, cholera, and other diseases broke out soon after the fighting ended on Christmas Day 1941. The high incidence of malaria was largely the fault of the Japanese, whose neglect ruined years of valuable anti-malarial work.[131] In the immediate aftermath of the fighting in 1941, services were disrupted. Anti-malarial squads stopped work and the scavenging labourers abandoned their rounds. Garbage accumulated in heaps, which in turn bred enormous numbers of flies and "the thousands of decaying bodies scattered on the hillsides were additional breeding grounds."[132] Mosquitoes bred in undrained pools, in the streets, and throughout the badly damaged and largely inoperable water reservoirs and distribution system. Flies and mosquitoes find barbed wire no impediment, and they swarmed through POW and civilian camps as freely as in the towns and villages. With them came dysentery, malaria, and dengue, among other diseases.

The anti-malarial work on the Island mentioned earlier was entirely of the drainage type; nothing was said about spraying or oiling ponds, etc. Nevertheless, the area of the Stanley Peninsula, where St. Stephen's College was located, and where Stanley Internment Camp eked out its existence for nearly four years, should have been a relatively malaria-free place. It was not.

The common occurrence of malaria produced problems for the prisoners as a group as well as for the unfortunate individual patients. The difficulty arose from needing to provide sufficient numbers of men for the work details. The Japanese demanded a fixed number of workers regardless of health conditions in the camps. And here the problem with epidemic malaria became acute. Sham Shui Po was at the end of the Kowloon sewer system. There was much malaria and much disease generally. A man who has a fever of 40/40.5°C should not be sent to work. Yet many patients with malaria and high temperatures had to work because the camp had to achieve its quota. Also, if a man didn't work the Japanese stopped his rations. The POWs would not permit the sick to go hungry; all rations were pooled and served in equal portions to sick and fit men alike. The consequence was that working men had scantier rations in order to feed the patients. And they still had to make the quota.[133]

For the men making "the water jump" to Japan, malaria continued to be a concern, though less so in that much less tropical country. Many POWs approved as "fit" for the trip were nevertheless malarial. Few drugs were supplied to the medical staff accompanying drafts. These had to be supplemented by private purchase via black market dealings, or with material supplied through Selwyn-Clarke's clandestine organization. Many men had attacks of malaria, and diarrhea and dysentery were usually epidemic by the end of the journey.[134]

In Japan, while there was less malaria than further south, and few new cases, relapses were not uncommon. In 1943, Capt. John Reid at Kawasaki received the results of tests done by the Japanese two months before. Seven diphtheria carriers were found, eight positive malaria smears, and 25 carriers of amoebic dysentery, plus seven who "harbored anal trichomonas."[135] A major problem in these camps in Japan was that the men had to do heavy work. The Japanese often forced sick men to go to mines or factories. A medical orderly at a camp in Yokohama testified that an Australian with a high fever was forced to go to work, and was later found to have malaria.[136] This occurred often.

In September 1945, a group of 325 ex-POWs was examined at Guam, on their way home from Japanese camps. There were 129 US

Other Ranks, 48 US officers, 135 Canadian Other Ranks, one Canadian officer, and 12 civilians. Of the diseases suffered during captivity, the top six were dysentery (184 cases – 56.4%), beriberi (136 cases – 42%), malaria (77 cases – 24%), non-specific avitaminosis (49 cases – 15%), diphtheria (40 cases – 12%, and all Canadians from Sham Shui Po), and pneumonia (37 cases – 11.4%).[137]

In the Hong Kong camps malaria affected over 40 percent of the men, whereas at a camp at Osaka, in Japan, the medical officers noted that only 15 percent of the men had malaria.[138] Allied medical officers discovered that malaria could display an impressive spectrum of symptoms. One group was in a camp in a malaria-free region in Japan on the island of Kyushu, from June 1944 through April 1945. The disease maximally caused one or two attacks with cold chills and then gradually disappeared, a clinical picture strongly at variance with the symptoms seen in tropical areas.[139]

Japan's less-tropical location may partly explain the difference. Limited immunity to malaria is possible after long exposure to the disease over several years, in the absence of treatment or protection. A degree of "acclimatization" may also be a factor here; after an initial period of high incidence of disease and high mortality, the survivors seemed to have less disease and much lowered mortality rates.[140] K.W. Todd, a medical officer captured at Singapore, Todd noted that many of the men showed minor or even grave symptoms of one or more potentially serious diseases. The medical officers lacked both the diet and the drugs to treat these patients adequately. Yet the threatened calamities did not occur. The diseases they experienced "became instead part of a picture of general ill-health; we became stabilized at a level of health not uncommon in the oriental villager or coolie whose life we were in effect living."[141]

Todd's arguments stem from observations of a variety of diseases that seem to have caused less severe sickness and fewer deaths than expected; he excepts the disastrous first six months on the Burma-Siam Railway when the rates were enormous. But that, in a sense, is his point: survivors adapt to the prevalent illnesses. These MOs came to regard benign tertian and sub-tertian malaria as diseases of health.

Of course, Allied servicemen and POWs were not the only ones to experience malaria. Admiral Ugaki Matome observed in his wartime diary how seriously Japanese servicemen suffered from the disease. For example, in December 1942 at Guadalcanal fewer than one-third of the troops were fit for combat: the rest were sick and wounded. Most of the sick had beriberi and malaria, and the losses from those diseases reached two to three times those by Allied bombing and bombardment. So serious was the manpower shortage that about 60 seriously ill patients were left in the jungle west of Mt. Austen. "As three hundred stretcher bearers are needed to remove them, they were left there lest fighting strength might be lost in so doing."[142]

By August 1945 anti-malarial work in Hong Kong was non-existent, and a new ward had to be opened in the Sham Shui Po Camp hospital to deal with combined malaria and dysentery cases that were pouring in.[143] Capt. Winston Cunningham, one of two dental officers in Canada's "C" Force, saw his dental orderly succumb to this double affliction. He had the combination himself, but fortunately only mildly.[144]

Why did this sudden and tragic upsurge in disease occur? Some post-war researchers believe that undernutrition in humans can decrease susceptibility to infection from some viruses and bacteria, and from malaria. Resuming normal feeding after starvation may diminish resistance to the same organisms and reactivate previously suppressed infection from them. These authors believe that this phenomenon is an important component of the ecological balance involving humans, their disease-causing predators, and their environment.[145]

Part of the historical background to this theory relates to prisoners—in this case, those inhabiting British civil prisons towards the middle of the nineteenth century. Food purchased by the prisons varied considerably. The investigators found an unfailing relationship between the amount of food consumed by prisoners and their sickness and death rates. "Those receiving the least food, 1 shilling and 10-pence farthing worth per week, had a morbidity rate of 3 percent per annum and a mortality rate of 0.16 percent. Those consuming the most food, 3 shillings and 2-pence worth per week, had a sickness rate of 23 percent and a mortality rate of 0.4 percent."[146]

In over a century since that study, extensive experiences of starvation and disease in concentration camps and ghettos has added little to our knowledge of how this phenomenon occurs. Certain diseases disappeared or affected inmates much less severely when nutrition was poor, the incidence usually reverting to "normal" when rations returned to more usual levels. The lack of rheumatic fever, glomerulonephritis (a kidney disease), and many common allergies such as hay fever and asthma in POW and concentration camps, and in ghettos, during World War Two are noted frequently in reviews of medical experiences during those years.

Directly related to the topic of resurgent malaria in POW camps are recent observations by two researchers that malaria in inhabitants in eastern Niger was suppressed by famine. However, the disease was reactivated within five days of vigorous refeeding with a diet of millet or sorghum.[147]

There is thus an apparent paradox of starvation. Increased resistance to viral infection and at least some bacterial infections exists despite an apparent decrease in immune function due to starvation. But increased susceptibility to infection occurs with refeeding when immune function might be expected to be returning to normal. There may still be much to be said for the adage, feed a cold and starve a fever.

Malaria was only one of several serious diseases that impacted heavily on the lives and contributed to the deaths of Allied POWs in Hong Kong, Japan, and elsewhere. When quinine was available, and when the strain of malaria was something other than the frequently lethal cerebral form, survival was the rule. But the rule could be broken when POWs suffered malaria in conjunction with other diseases and the combination proved overwhelming.

Dengue

A medical officer suffering through an attack of dengue fever in New Caledonia wrote a vivid and illuminating account. A severe throbbing headache began suddenly. Towards nightfall the headache localized over the forehead, became continuous, and was "in the nature of a boring ache, as though two screws on either side were being slowly rotated into the right and left frontal sinuses." He was perspiring heavily and felt very weak. Within a few hours he had excruciating pains in the bones of the arms and legs, worse than anything he had experienced previously. This lasted about four days. Then he was tormented by depression and suspicion of the capabilities of his medical attendants. After six weeks he was fully recovered and able to work.[148]

Dengue was common in Rabaul, New Britain generally, and Japan itself, according to captured Japanese documents.[149] But it occurred in Hong Kong as well, where several Canadians came to know its bite. Joe Ateah, 40 years after the event, recalled its symptoms as very like malaria: "You sweat and get a temperature pretty high, but you're not quite as sick. It's a lingering thing, I had it after I came home too. They treat you the same. They gave me quinine."[150]

There is no relationship between dengue and malaria except some similarity of symptoms. Unlike malaria, which is a parasitic disease, dengue is caused by a virus that is carried to its victims by mosquitoes, most commonly *Aëdes aegypti*. There is often a rash lasting a few days. In general, full recovery occurs.

Worms and Other Parasites

Parasites of all kinds abounded in the camps and, of course, in the surrounding population. On one occasion Bill Ashton passed 180 worms, according to an orderly's tally, "and that was just large ones and not counting the small ones."[151] Many of the men carried unwelcome guests home. In one group, 343 of 400 (83%) had parasites of various kinds.[152] In another large group of American ex-POWs, 70 percent of 4,618 had intestinal parasites.[153] And Geoffrey Gill, studying British ex-

POWs long after the war ended, found 88 instances of strongyloidiasis (a parasite) in 129 men.[154]

Dr. Coombes remembered one of the unusual side-effects of giving the men anesthetrics. "Lots of worms...it used to cause people to bring up a lot of worms from their stomach. I suppose the chloroform irritated and anesthetized them, and people used to vomit quite a packet of earthworms—looked like earth worms, Ascaris."[155] But no POW medical officer would waste chloroform to treat worms.

Venereal Disease (VD)

Perhaps no condition was so ubiquitous during World War Two as the venereal diseases, particularly gonorrhea and syphilis. The Winnipeg Grenadiers felt the sting long before they arrived at Hong Kong. In 1940 at Kingston, Jamaica, condoms were issued freely in an effort to curb the increasing toll from VD. In January 1941, the average daily strength of the regiment was 653 men; VD prophylactic cases numbered 233, and 25 cases of venereal disease were under treatment.[156]

At Hong Kong, the Japanese guards acquired the habit of bringing ampules of anti-venereal medicines to the POW medical officers, requesting that they—the guards—be treated. If a Japanese soldier got VD his whole group was penalized and their leave stopped, so reporting infection was not popular.

According to one American medical officer, the usual Japanese treatment for venereal diseases was "a good face-slapping and confinement in the guardhouse, if the disease was discovered."[157] This seems to have been the case. In the Imperial Japanese Army there were monthly "short-arm" inspections of the penis, and severe penalties faced any soldier found to be infected. Venereal disease was categorized as less serious than wounds and other diseases. Men found with the tell-tale penile pus usually had to endure loss of rank. This penalty could extend to the unit CO if he was seen to have failed to provide proper discipline or not to have stressed precautions. "There might be spells of confinement in the guardhouse or even beatings in the hospital for men with a long history of venereal disease. The island of Ch'ungming on the Yangtze was used for isolating serious cases, recalling the legend among Allied troops in Southeast Asia that there was an island where sufferers of the quickly fatal 'black pox' were sent to die."[158]

A 1942 Japanese document reported on hygiene in Hong Kong: venereal disease was spreading. Plans were underway to concentrate all comfort stations (official brothels) in one district of Hong Kong, Wan Chai, on Hong Kong Island. This area had been appropriated as a residential area for Japanese only.[159]

At Hong Kong, care was taken by the POWs that no actually beneficial therapy was ever given to their captors; one cynical medical officer believed that the "ethics of this are debatable only until you know the Japs."[160] This Japanese fear of revealing the presence of venereal disease was often taken advantage of by POWs, particularly medical officers, to blackmail the enemy into smuggling needed medicines into camps.

Venereal disease was not a common problem within POW camps. There was little opportunity to acquire fresh infections. Some chronic cases entered the camps, but gonorrhea tends to burn itself out even without treatment, and syphilis enters a phase of seeming cure when all symptoms and signs disappear for long periods. Thus even without treatment the diseases were not a source of major sickness.

Inevitably, when the war ended, thoughts of what they had been missing for 44 months rested heavy on the minds of some of the ex-POWs. At Sham Shui Po, where there was a lengthy delay between war's end and freedom to leave the camp, some could not wait. At least by the night of 26 August, women were being smuggled into camp.

Other Medical Problems

Skin Diseases

One POW recorded a picturesque if homely account of problems he had with his "bum" in August 1942. Most POWs could relate similar stories of affliction in various parts of their bodies. These were nuisance disorders, though not less painful and worrisome for that. This single example can serve to represent many. The notes cited were made between 9 and 19 August 1942: "Boiled water in pail & bathed my bum." "Went sick & missed PT. MO says he is very sorry for me but can't give treatment. Excuses me from marching!" Next day: "Bathed myself with hot water, my sores look cleaner but my crutch is very painful." Two days later: "My bum is like a close up of the moon, all craters and peaks." Finally, on 19 August 1942: "Officer and Staff Sgt look at my bum, taken off Eusol baths and have tarpaste instead, but my hip sores are still full of sores and pus."[161] And so on. What was the disease? Ultimately it disappeared.

Ray Squires wrote, in the middle of 1943, that he was then in charge of the Canadian skin ward. There, they seem to have treated their patients with four agents: bichloride of mercury (corrosive sublimate), calomel (mercurous chloride), potassium permanganate, and iodine.[162]

Typhoid Fever

This disease is usually caused by contamination of water or food by feces containing the typhoid germ. Billings wrote in August 1943 about what evidently was a small epidemic of the disease: "Another typhoid death—Sgt Woods, D.D.C., foreman of R.N. Dockyard. Four more cases in hospital; hope we are not in for another epidemic."[163] And 15 months later they were inoculated because of suspected typhoid.[164] Fortunately, this disease never became epidemic at Hong Kong.

Scarlet Fever

I have found a single reference to this disease, caused by streptococcal bacteria and then much commoner than it is now. The date was New Year's Eve 1944: "I forgot the Batmen got a case of scarlet fever on Christmas Eve, so one of their huts (not the cooks fortunately) was put in isolation."[165]

Tuberculosis

One of the ironies of POW medical conditions in the Far East is that tuberculosis was relatively frequent but was less documented in the surviving records than more dramatic and frightening diseases such as cholera or diphtheria. The long drawn-out illness associated with tuberculosis is one reason why it has rarely been seen as a major "epidemic" disease, even though tuberculosis may over a prolonged period kill far more people than smallpox, or dysentery, or malaria.

Another reason is that tuberculosis tends to affect its victims gradually, often over a long period of time. At Hong Kong, for example, one of the medical orderlies looked after tuberculosis patients, of which there were only a few relegated to one corner of a ward. He remembered clearly hearing the medical officer warn him that he stood an increased chance of developing the disease in the next 20 or 30 years.[166] This man did not, but many of his fellow POWs did.

The evidence shows that tuberculosis existed in all the camps, but that the incidence was low, or seemed to be low. One immediate post-war study examined 325 men; 20 had active tuberculosis and another 23 had findings suggestive of this disease (6.2% and 7% respectively).[167] Similar studies showed 101 tubercular patients among 3,742 ex-POWs (3.4%),[168] and 66 cases amongst 1,507 (4.3%).[169] In a camp on Formosa (Taiwan) just at the end of the war, there were 14 men with tuberculosis among 60 cited as being ill enough from any disease to be in hospital.[170]

At the camp designated as Fukuoka 17, in Japan, there was a total mortality of 122 over two years. Tuberculosis was the cause of six of these deaths. The first case of tuberculosis was seen in March 1944, eight months after the camp opened. A total of 11 cases were proved to be tuberculosis in the next year and a half, plus four suspects. The only treatment possible was rest in bed.[171]

Even this boon was sometimes denied. In Kamioka Camp one Allied soldier was forced to work until he died of his tuberculosis.[172] In Sendai Camp 3 it was equally difficult to be excused from work; one POW recalls comrades sick with tuberculosis and coughing up blood who were nevertheless sent to the shipyards.[173] And at a small camp near Yokohama, similar treatment of a tubercular patient caused a sit-down strike organized by the indomitable W/C Leonard Birchall, RCAF. In this instance, although Birchall was beaten up yet again, the sick men were permitted to stop working.[174]

The best records on tuberculosis among POWs in Japan were found in Shinagawa Hospital. Data exist because it was one of the few places International Committee of the Red Cross (ICRC) representatives were allowed to visit, and because of evidence given at the post-war trials of the senior member of the Japanese medical staff and of his medical sergeant.

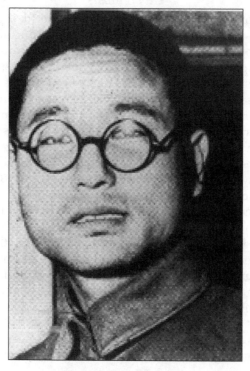

Figure 6.3. Photograph of Dr. Tokuda Hisakichi, commandant and senior Japanese medical officer at Shinagawa Hospital, Tokyo, 1943-1945. (*The Sphere* newspaper, 24 November 1945; photo supplied by Wellcome Institute Library, London, RAMC Box 143, File 237/9.)

In 1942, Shinagawa was an ordinary POW camp. That December, of 400 men there, 29 were seriously ill, several (number not noted) with tuberculosis.[175] The camp became a POW hospital in August 1943. By February 1945 there had been 53 deaths, mainly from tuberculosis, amoebic dysentery, pneumonia, and beriberi.[176]

Given the many thousands of Allied POWs in Japan by 1943, and the ongoing malnutrition, inadequate clothing, overwork, and brutality with which they struggled to cope, it is not surprising that tuberculosis occurred. But at Shinagawa, from March 1945 on, unfortunate patients with tuberculosis had another hazard to confront, one that cost some their lives. They suffered from medical experimentation carried out by Dr. Tokuda Hisakichi, who may well have been psychotic at the time. After the war, and especially during and after his trial, he became overtly psychotic and died in that condition.[177] But as commandant at Shinagawa he took overall responsibility for the care of these very ill men from the Allied medical officers. He then undertook completely unscientific experiments on the miserable patients.[178] Tokuda gave substances to them that had no known benefit in tuberculosis. One of the procedures he carried out, artificial pneumothorax, was itself standard therapy at the time, but he did so ineptly, risking the health of the patients.[179]

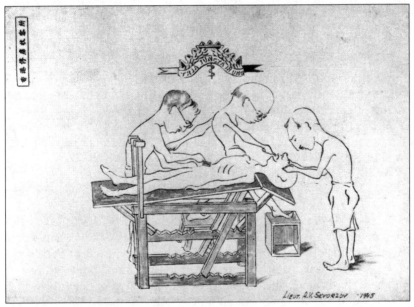

Figure 6.4. Surgeon, dentist, and anesthesiologist with a mock patient, using POW-made operating table, Sham Shui Po POW Camp, 1945. (From: A.V. Skvorzov, *Chinese Ink and Brush Sketches of Prisoner of War Camp Life in Hong Kong, 25 December 1941-30 August 1945.* A.V. Skvorzov, 1945.)

Tuberculosis apparently was common among the Japanese also. According to documents captured during the war, tuberculosis was prevalent in Japan; 5 percent of those in the army had "a touch of TB." For example, in June 1943, in the 238 Infantry Regiment, there were 340 cases of tuberculosis. If this figure is accurate it means that close to one-third of the men had the disease. Commenting on captured Japanese medical documents, an Intelligence officer wrote:

> There is a record of cases of TB being evacuated to Takao and then returned to the field again....It is difficult to understand the Japanese policy in regard to these cases. It must be obvious to them that the retention of TB sufferers must lead to their deterioration and also be a very big factor in causing a spread of the disease to troops who are weakened by the hardships of warfare.[180]

The civilian population of Japan also suffered with tuberculosis. The Welfare Ministry surveyed the country in 1943 and noted a marked increase in tuberculosis as well as various vitamin deficiency diseases.[181] This topic will be discussed in a later chapter.

Immunizations and Tests

The Japanese medical department was active in most camps in injecting or causing Allied medical officers to inject various immunizing agents. Many POW medical officers expressed concern about the potency and sterility of these materials, but they were given. This was particularly likely to occur immediately before a draft of POWs was shipped to Japan, but immunizations and various tests were carried out intermittently throughout the POW years. One man kept a record of those he received during 1942: 2 February: "Cholera & TAB[182] jabs"; 27 February: "Innoculation [sic] for cholera at 12"; 15 September: "Paraded for swabs at 1:30"; 18 September: "Battn Parade for swab & stool test at 4 pm."[183]

Injuries

Injuries of all kinds occurred. Most of these will be discussed in the chapter on camps in Japan because most serious injuries happened there, a result of the more severe work duties required of POWs. At Hong Kong, a particularly grim case of injury came about because of Japanese disciplinary measures. After a long period of being held in a cage about 6' x 6 'x 9' in Sham Shui Po, Walter Spencely, RRC, was left paralyzed. He had been a chronic troublemaker, at least in Japanese eyes; fortunately for him their eyes did not see everything, as Spencely may have killed a guard. After his release from the cage he developed both dysentery and diphtheria and was expected to die. However, he had enormous willpower. "Somewhere he found a pair of roller skates and attached them to a board. He would push himself around camp laying on his stomach. After a while he could sit up on the board and then he started to walk. No other man could have pulled through. Spencely made it back to Canada and became a clown in Toronto."[184]

Surgery

Ideally, major surgery for POWs at Hong Kong would have been done at Bowen Road Military Hospital. That sometimes occurred, but due to Japanese refusal or procrastination in arranging transport, much surgery was done in Sham Shui Po and some in Argyle Street Camp and the nearby Ma Tau Chung Camp.

Luigi Ribiero had his appendix removed at Sham Shui Po and left an account of the experience. His MO was Capt. Albert Rodrigues. Because Ribiero's appendicitis was chronic, not acute, Rodrigues consulted with Maj. Ashton-Rose. With so few drugs available, the medical team urged removal of the appendix to avoid any possibility of later flare-ups and fatal abdominal infection. Ribiero agreed and the operation was done without any problem. Afterwards, though, he experienced wound infection and an abscess. Then his bowel obstructed, and he developed both benign and malignant malaria simultaneously—a major complication to convalescence.[185] Nevertheless, he survived all these complications. Poor healing commonly follows poor nutrition.

In May 1943, medical orderly Sgt. Ray Squires noted that there had been five appendectomies in his ward recently.[186] And as late as 29 October 1943 he was coping with Les Canivet's shoulder wound, dating back to December 1941, "which is sprouting loose bone."[187] Wounds often did badly because of poor nutrition and inadequate medical supplies. In June 1942, an NCO's open wound was "running with yellow matter, afraid to operate for hidden shrapnel, too near the backbone."[188]

Anesthesia was available much of the time in the Hong Kong camps. Capt. Winston Cunningham, Canadian Dental Corps, had supplies of a powdered anesthetic substance—Novocaine hydrochloride—that he had retained in his kit when captured. By careful rationing, this lasted until 1945.[189] The hypodermic needles were another matter, becoming painfully dull despite efforts to sharpen them. Bowen Road Hospital was also able to make its pre-war stocks last, though it was a close thing at the end.

Chloroform was available, as part of the army field medical kit. "I gave a lot of anesthetics and I was very impressed with chloroform, partly because you had all the time in the world to give it. You just did it gently, drop by drop, took your time about the whole thing until they were well under and never overdosed or anything like that."[190] There were no complications, though some liver damage might have occurred, eventually. Chloroform worked, but no one would use it today except in an emergency, it having been replaced by far safer and more effective anesthetic agents.

Dentistry was performed in Sham Shui Po. Capts. Winston Cunningham and James Spence were the Canadian dentists; "Willie"

Wallis was the British dental officer. Unlike the Canadians, he had no anesthetic. "Don't come and see me unless you can't stand the pain any longer. Then I will take it out without any anesthetic." He would seat the unfortunate sufferer and then tilt the chair-back against a wall. Then he would just make a "quick grab." He became quite ill in camp, and would lie on a mat and extract teeth by making his patient lie down beside him. "He used to still go on pulling teeth, lying on the floor!"[191]

Psychology, Psychiatry, and Suicide

Only a few men experienced mental disorder severe enough to incapacitate them. With some, the problem might have arisen regardless of the war or captivity; for others, the strain of their peculiar and threatening existence proved too heavy. Most often the difficulty was temporary. Some went into a sort of shell and wouldn't talk, while others talked compulsively. A particularly well-known individual in one camp walked around asking himself questions and singing: "he was the most well-fed man in camp because the Japanese had a certain respect for mentally disturbed people."[192] Another Hong Kong POW had similar recollections, particularly of a man who had let his beard grow long and was "quite obviously mental"; the Japanese seemed to let him get away with much because they either respected or feared him.[193]

That the Japanese were frightened of people with mental problems, or were repelled by them, could be used to the POWs' advantage. "One guy really was very strange—'nutty'—and if we wanted to be sure of getting something into camp we'd give it to him because the Japanese wouldn't go near him."[194]

There were remarkably few instances of suicide among western POWs generally, and this held true at Hong Kong. Hope supplied the prisoners with remarkable resilience. Indeed, even in the profoundly more brutal and certain blackness of Nazi concentration camps, suicide was less common than outsiders might have anticipated. Primo Levi, who survived Auschwitz, credited this to the "last senseless crazy residue of unavoidable hope."[195]

A Canadian at Hong Kong could remember hearing of only four successful attempts at suicide among the several thousand POWs there. One man crawled up the sewer to touch the electric wires that covered the opening. One POW slit his wrists, one jumped off the top of the latrine head-first onto the concrete, and one deliberately climbed onto the electric wire around the camp.[196] T.J. Dewar knew some of the details about the unfortunate man who leapt from the latrine rafters. Some men were cleaning the washroom in Sham Shui Po "and this fellow got a letter from home which contained bad news and he just climbed up in the rafters and crashed down head-first."[197] He fractured his skull and died during the night.[198]

In August 1943, in Sham Shui Po, an RAMC sergeant "went mad"—whatever that may have meant at the time. "He's quite mad, but harmless."[199] Another man decided to go home one night. He took his bag and walked as far as the gate. The Japanese guards started shooting at him and he turned back. He then said he was going to wash his clothes, but instead of taking the clothes out of the top of the bag, he cut the bottom out of the bag and started to pull them out. In August 1944, a Canadian cut his throat but, according to one diarist, "made a poor job and has recovered."[200] And just four months before the war ended: "Carl Henson, U.S. merchant seaman, had a coma yesterday. Just now, during an air raid, he turned in and slashed his wrists. When they shook him to eat his food they couldn't rouse him and, upon investigation, when they pulled back the blankets, the bed was soaked in blood. (Funny how blokes reached the end of the line.)"[201]

A lot of the men just gave up.[202] This was not an uncommon occurrence in camps throughout the Far East: "I remember a chap who was sick and they were taking him to Bowen Road. When he was leaving he came and shook my hand and said, 'It was nice to know you.' He was dead in 48 hours—but he wasn't that sick, he just turned the switch off."[203] Raymond Sellers saw this phenomenon also. He observed both the giving up and the more common signs of mental distress:

> I never saw anyone directly commit suicide. I saw several who "turned off the switch." In particular, one man called Lavery [Pte. Cecil F. Lavarie, WG, d. 13 February 1944], a friend of mine who, within ten days, said 'I've had enough of this' and he just up and died. It seemed he wished himself to die. His health was no worse than anyone else, but he just said "I don't want to live any more," and he died....It seemed to be after about the three-year mark we noticed people doing stupid things like nurse their pillows and do things that ordinarily they wouldn't do. They would start talking about food. They would talk to themselves. Maybe we all did. Maybe I did.[204]

Randy Steele worked as an orderly in the "agony ward." Some of the worst cases were there; blind men, men who had lost their memory. He used to feed them with watery soup, or try to get them to eat, and to help them the best way he could. The patients sometimes seemed to be like babies. "If you gave them a kind word, they would cry and give up and in a few days they would die. If you told them they were not trying, they would get mad and really put up a fight and in a few weeks they would be up and around. This seems funny, but it's true."[205]

Luigi Ribiero remembered one man whom he termed an apparent schizophrenic. This man haunted a derelict hut where Ribiero once saw him dancing and chatting with what seemed to be a phantom woman. On occasion he also simulated the motions of a fighter plane attacking, his arms representing the wings while he made sounds imitating machine-gun fire.[206]

Men outside the camps also succumbed to overwhelming stress. Two professors in the Hong Kong University medical department were allowed to stay outside the internment camp at Stanley because the Japanese needed their medical expertise. One, Gordon King, escaped in 1942. The other, R.C. Robertson, remained at work at the Bacteriological Institute under Japanese supervision. His work in the laboratory benefitted the Japanese. This forced collaboration was a source of anguish. Despite the fact that members of the Chinese community were aided also by his work, "he became depressed....Eventually on 4 August 1942 his body was found lying on the ground outside the Institute; he had apparently fallen from a verandah, and had apparently committed suicide. Such were the stresses to which sensitive minds were subjected during the occupation in trying to decide where their duty lay."[207]

Agnes Keith, an internee, summed up the problem of mental strain succinctly: "In the end I learned that it isn't the outward circumstances which determine what one can endure, but something in oneself which either breaks, or stays intact, under strain. It isn't the difference in strain, it's the difference in tensile strength of people."[208]

The medical teams had little to offer. What was most needed was normality, and that vacuum they were powerless to fill. Most of the men made do with comradeship; combines of three or four men formed strong bonds of mutual support, dividing the good and the bad and stretching out better hope for survival than could be anticipated for most of the "lone wolves."

After the war, Dr. Selwyn-Clarke commented on the local mental hospital: "Forty Japanese military patients were handed over to the Military Authorities for repatriation to Japan, one having died out of the original number transferred to the Mental Hospital from dark and overcrowded cells in Kowloon at the time of the liberation."[209] The fact that they kept their own mental patients locked in jail gives some insight into how the Japanese viewed mental disease. Not surprisingly, they were not sympathetic to similar disorders amongst the POWs.

Orderlies

I do not ask the wounded person how he feels,
I myself become the wounded person.[210]

The work of medical orderlies, both regularly trained men and volunteers, warrants particular attention. Some of the trained RAMC medical orderlies were looked down on, serious questions being raised about the honesty of at least a few. "Nursing in a prison camp is apt to be of varying standards," Bertram noted, "and the traditional British Army rendering of the initials RAMC [Rob All My Comrades] was not altogether unjustified in Shumshuipo."[211] And another prisoner noted, on visiting a friend in hospital, that his friend complained "of RAMC relieving him of $27, 16 Pkts of fags, 2 bars of soap, ½ lb tea & pair of cuff links. The dirty robbing Bastards." Revising his diary in 1966, he added that the RAMC were referred to as Rob All My Comrades, or Can't Manage A Rifle (backwards).[212]

Another POW, an Australian captured at Singapore, found—unsurprisingly—that there were good orderlies and some not so good: "The orderlies of this Field Ambulance Unit look almost incorruptible, the General Hospital orderlies we had up north were not properly trained medical staff and, to say the least, were 95% robbers and thieves, their main profession being the robbing of dead men's kits and the second profession robbing the patients of their food."[213]

There must have been some fire to generate such acrid smoke. Capt J.J. Woodward, an MO in the IMS, testified to his observations of such behaviour: "One had become accustomed to the cases of medical orderlies looting a dying man's kit before his eyes or indeed removing the valuables from any patient too ill to resist."[214]

Yet some POWs were able to rationalize even this kind of shadowy activity, at least in remote and rigorous camps such as that on Haruku in the Javanese islands near Ceram:

> As soon as I was well enough I went to ask the medical orderlies what had happened to Bert's possessions. He had often shown me a gold pocket watch that had been presented to his father on retirement. He had prized it so much that he had refused to part with it even though its sale would have brought him some of the food he so desperately wanted. I felt that some effort should be made to get it back to his widow. But the watch, along with the rest of his pathetic possessions, had vanished. The orderlies had a dreadful job caring for dying dysentery patients, many of whom had lost control of their bodily functions. And whereas a man on the outside working party always had at least the hope that he might find or steal something more or less edible, the orderlies, confined within the camp, had no such opportunities. So if some came to regard the dead's possessions as perks of the job it would be hard to judge them too harshly. There were always Nips ready to buy watches or rings. And with cash in hand you were ready to buy smuggled food when the opportunity presented itself.[215]

One ex-RAMC medical officer thinks that the Rob-All-My-Comrades talk stemmed from World War One, and that there may have been more truth to it then. But WWI medical orderlies were dealing with casualties in the field that needed to be carried to a casualty clearing station or a regimental first-aid post. "I expect some of the types in the army in those days used to pinch a ring, or a wristwatch, or even a wallet. And it was translated into 'Rob All My Comrades.'

But it was First World War stuff. It was different in the Second World War." The orderlies were much better trained and had a much improved reputation.[216]

Alsey made numerous digs at the medical orderlies. The antagonism is evident: "The skin ward is crammed with patients as the RAMC orderlies dodge treatment."[217] And another time: "No more War Paint available in M.I. Room, and how that orderly loved to tell me so!"[218]

Yet negative comments and innuendoes, while they must be acknowledged, should not be allowed to blot out the honourable, often selfless, and occasionally heroic behaviour of the vast majority of the medical orderlies. Their devotion to service was legendary and genuinely appreciated.

At Hong Kong a group of Canadian volunteer orderlies were widely praised by their former patients as well as by medical officers. The Japanese even permitted the transfer into Bowen Road of a group of volunteer POW medical orderlies to supplement an overworked staff of trained orderlies. Ken Cambon, who became a physician after the war, observed: "In August, 1942, when Bowen Road Hospital asked for men to work as orderlies, I was one of the half dozen chosen...probably saving my life."[219] He believed this because later, in 1943, in a camp requiring brutally hard labour, he was able to continue his less strenuous work as a medical orderly.

One memorable British medical orderly was Hyacinth D'Arcy, an Irishman. Before the war, whenever he left the barracks on leave he was followed by military police because, customarily, he started a fight with any American personnel who were visiting the port. But in the POW camps he was a different man. "I've seen him with a dying chap, bending down by him pretending to be his old mother, and comforting him, that sort of thing. Anything looking less like his own mother was old D'Arcy! But the chap was half demented and everything else, and there was old D'Arcy patting him on the head and saying, 'It's all right my dear.' He really was a first-class orderly."[220] Peace to the D'Arcys, of whatever name, who graced camps around the globe.

International Committee of the Red Cross (ICRC)

In general, Far East ex-POWs find little cause to applaud the help they received from the Red Cross. Generally, they realize that the Japanese were the stumbling block, not the Red Cross, but nevertheless they felt abandoned, a sensation much intensified after they came home from captivity to hear about the food parcels that reached western POWs in Europe weekly throughout most of the war.

The few parcels that were received in the Far East were precious. One ex-POW remembers receiving less than one parcel a year, but each parcel, when it arrived, "was a heaven-sent miracle, a radiant dream image that sat before us, shimmering, new, unbelievable, threatening at any moment to vanish as we gazed."[221]

When Hong Kong fell, the ICRC appointed as their Hong Kong representative Mr. Rudolf Zindel,[222] a Swiss businessman resident there. However, his appointment received Japanese assent only in June 1942.[223] Dr. Selwyn-Clarke was eventually able to pass most of his multitudinous welfare duties on to Zindel. "Although I was glad to do so, I gained the impression that he had heard rather too much about Japanese severity to act with the necessary boldness on behalf of the prisoners and internees. And from what I was told after the end of the war my foreboding had been justified."[224] Selwyn-Clarke, it is fair to say, set a very high standard for boldness.

Once the Japanese recognized Zindel he visited Bowen Road Hospital for the first time that same month.[225] Red Cross parcels finally arrived there in late November 1942, one food parcel for each patient and staff member. There were 392 parcels, all but about 10 intact; each weighed 12 lbs (5.5 kg). Bowie commented, "The value of the contributions made by the Red Cross Society to the well-being of patients and staff can hardly be overestimated."[226] Further parcels were received at Bowen Road in May 1943, and on 1 and 4 September 1944, a total of four-and-a-half parcels per man. In addition, beginning in January 1943, the Hong Kong Red Cross sent in bulk stores of foods such as tinned meat and vegetables, sardines, condensed milk, shark liver oil, marmalade and jam, sugar, tea, and cocoa. Between that time and the end of the war, a total of 18 shipments was received at Bowen Road, of varying size and contents.[227] In parcels received, and in visits from an ICRC representative, Bowen Road Hospital was treated more generously than were regular POW camps.

Dr. Uttley reported on a visit to Bowen Road on 19 August 1942:

> Yesterday, after nearly six weeks of his appointment as International Red Cross Representative, Mr. Zindal [sic] came to have a look at the hospital. He looked for about ten seconds and then pushed off. Mr. Egle [sic], his colleague, has already published in the papers, among other things, that the hospital was well run and well equipped. I don't know how he could say this as he had not been near us. However, the Japanese have only appointed as Red Cross Representatives such men as they can intimidate into saying what they wish to say.[228]

This could be correct but certainly was unkind towards men doing difficult and largely thankless jobs.

Mr. Zindel apparently was unable to enter Sham Shui Po until 21 December 1942. Then he could spend only about 20 minutes in the camp, obviously being hustled along by the Japanese. He did manage to speak briefly to one or two POWs, though no one was allowed to speak to him officially.[229]

The difficulty of getting individual parcels to POWs in the Far East cannot be overstated. There was Japanese reluctance at high levels, and there was the problem of ensuring that shipped parcels actually arrived. Before April 1945, five ships carrying more than 225,000 parcels designated for POWs and internees were dispatched to the Far East, and are known to have reached their destination. The unfortunate sinking of the *Awa Maru* on 1 April 1945 (described below), by an American submarine, was the reason given by Japanese spokesmen for forbidding additional consignments. "Thus, no relief supplies reached Japan or the occupied territories after those which had been brought by the *Hakusan Maru* in November 1944."[230]

Table 6.2
Sources of Funds to Purchase Supplies for POWs (in Swiss francs)

Use	Govt & RC Soc's	Local funds	Total
Drugs, instruments	953,032	38,568	991,600
Soap, disinfectants	289,894	6,859	296,753
Food	8,784,470	547,737	9,332,207
Clothing, footwear	601,196	89,197	690,393
Toilet articles	134,809	2,440	137,249
Books, games, music	44,060	28,354	72,414
Beds, blankets, towels	126,899	37,359	164,259
Utensils, brooms, toilet p.	104,476	5,024	109,500
Office supplies, stationery	37,213	74	37,287
Allowances (civilians)	831,644	-	831,644
Pocket money	1,518,161	50,080	1,568,241
Relief packages	371,161	-	371,161
Tobacco, cigarettes	486,265	177,307	663,573
Officers' mess (Shanghai)	18,281	-	18,281
Rent, telephone, etc. etc.	899,099	44,891	943,991
Misc.	913,338	155,512	1,068,851

Source: *Report of the International Committee*, Vol. 1, 461.

Two hundred and twenty-five thousand parcels sounds like a lot, but there were nearly that many western POWs and internees. So the total might mean only one parcel per person, if distributed evenly. Evidence from a series of war-crimes trials after the war indicates that many parcels were stockpiled until August 1945, against some contemplated future need, and that others were pillaged by the Japanese.

Because so few individual parcels got through, local purchase became vital. Table 6.2 shows money spent on various items for prisoners of war throughout the Far East. Considerably more than half these funds were used to provide food for the prisoners. Most of the money came from governments or from Red Cross societies.[231]

The ICRC representative reported to his headquarters in Geneva that the POWs at Hong Kong were housed in two camps and in the Bowen Road Military Hospital. This implies that he visited Sham Shui Po and Argyle Street camps and, by inference, that he did not go, or was not permitted to go, to the Indian camp at Ma Tau Chung. His first visit took place after the closing of North Point Camp.

Any visit to the camps by the delegate was contingent on the approval of the authorities in Tokyo, a sanction that was invariably slow in coming. Regular visits to camps by ICRC representatives apparently were permitted only in Japan, Korea, Formosa, and Manchuria, and even in those countries only 42 of 102 known camps were ever visited.[232] When visits did occur they were rendered still more difficult by the measures the Japanese military took to prevent the POWs from talking to the delegate and thereby betraying their true situation.

> The delegate was always accompanied by at least six Japanese, and the PW, especially the officers, had to resort to ingenious, but risky devices for conveying information to him. Once, for instance, during a visit, a French PW who had been a member of the Hong-Kong volunteer defence forces, shook hands with the delegate, and at the same time slipped to him a small piece of bamboo containing a minute piece of paper on which was written valuable information regarding the prisoners' needs, especially in medical stores. Another time, a PW who openly told the delegate that he and his compatriots were starved, was severely beaten.[233]

We have considerable information about the first visit to Sham Shui Po, since Zindel was accompanied by Mr. C.A. Kengelbacher, an ICRC official from Japan. The detailed report of the latter is informative, displaying for the reader the insight these selfless men were acquiring into the complexities of working with the Japanese:

> Early on Monday morning, December 21st [1942], we ferried over to Kowloon from where an Army car, escorted by Lt. Tanaka, brought us to the headquarters of Camp Commander Colonel Count Tokunaga, located just opposite the Argyle Street Camp. Count Tokunaga speaks only Japanese, which suited me perfectly. Consequently, the reception as well as the ensuing conversation lacked the stiffness so common on such occasions. Cocoa and cakes were served, and in an easy flowing atmosphere we went through our agenda, as prepared by Mr. Zindel for questioning. Count Tokunaga, however, soon turned out to be extremely touchy at times, requiring all my skill and knowledge of Japanese men-

tality to avoid his irritation reaching the danger point. He principally disliked our repeated mentioning of the Geneva Convention, and right there I began to realize how helpless the Red Cross organization really is when dealing with the Japanese Military authorities; even the slightest hint at desired improvement or criticism of the mildest form was turned down.[234]

Lt. Harry White noted Japanese preparations for Zindel's visit in May 1943. They arranged the POWs on parade so that the sick and the most badly emaciated men were in the rear, out of sight. The Japanese would not allow Zindel to get closer to the prisoners than about 30 feet. He did approach one group as he walked past, but Col. Tokunaga called him back. He was not allowed to visit the hospital or enter the huts.[235]

Though understandably dissatisfied with the amount of aid they received, in the end the prisoners seemed to recognize Zindel's efforts and those of the Red Cross generally, despite Japanese obstruction. On 18 August 1945, Zindel "got quite a cheer from the boys when he came into camp today."[236]

The risks to the Swiss volunteers attempting to mediate between often arrogant Japanese administrators and hungry, confused, frightened POWs were real. For example, the ICRC delegates appointed in Borneo, Dr. Mattheus Fischer and his wife, were never recognized officially. They were arrested in May 1943 and charged, sentenced, and executed in December of that year. "One of the charges against them was that they had 'criminally' sought to learn not only the number of prisoners of war and internees in Borneo but also their name, age, race and condition of health, and had tried to send them food."[237] If these activities were judged criminal, then all Far East ICRC representatives were felons in Japanese eyes.

Indirectly, the struggles with the Japanese had other costs. Among a list of ICRC members who died during World War Two is listed Dr. S. Paravicini, "Chief of the delegation in Japan, worn out by the difficulties of his position and duties."[238]

Nor was the visiting of camps by ICRC representatives always productive for the prisoners they were attempting to aid. Page has pointed out one major problem connected with being in a "favoured" camp that had regular visits. He was then at the POW hospital in Kobe. Unfortunately, because this hospital was known to and sometimes visited by Red Cross delegates, and was thus apparently designed as a propaganda affair or "shop window," the Japanese authorities kept the mortality down by seldom admitting seriously ill prisoners, or at any rate, those who would probably die. As a result, many deaths continued to occur in the nearby but unvisited camps.[239]

In an obvious understatement, an ICRC historian noted that "up to the capitulation of Japan in August 1945, the activities of the ICRC met with the most serious difficulties in all areas under Japanese domination."[240] The governmental agency with which they tried to deal was the POW Information Bureau (*Furyojo-hokyoku*). Relations with this Bureau were so difficult that it was only after the end of the war that the ICRC delegation was able to discover exactly how the Bureau was organized.[241] In the Japanese Home Islands, ICRC delegates found 34,000 Allied prisoners of war after the surrender of the Japanese forces, but only 27,000 names had been provided by the Japanese to be forwarded to Geneva.[242]

The ICRC delegation in Japan had its headquarters in Yokohama from 1942 until 1944. They then moved to Karuizawa, a small hill town not far from Tokyo, at that time under constant bombardment by the Allies. "From the outset, the delegation of the ICRC met with many difficulties in the execution of its task. In spite of these, however, it successfully acted in behalf of the American, Australian, British, Canadian, and Dutch PW, of whose presence in Japan, Korea, Manchuria and Formosa notification had been received." The delegation was able to visit 63 camps, 42 for prisoners of war and 21 for civilian internees. They tried to assist the prisoners and internees in corresponding with home. They also attempted to give them food and clothing bought on the spot, to supplement the supplies from the exchange ships. "These attempts however met with the opposition of the Japanese military authorities, who refused to sanction any purchases other than medical supplies."[243]

The Japanese were reluctant to permit relief packages to be sent to their prisoners. But the USA had relocated thousands of Japanese citizens and American citizens of Japanese descent into camps distant from the supposedly sensitive west coast, and the Japanese wished to send aid to these individuals. After lengthy, painstaking negotiations, an agreement was at last reached whereby food and medicine would be shipped on Russian ships from Portland, Oregon, to the USSR. But it had taken until the end of 1943 for this stage to be reached.[244]

The negotiations had been much prolonged because the USSR was reluctant to be involved. The Japanese had, however, made maximum use of the opportunity by insisting on their right to include war materials of various kinds in the cargoes of the Japanese ships that were to pick up the relief supplies. This was highly unusual, but the Allies were so concerned with the imperative need to get aid to their nationals in Japanese hands that they agreed.

The first Japanese ship to pick up aid for POWs and internees was the *Hakusan Maru*, which left Nakhodka, USSR, early in November 1944.[245] She was followed by the *Hoshi Maru*, which delivered supplies of relief food and medicines early in January 1945. A third vessel, the *Awa Maru*, also delivered supplies to Hong Kong and Singapore in March 1945.

But in one of the tragedies of World War Two, the *Awa Maru* was sunk by US submarine *Queenfish* on 1 April 1945, despite being under international protection because of her special status. That event has been chronicled in great detail,[246] but the main problem for Allied POWs in the Far East was that the sinking ended all possibility of further aid reaching them in this manner.

International law lays down that a country not ratifying one Convention is still liable to the full obligations of any previous Convention or treaty of the same class. Japan ratified the 1907 Hague Convention, to which it was thus bound to adhere. Had it done so, many difficulties would have been circumvented and deaths prevented.

Medical Experimentation

For the Hong Kong POWs there was blessedly little of what might be called medical experimentation. Those who went to Japan were, in a few instances, confined to Shinagawa Hospital near Tokyo; there some "experimentation" was done. Of the truly horrendous projects such as the bacteriological warfare experiments conducted by the Japanese army in Manchuria[247] (Unit 731 and others) there seem to have been no instances in Hong Kong, Singapore, Malaya, Java, or the Philippines.

Indeed, the only instances of this sort at Hong Kong seem almost laughable in comparison with what was going on in Manchuria and in Nazi concentration camps. Hong Kong's "medical experimentation" seems to have been limited to the "Happy Valley Garden Project," conducted at Happy Valley race track in spring 1945, and to one other short-lived and inconclusive investigation.

The Happy Valley project was supervised and, presumably, devised, by the Japanese medical officer, Capt. Saito. It was his "inhuman" plan to run a physical endurance study on the 100 Canadians assigned to his project.[248] Sgt. Brady, the NCO in charge of the men, regarded the experience as a real test of the human body's breaking point. They laboured for "thirty horrible days and nights," with no excuse permitted for absence from the worksite. It was a painful sight to witness 100 Canadians, already weakened by more than three years of malnutrition, "electric" feet, malaria, and dysentery, wielding hoes and shovels to dig up the oval race track still so familiar to visitors to Hong Kong. Why the Canadians were selected for this so-called study is a mystery. Any conclusions reached by Dr. Saito are unknown.

A more obvious "research" project was carried out by this same officer. Saito occasionally came round the wards with a stethoscope (handy for beating patients and staff); he was "obviously guilty of criminal neglect in his own job, but he had a keen interest in medical research." One day a strange order came from the camp office. One man from each national group represented among the prisoners was to report for specific duty. More than 20 men were picked, one Englishman, one Frenchman, one Canadian, one Dane, one Dutchman, and so on. They were taken to a Japanese military hospital, kept waiting interminably in corridors, and finally were put through a series of elementary physical tests. "'Ach, they measured our toes!' grunted a Norwegian gunner. 'So many millimeters' difference in the spaces....And they measured our ears and our fingers.'...So much for Dr. Saito's research."[249]

Bush has written about the same project. In May 1943, a truckload of POWs of several nationalities was taken from Sham Shui Po to the Japanese POW HQ at Argyle and Forfar streets. A Japanese beckoned one of the POWs to come forward, and suddenly nicked his earlobe with a sharp knife. The blood from the wound he put in a test tube. "We were then weighed and measured all over, our teeth were inspected, and all the time one of the Japanese would be making notes on filing cards. We soon got used to it and in fact it was good fun, especially as we were given cigarettes, and, when it was over, a large plate of curry and rice."[250]

These so-called experiments, which don't really qualify as such, were overshadowed by events that were to come in Japan.

Death and Burial

> Our hearts, though stout and brave,
> Still, like muffled drums, are beating
> Funeral marches to the grave.[251]

Longfellow's stately, sonorous lines conjure up a picture of dignified interment. In contrast, the grim reality in Far East POW camps was never stately, but frequently squalid, often disgusting, and invariably degrading.

Death became a commonplace event to the prisoners. Burials were routine duty, though no less difficult both psychologically and physically, as the POWs steadily and inexorably weakened. One of the early deaths from disease among the British at Sham Shui Po occurred on 13 February 1942. Cpl. Jack Smart died in hospital after a 10-day illness with dysentery. Six men, including Carden, the diarist who recorded the event, were detailed as grave-digging party and left the camp for the first time since their capture. A piece of waste ground about a mile from the camp, quite near the Argyle Street Camp, had been set aside as a cemetery. "It was a queer experience to be digging a grave on a windy hillside under the eyes of two Japs with fixed bayonets. They were good lads, however and gave us a fag each. One could speak a little English and told us about his family in Japan, whom he had not seen or heard from for five years (Jap soldiers are not allowed to write or receive letters)."[252]

In August, one man who died in Sham Shui Po, a man from the Royal Signals, purportedly weighed only 50 pounds (23 kg).[253] In September one POW returned after digging a grave. "Given a cigarette each coming back from Argyle St. All wooden crosses stolen from graves."[254] Another man found it curious that the Japanese would not spend a military yen on medical supplies yet always provided a wooden coffin and a wreath of flowers for a funeral.[255]

Pte. George C. Badger, Winnipeg Grenadiers, died of malaria in November 1942. A full-blooded Indian from Kamsack, Saskatchewan, he had been taught some arithmetic, in the earlier days, by his officer, Lt. White. White was in charge of his funeral. "We hold a quiet service in the chapel, then the Japs bring a truck and we load the plain wooden box on board, an Officer and 6 men as bearers, with a couple of shovels, and a rope, and away we go to the cemetery near Argyle St. camp."[256]

Harold Englehart, a member of the Royal Rifles of Canada, had the eerie experience of waking up in the "death house" at Sham Shui Po. He had been ill for several days with dysentery, and finally was moved into one of the makeshift hospital wards, which he found a discouraging place: "Some guys would get up at night and go to the window and order all kinds of food; they seemed to be delirious or something. In a day or two they would be dead." Englehart couldn't remember how long he was there because he became delirious himself. In the compound at Sham Shui Po there was a small shed about 10 ft by 10 ft that had something to do with the hospital, though he didn't know exactly what. His next recollection was waking up in the middle of the night with a terrible burning in his throat. He didn't know where he was, but it was obvious that the man on the stretcher alongside was dead.

> I thought, "They used to call this the death house; they put me out here to die!" I tried to get a drink of water out of my water bottle, and I was too weak to lift it so I had to spill most of it before I could get a drink, but the burning in my throat wouldn't go away. I stayed there until almost noon the next day, and it was very hot in that little building. The guy next to me was dead—one of the Winnipeg Grenadiers. And then I heard somebody coming. Well, all I can remember was seeing some hands come in the door, and they had some strips of cloth in their hands, probably to tie our feet together. I started yelling and cursing at these people, because I knew that they were coming to bury us. So they ran back and brought Dr. Banfill. He came and said, "You're still alive!"[257]

That he was. He lived for another five decades, savouring his escape from a remarkably close acquaintance with death.

Some deaths were tragically unnecessary. One of these took place on 27 August 1943, when Mattseau, an HKVDC POW, was killed on the electric wires around the camp. He was cleaning grass from between the fences on Japanese orders; apparently they forgot to turn off the electricity.[258]

These reflections on disease and death in the Hong Kong POW camps serve as an introduction to the next phase of life for the majority of the survivors. Those few who were reasonably healthy, and a much larger group who were judged by the Japanese as healthy enough, were sent to Japan, Korea, or Manchuria as labourers. The next chapter will describe the hazardous and often tragic voyages these men made between summer 1942 and the late months of 1944.

Chapter 7

The Overseas Drafts

*D*uring 1942 and 1943, the number of POWs at Hong Kong fell rapidly. Group after group, generally referred to as drafts, were shipped out to Japan, Korea, and Manchuria. This chapter will relate some of the events connected with these movements, and give a general summary of POW life in Japan. The following chapter will describe in more detail the subsequent history of the men in Japan. There were many dozens of POW camps there; only a representative handful will appear in these pages.

The fundamental explanation for the POW drafts to Japan is straightforward. Japan desperately needed able-bodied men for labour, most particularly in the mines, on the docks, and in various manufacturing plants. The drain on manpower by the war, which for Japan had begun in 1931, was immense. Casualties were high, and success in the early years carried its own burgeoning demands for garrisons scattered across tens of thousands of square miles of China and southeast Asia.

As early as August 1942, the Home Ministry reported that the need for labourers had become acute. A conference was held, and one conclusion was that POWs would be employed in mining, stevedoring, and engineering and construction "for national defense."[1] Thus the Geneva Convention interdiction of POWs working on projects that would contribute to the war effort of the capturing nation was disregarded officially from this date, if not before. Actually, beginning 12 June 1942, American POWs from Zentsuji Camp in Japan had worked as stevedores.

Given the needs, it was quickly obvious to the Japanese that there was little to gain from feeding (no matter how inadequately) tens of thousands of POWs without enforcing payment by work. Thus, from Singapore and Java, men were sent to the Burma-Siam Railway, while

---

from Hong Kong, the Philippines, and other sites, forced labourers were sent to Japan, Korea, and Manchuria.

Nor was the importing of POWs the only step taken by the Japanese to solve the manpower shortage. Far from it. The ongoing efforts to maintain and supplement the labour force were prodigious:

> [I]t was determined in 1942 to use all students over 14 years of age for short period assignments through the Patriotic Labor Corps for Students and this program was intensified in 1943. Additional measures to expand the size of the labor force in Japan proper included limitations on the exportation of workers, efforts to import additional Koreans and other aliens (along with attempts to use more local labor in the exploitation of overseas territories), employment of prisoners-of-war, greater utilization of inmates of penitentiaries, and some effort to stimulate the employment of women.[2]

Another reason that manpower—a significant part of which was womanpower—was needed so desperately was that the ravages of disease among the Japanese people became manifest early in the war. Beriberi was a major health problem, indicating how poorly the civilian population was fed. For example, between 1942 and 1944, absenteeism because of beriberi increased threefold at the Tsurumi plant of Mitsubishi Kasei, and by August 1944 about 30 percent of the women workers and young apprentices at this glass factory were suffering from beriberi to some degree.[3] Other working places were similarly handicapped.

The total number of prisoners of war imported to Japan proper was never large enough to assist the war effort significantly. (Indeed, in light of what is known of various types of POW sabotage, their contribution may well have been negative.) A survey in June 1944 showed that about 16,000 POWs were engaged in productive work such as mining, shipbuilding, stevedoring, freight handling, iron, steel, and other manufacturing, and civil engineering work. These figures should be contrasted with Germany, where by early 1943, 1,170,000 Allied POWs (excluding Soviet prisoners) were integrated into the war economy of Nazi Germany.[4]

Requests for prisoners as workers were submitted to the War Ministry in Tokyo, which stipulated the number of workers allotted, the type of work, and the wages. Two yen per man per day was paid by the employer. These funds did not, however, go directly to the prisoners; rather, the money "is either handed in to the Army, used for the expenses of the prisoner of war recreation equipment, or for national defense offerings and general expenses."[5] The wage actually received by a working POW ranged from 10 to 25 sen a day. Prisoners doing heavy labour, the Japanese said, received the same food as a civilian heavy labourer. An official admitted, however, that as the air raids increased it became more and more difficult to supply food.[6]

The US Strategic Bombing Survey was carried out immediately after the war. The book included Table 7.1, which shows that there was a major shift of POW workers into mining as the end of the war neared. Without coal and ore, the Japanese economy was strangling. This table excludes those not assigned to regular work. The total number of prisoners of war in Japan proper was reported as 20,828 in May 1944 and 32,418 in August 1945. In the period 1 January 1942 to August 1945, 3,432 were reported to have died in prison camps on the four Home Islands[7]; 99 prisoners were killed in Japan proper by bombs and naval gunfire, and 113 were wounded.[8]

Table 7.1
Work Performed by POWS, by Industry, May 1944-August 1945

Industry	May 1944	Aug 1945
Ship building	3,837	2,037
Iron and steel	2,421	2,211
Other manufacturing	1,780	2,133
Mining	4,698	9,810
Transportation	2,564	2,317
Construction & civil engineering	783	596
Total no. of POWs	16,119	19,184

Source: US Strategic Bombing Survey, *Japanese Wartime Standard of Living*. From Table HHH, "Utilization of Prisoners of War for Work, by Industry, Japan proper, May 1944 and August 1945"

Coal mining employment is a representative category. Listed by origin of worker, in January 1945 there were 244,571 Japanese full-time coal mine workers, 28,047 Japanese short-time workers, 133,515 Koreans, 6,423 POWs, and 7,750 Chinese in a total work force of 420,306.[9] Thus POWs made up only 1.5 percent of coal miners. Clearly, the relative contribution to the labour pool by POWs was minimal. Nevertheless, the demand for workers was endless, and more and more POWs were shipped north to the Home Islands.

Transporting Hong Kong POWs to Japan

Drafts for what the men called "The Water Jump" began in the summer of 1942. A first draft of about 650 men, purportedly culled from the so-called undesirables of Sham Shui Po, left the camp in the first week of September.[10] This demand for men to labour in Japan was seen in largely optimistic terms by the POWs. Their fond hope was that being a prisoner in Japan would be an improvement over being one in Hong Kong. The rationale was that being in the Home Islands, the food supply should be better. Moreover, the Japanese spoke eloquently of the beauty and culture of their homeland, suggesting that those who were selected for the trip were most fortunate. The Japanese officers assured the men they were lucky to be going. But most of all, perhaps, the trip represented a change. They had had several months to become thoroughly bored with imprisonment, to learn what true hunger was, and to see with foreboding the increasing ravages of disease.

Thus when the process began on 27 August 1942, one POW wrote in his diary: "GREAT EXCITEMENT. 600 men shifted into Jubilee, ?undesirables?" Three days later he noted that the padre had prayed for the 648 about to go on a sea trip.[11]

The second draft from Hong Kong took place at the end of September 1942, when 1,800 men left on the ill-fated *Lisbon Maru*. Almost half were lost at sea. No Canadians were aboard. Diary notes made by a Royal Scots sergeant who survived, Arthur Alsey, give some glimpses of the tragic journey:

> 25 Sept 42: Awake at 2 a.m. with Happy feet....Reveille at 4 a.m...."Fat Guts" [Col. Tokunaga] says farewell at 7:30....Moved off in stages & eventually boarded "Lisbon Maru" at 10 a.m. By 3 pm 500 are crammed in bottom hold, 600 on top. No washing arrangements. 12 W.C.'s on top deck, 4 urinal pipes, no leaning over the side.[12]

The next day he described feelingly the tantalizing smell of steaks frying in the Japanese galley. On 30 September he noted that the diphtheria patients were being kept on deck covered with tarpaulins. Then catastrophe struck in the form of torpedoes from what we now know was an American submarine, *USS Grouper*:

> 1 Oct 42: Frantic shouts from Bridge and bow gun fires about 30-40 rounds. Applause from Bridge gives impression of hit on sub which fires another torpedo, luckily going past bows. No food all day, no one allowed on deck for latrine, 2 Boards are pulled up from bottom of hold and 1100 line up for piss, men use their mess tins for shit pans.[13]

Miraculously, on 2 October they were still afloat. Repeated requests from the holds for air and water had been disregarded. The noise in the next hold gave the impression that the ship was sinking. At 8 a.m. there was a desperate scramble for ladders leading out of the death trap in the hold. There were no lifebelts. Alsey found a length of 4" x 3" timber that supported him until he was picked up by a Japanese patrol boat.[14]

The *Lisbon Maru* was armed. When it left Hong Kong its major cargo was Japanese troops, and the ship bore no indication that there were POWs aboard. When she was torpedoed, the hatches were fastened shut and the prisoners confined below. Eventually, when it became certain that the stricken ship was sinking, the prisoners broke out of the holds. Japanese guards opened fire but many of the men got over the sides. Of the more than 1,800 POWs aboard, 843 died in this disaster. A handful escaped to China. The remainder continued their traumatic trip to Japan in other ships.

Back in Hong Kong, rumours of this catastrophe spread quickly, as shown by this diary entry made by Barbara Redwood, a young woman in Stanley Camp, on 8 October 1942:

> For the third night in succession I've dreamt of meeting Arthur....Rather worrying news that a ship "Lisbon Maru" carrying British and Australian prisoners of war had left a southern port and was torpedoed by American subs. Some were able to swim to a nearby island, others were rescued, and a few drowned, and every one worried about their men, but rumour is that Nakazawa has given his word that no soldiers have left Hong Kong yet.[15]

The last rumour was wrong, of course. *Lisbon Maru* was packed with Hong Kong POWs, including the diarist quoted above, Arthur Alsey, about whom Barbara had dreamed. He survived the sinking. On 12 October 1942, Japanese newspapers correctly announced that the *Lisbon Maru* was full of Hong Kong POWs.[16]

Dr. Anthony Coombes was slated to be part of this draft. Fortunately for him, he was removed because he was a dysentery carrier. The Japanese gave everyone a stool test. As a further part of the selection process, they made the men run in a wide circle around a Japanese medical officer, who picked out POWs "unfit" to go:

> They were often well enough. They were too thin or they were falling about and they were obviously no good for work. Of course you got a lot of people developing what we called "daylight limp," pretending they couldn't go around. And they would be falling over just as they got in front of these fellows, and that sort of thing, and went over in a fall, holding their leg. Then when they were taken off the draft they were just ran off and having a bit of laugh. Perfectly fit, good. They were called daylight limpers, but the "limp" disappeared after dark![17]

Four drafts from Hong Kong to Japan included Canadians either predominantly or in substantial numbers.

First Canadian Draft

Six hundred and sixty-three men sailed 19 January 1943 aboard the *Tatu Maru* or *Tatsuta Maru*.[18] These men went largely to Kawasaki. This was the so-called "Show Draft." Instead of travelling, as most drafts did, in filthy, decrepit tramp steamers, the men were conveyed in "the newest and fastest of the Japanese luxury liners, and made the whole trip in three days."[19] See the chart outlining these travels.

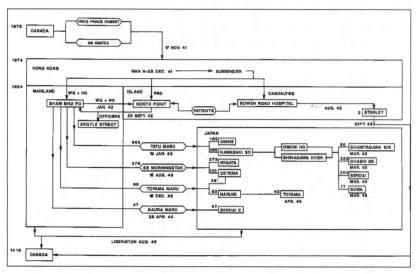

Figure 7.1. Flowchart of movements of Canadian servicemen captured by the IJA at Hong Kong, December 1941.

CSM William Ebdon kept a diary. It allows insight into how the Japanese organized a draft and how determined they were to avoid importing infectious diseases along with the Allied POWs. By 11 January 1943, the prisoners making up the draft were segregated into various sections. Ebdon was in charge of 50 men, including most of his own Company D.[20]

The men underwent many tests, especially the loathed rectal rod, and some inoculations. The draft included 610 Canadian, 510 British, and 200 HKVDC POWs, a total of 1,320. The medical officers accompanying the group were Capt. John Reid, RCAMC; Surg/Cmdr. J.A. Page, RN; and Maj. J.E.C. Robinson, RAMC.[21] Five days before departure the men in the draft were vaccinated again, throats were inspected, and then they were isolated from the rest of the camp. The isolation was enforced with barbed wire and armed sentries. On 15 January there was another swab and a stool test for all members of the party. And so it went: next day another inoculation, larger than the last, producing sore arms and fever.[22] January 17: "Another Inoculation this morning for Dysentery. I had this one on the same arm as the Vaccination yesterday. Three needles & Vac. in four days going some. I feel pretty rotten tonight....My Party is now No. 15, we are 49 strong, some out as Dipt. [diphtheria] carriers."[23]

Finally, the ordeal of preparation was over. On Tuesday 19 January 1943, Ebdon drew 500 military yen for his party, 10 yen per man. They marched out of camp at 0730 hrs, "the *Silent Army* until we started to sing & then we let our feelings go. We all wore Rubber running shoes....Wharf at 0930 hrs, board Japanese S.S. TATUTA MAROU 19000 Tons. We are in No. 1 hold 'C' deck with four other Party's [*sic*] making a total in this hold of 250."[24] Two days out, after yet another throat inspection and gargle, the draft was divided into three parties. There were 500 Canadians in "A" group, 400 English in "B" group, and 300 Canadians and the members of the HKVDC in "C" group. Ebdon's Section 15 was in the last grouping.

Whatever else can be said for Japanese methods, they were unquestionably thorough with regard to public health measures, although techniques often seemed slipshod. The draft was tested, vaccinated, inoculated, and gargled to a remarkable degree. This flurry of medical activity probably represents both a desire to have potentially able-bodied labourers arrive in the Homeland, and a further desire to keep that Homeland as uncontaminated as possible by exotic diseases that the new arrivals might bring with them. Typically, however, the actual voyages were so lengthy, so poorly supplied with all necessities, and so desperately overcrowded that the men arrived in Japan much sicker and less fit than when they left.

On arrival in Japan, the Canadians were divided. One hundred and sixty-three were sent to Omine (which is located on the far western tip of Honshu Island near the Shimonoseki Straits), and 499 travelled to Kawasaki Camp 3D, in the Tokyo-Yokohama industrial area along Tokyo Bay. These camps will be described in some detail in the next chapter.

Second Canadian Draft

Three hundred and seventy-six men sailed 15 August 1943 aboard the *SS Morning Star* or *Manryu Maru*. Conditions appear to have been remarkably good on this voyage also, relative to most others made during the war by POWs. Lewis Bush, whose book portrays him as an upbeat person tending to see the positive side of everything, has much good to say about the IJA officer and the NCO accompanying the draft, and about the ship's company. For example, on the *Manryu Maru*, interpreter "Cardiff Joe" Matsuda gave up his cabin accommodation to Bush and other POWs, saying he would sleep on the saloon settee.[25] Also:

> Considering the condition of over half of the men when we left Hongkong, [*sic*] it seemed nothing short of a miracle that we had not suffered a single death, thanks in great measure to Matsuda, "Cardiff Joe," to the medical orderlies, and to the considerate captain and officers of the "Manryu Maru" who had done everything possible to assist. Captain Ito and the sergeant-major had also been quite good to us, and if the army officer had been rather stiff and formal in the early days, I could realise that his was no light responsibility.[26]

Nevertheless, when this draft reached Japan a Japanese medical officer did a medical examination of the men as they left the ship, and his question to the accompanying officer was: "Who selected these men? Most of them are not fit to work."[27]

Though judged unfit, these POWs were in fact to work to total exhaustion—those who survived. Of the group of 376, 276 went to Camp 5B at Niigata, on the coast of Honshu north of Tokyo, and the remaining 100 went to Oeyama, north of Kyoto.

Third Canadian Draft

Ninety-eight Canadians sailed 15 December 1943 aboard the *Toyama Maru*. Rumours of this draft were first recorded on 2 December 1943. The clues were obvious: a day or two before this, the whole camp was mustered on the square and all men had to perform a physical fitness test involving running 100 yards and chinning a bar four times. The wounded and the disabled were excused. "A farce. Dr. Saito conducted affairs. I was categorized 'C.'"[28] On 15 December, this man noted that the draft left that morning. There were a total of 504 sent to Japan, leaving approximately 1,100 in camp plus 450 in hospital.[29]

The reasons for selection to this draft varied. At least one man was sent as punishment. For several months James Bertram had edited an illegal news-sheet that circulated within Sham Shui Po. Compiled mostly from Japanese papers, it filled a definite need, both for information and as a morale booster.[30] Bertram was sent to Tokyo because of this activity in December 1943. And, as always happened when any prisoners left Sham Shui Po for "the sacred and unpolluted islands of Nippon, our 504 men were segregated, swabbed, injected, and generally given more medical attention in a week than we had had previously in two years."[31]

Of the 98 Canadians on this draft, 48 were sent to Oeyama to join their fellow Canadians already there, while 50 went to Narumi.

Fourth Canadian Draft

Forty-seven Canadians sailed 29 April 1944 aboard the *Naura Maru*. Also on this draft were 10 medical officers (none of them Canadian), 10 medical orderlies, and a total of 153 additional Other Ranks.[32] As was the customary practice, the draft was isolated for two weeks while inoculation against typhoid fever, dysentery, and cholera was carried out, together with stool tests. The results of the latter were presumably cultured and examined "as we were told later in Japan that one of the 220 men (name unknown) was a cholera carrier."[33]

The 220 officers and men were transferred to a Japanese transport on 29 April 1944. They were accommodated in the rear hold, one deck below the main deck. This hold was indescribably filthy. In addition to British and Canadian prisoners, the hold contained a cargo of dried fish and soya beans. Throughout the trip the area was thick with flies. A few drugs were supplied to the group before leaving Hong Kong; these were supplemented by private purchase—i.e., the black market. Several men suffered from malaria, and diarrhea and dysentery were rampant by the end of the journey. "No provision whatsoever was made for the care of the sick. No deaths occurred however."[34] This, the final draft that included Canadians, was sent to Sendai Camp 2.

Of course, much that was and is Japanese depends on a belief system profoundly different from western ideas. A letter by Lafcadio Hearn, in April 1893, from Kumamoto, illustrates one such gulf between western and Japanese concepts. Apparently a peasant consulted an astrologer because his mother had become blind. The astrologer said that her sight would return only if she could obtain and eat human liver, which must be fresh and taken from a young body:

> The peasant went home crying, and told his wife. She said: "We have only one boy. He is beautiful. You can get another wife as good, or better than I, very easily, but might never be able to get another son. Therefore, you must kill me instead of the son, and give my liver to your mother." They embraced; and the husband killed her with a sword, and cut out the liver and began to cook it, when the child awoke and screamed. Neighbours and the police came. In the police court, the peasant told his tale with childish frankness and cited stories from the Buddhist scriptures. The judges were moved to tears. They did not condemn the man to death; they gave only nine years in prison. Really the man who ought to have been killed was the astrologer.[35]

And, as Hearn points out, all this took place only a few miles from the university, where they were teaching integral calculus, trigonometry, and genetics. Yet he was correct in observing that western science and religion could never have inspired the devotion to a mother that the old peasant and his wife had. The latter thought it her sacred duty to die for her mother-in-law.

The Japanese proved equally willing to die for their treasured country. And if they would labour, and perhaps die, why should the lowly, despised prisoners not labour and, perhaps, die also?

The Japanese located POW camps on all four of the main islands. The situations were related to their increasingly desperate need for labourers, so many camps were in large cities where there were factories and shipyards while others were placed in proximity to mines and other sites in isolated areas.

The main diseases encountered by POWs in Japan were dysentery plus the confusing mix of signs and symptoms that occurred because of long-term malnutrition and lack of vitamins; beriberi and pellagra were common diagnoses, though these diseases were seldom seen in uncomplicated clinical situations. Respiratory and skin diseases, as well as climate- and work-related traumas also occurred, injuries being common at workplaces associated with certain mining and heavy manufacturing camps. The chief difference noted when comparing this with the Hong Kong or the Philippines experience was the almost total absence of new cases of malaria in Japan.

Trying to cope in these camps, the medical staff dealt with the specific diseases and traumas as best they could. In addition, they struggled with the interrelated problems of inadequate housing, grossly deficient sanitation, and the inadequacy of diet, drugs, and medical supplies. In prison camps in Japan as elsewhere, the food supply was so limited and the food itself so poor that illness was inevitable. Because the food was always calorically inadequate, the prisoners were constantly hungry. The prisoners' weights had dropped to about 110 pounds, an average weight loss of 60 to 80 pounds per man.[36]

An accurate description of the prisoners' diet is difficult because it varied from time to time and camp to camp. In broad terms, the ration consisted mainly of polished rice, sometimes replaced or supplemented by barley, corn, and millet. There was little or no meat or fish. A ration consisting solely or largely of white or polished rice seemed especially damaging to the POWs.

> Our standard ration at Omori was always called "rice," but this was a courtesy title. In fact it was a cereal base composed of North China millet, barley, and perhaps 10 per cent of white rice....But though it was a harsh staple, and cruel to a tender stomach, it was probably much better balanced, from the point of view of nutriment, than the Japanese white rice and barley. The comparative rarity of beriberi and the deficiency diseases among prisoners in Tokyo bore witness to its vitamin B content.[37]

According to a detailed survey carried out by American personnel immediately after the war, Japan depended upon imports for 17 percent of its caloric supply from rice, as well as for 67 percent of calories from soybeans, for 84 percent from sugar, for 21 percent from wheat and other grains, and for 37 percent of its requirements from beans. Other foods were produced almost entirely domestically.[38]

Most of the rice the Japanese issued was second or third rate. They would not eat it themselves because it was often heavily contaminated with rocks, dirt, broken glass, rat droppings, and worms.[39] The caloric intake for each prisoner per day was roughly 1,800 to 2,500 calories, usually closer to the lower figure than the higher. These are approximate figures; caloric intake varied from camp to camp. The sick ration was even lower because the Japanese believed that by denying food to the sick, they would be forced to return to work quickly.[40] The insufficient quantity of food resulted in constant hunger and weight loss, while the insufficient quality contributed to vitamin deficiencies, weakness, and many deaths.[41]

Japanese food supplies were getting low throughout the war and were especially limited from 1943 on. Allied successes in the submarine war meant that Japan had less and less capacity to transport food, or anything else. Thailand, from the outbreak of war, had been a rice-bowl for Japan, China, and Malaya. The annual export capacity of Siamese rice had risen from 800,000 tons to 1,100,000 tons. But from the beginning of 1945, these figures "dropped spectacularly, and the export capacity was soon down to 300,000 tons."[42] Thus there was much less rice that could be imported into Japan even if freighters had been available to carry it.

At Oeyama they were given maggoty rice daily, with barley mixed in, and yam leaf stew that occasionally contained a little meat or fish.[43] They also ate snakes, frogs, sparrows, and daikons. One POW saw a couple of seriously ill prisoners in desperation eating the lice off their blankets.[44] "The furnaces in the factory [at Oeyama] gave us the opportunity to light small fires around midnight when the frogs and also sparrows, stuffed with rice, were roasted."[45]

Japanese experts estimated that the daily per capita average requirement was 2,160 calories, and consumption was about 2,200 calories. Men working at heavy labour required from 2,700 to 3,400 calories daily. These figures are less than the accepted levels in the western world. According to a US report, both foreign and Japanese authorities had recognized the meagre and poorly balanced nature of the Japanese diet. "It contains too high a proportion of cereals, principally rice, which normally accounts for more than half of the entire calorie intake, and is deficient in animal proteins, fats, vitamins, and minerals."[46] During the early 1940s, Japan had undergone a period of remarkable military and economic expansion, on a national diet that did not conform with accepted scientific standards, either in quantity or quality.[47]

The mountainous terrain of Japan restricts the amount of land capable of being brought under cultivation to roughly 16 percent of her total land area.[48] The decline in Japanese agricultural production between 1941 and 1945 was further influenced by a shortage of able-bodied farm labourers. By 1944, women, children, and old men made up the majority of farm workers, with a considerable increase of women in all age groups except late teenagers. There was a net decrease of agricultural population from February 1944 to February 1945, totalling 701,000 men and 167,000 women.[49]

Moreover, the fishery yield decreased from 4,800,000 tons in 1939 to 2,080,000 tons in 1945, a decline of 57 percent. According to figures released after the war, the daily per capita supplies of fish actually distributed in Tokyo, in grams per day, was 36.6 grams in 1942, and only 9.6 grams in 1945.[50]

In pre-war times, Japan typically had one to 1.5 million tons of rice on hand on 1 November, the beginning of the rice year. On

1 November 1941, the beginning of the 1942 rice year, Japanese stocks of rice amounted to 1,178,000 tons. This quantity decreased to 392,000 tons on 1 November 1942 and fluctuated around this figure for the rest of the war. "With total annual requirements of staple food in the neighbourhood of 13 million tons, it is apparent that this carry-over stock was tantamount to a 10-day supply."[51] Customarily, the staple ration consisted entirely of rice. But as early as 1942, the government had to begin substituting wheat and barley for a portion of the rice in the ration, in order to maintain the system despite inadequate rice supplies.[52]

So far as the POWs were concerned, they knew all too well that it was entirely possible for Tokyo to issue orders about POW diet without creating an organization for carrying out these orders.[53] We may know a theoretical figure for the quantity of food representing an individual ration, but this figure may not represent what each man actually ate, or received to eat. For this fact two main factors are responsible. First, there was an almost universal craving for tobacco. Depending on the cigarette supply a bowl of rice might trade for one to five cigarettes. No amount of warning could suppress the practice. Secondly, gambling with the contents of Red Cross parcels was a popular activity and trading items was a close second. This often resulted in a seriously unbalanced distribution of food. "One or both of these latter habits seemed to be universal amongst the American troops."[54]

At Hanawa Camp, in September 1944, Dr. Calvin Jackson recorded that dinner and supper consisted of cabbage and mongo bean soup. By this time the POWs were getting only 20 percent rice and 80 percent millet. The interpreter told Jackson that only low-class Japanese ate millet.[55]

The Japanese armed forces reduced the loss sustained in milling rice in order to increase both quantity and quality. White rice (in which 100 percent of the bran from brown rice has been removed) was provided to military personnel until 1933. After then, until April 1943, the standard issue was 70 percent polished rice—that is, rice with 70 percent of the bran removed. From April 1943 until September 1944, 30 percent polished rice was adopted. Then, in September 1944, the use of wholly unpolished rice (brown rice) was begun; "however, because of its unpalatableness and the digestive disorders it caused, its use was discontinued in October 1944. From then until the end of the war, 20 percent polished rice was used in the ration."[56]

By 1944 it had become a necessary routine for urban Japanese to make food-foraging expeditions into the countryside. These outings became more frequent when bombing attacks destroyed stocks of food in households and stores. "Food foraging by workers became an important cause of industrial absenteeism in 1945."[57]

Disease Among POWs in Japan

Disease was abundant. Fever, chills, pain, anorexia, abdominal cramps, and dysentery plagued nearly all. Many died. Medical care was inadequate. At best, drugs and medical supplies were always limited. Red Cross supplies were rarely permitted into the camps, and when they were, it was most often in small amounts, even though much more seems to have been available.[58] Surgical supplies and instruments were never adequate to carry out major surgery; there was always a shortage of dressings, bandages, and antiseptics. Sometimes, drugs were smuggled into camps by hiding them on patients discharged from hospitals.[59] Treatment being so often inadequate, numerous POWs died helplessly and unnecessarily.

One method of prophylaxis that the Japanese believed in was the use of medicinal gargles. Here is one account of their use, in this case at Omori POW Camp:

The parade inspection passed off without incident. Orderlies went down the ranks with iron kettles, pouring a weak solution of Condy's into each man's mug. Then the familiar order: "Prepare to gargle. *Gargle!*" The Japanese Army has great faith in this ceremonial gargle, which was the token of expert medical attention. If a prisoner gargled regularly, how could he ever get ill? Surprisingly, they still did.[60]

Physical work was required, often including prisoners suffering from major physical illnesses. POW camps in Japan were created expressly to provide manual labour. The labour—hard physical work on farms, in factories, shipyards, coal, nickel, and copper mines, and other sites—was often harsh for malnourished prisoners. As a result, many accidents, some of a serious nature, occurred. One report has shown that the peak period for accidents paralleled the peak period for diarrhea, vitamin deficiencies, and other diseases.[61] Numerous accidents were caused by faulty machinery and improper working conditions. For example, arc-welding torches were used by the prisoners without protective goggles, and injuries to the eyes were common. Septic infections of the hands were also frequent.

At times, in order to get a few days rest from work, a prisoner would intentionally encourage or seek out a minor injury. This was risky, however, because a serious condition often resulted. Deliberate injuries were self-administered in certain camps where the work was especially difficult, and in a few camps injury was a commodity purchasable from a fellow-POW—in camps along the Burma-Siam Railway as well as in Japan. At Fukuoka 17, a Japanese camp with an especially vicious reputation, this sort of activity was not uncommon. Methods included applying lime or other irritant chemicals to ulcers, and fracturing one's own upper or lower extremity."[62] One medical officer described an epidemic of self-inflicted or purchased arm fractures to escape brutal working conditions in the mines.[63]

An American in another camp in Japan, Wakasennin, near Sendai, saw a fellow-POW deliberately injure his foot with a large piece of iron, "in order to get out of work for a few days. It's a 'mizzerbul' life that will lead a man to do something like that."[64] And a POW named Scott hired himself out as a professional "bone-crusher," breaking limbs on demand at Omuta Camp 17, on Kyushu Island.[65] Garrison also recorded men deliberately breaking an arm to get off work.[66] On the Burma-Siam Railway, Dr. Huxtable wrote about his roommate, the cheery and gallant young Mac, whose foot was still in plaster because of a fracture of a metatarsal bone. Mac had asked Huxtable to break his leg so that he would be able to stay in hospital. Huxtable refused to do this "but agreed to fracture a metatarsal bone with a sledge-hammer as the only means of keeping him there."[67] The significance of this differentiation is difficult to interpret. Also on the railway:

> I buried another ol' boy who committed suicide. There's no way that I'd mention his name, but he just in effect committed suicide. I believe he was the laziest man that I've ever met anywhere, anytime, anyplace. As we worked on that railroad, the rest of the people who worked in his *kumi* usually had to do his work because he just wouldn't put out. Then when he saw that the Japanese weren't making some of the people with ulcers work, and they'd let them stay in and have the doctor treat them, well, he began to cultivate one. We'd catch him sitting there picking at a raw sore with a sliver of bamboo, and that bamboo was just as poisonous as could be. He'd pick at that thing, and you'd find him rubbing old mud in it. I was not surprised after I'd been sent to 80 Kilo to see him come down with one of the following groups, and he had an ulcer that didn't need any cultivation then. It was tremendous, and he didn't last, I think, only about four days after they sent him down there.[68]

Lack of proper clothing during the winter months was also a contributing factor to work-related traumas, as well as to influenza, pneumonia, frostbite, and in some cases gangrene of the toes. Living conditions were uniformly miserable. Clothing, bedding, and housing were insufficient and contributed to the general suffering. Living quarters were crowded, sometimes as many as 50 men in one small room. Lack of soap and warm water led to troublesome skin lesions; lice and fleas multiplied prodigiously.

Surgery

In some situations, surgery had to be performed without anesthesia. For example, at Fukuoka 2:

The Japanese hospital was a place of horror that appalled our Western eyes. The dockyard workers lived in shacks provided by the Company, and if they were admitted to the hospital their whole family moved in with them and lived around the hospital bed. We often had to carry the accident cases to this charnel house, where the doctors were covered in blood like slaughter-men, and the nurses slopped around the wet, slush-covered floor in bare feet. Hygiene was non-existent, drugs and anaesthetics were seldom available, and hot water was regarded as harmful and its use avoided. A primitive toilet leaned against the dispensary, and from the toilet came maggots that crawled up the passage and on to the bandages that littered the wet floor.[69]

An Australian POW in Japan described an operation on an injured comrade. This accident occurred in a Japanese mine. When the whole group of POWs joined the injured man on the surface, four of them were given a stretcher; the direction of the hospital was pointed out, but no guard accompanied them. At the hospital they were shown to an operating room, and the four put Pratt on the table. A surgeon, an assistant, and two nurses arrived and set about their work. The doctors wore neither masks nor headgear; their white coats buttoned up the front. The small young nurses wore white smocks, and had round caps over their hair, coming down over their ears.

The four POWs were told to stay and assist the surgeon by holding Pratt down. The flesh had been rolled back so that the shin bone could be seen. The patient had not been prepared in any way for the operation, still lying on the table in his working clothes. The four who had carried him to the hospital were in their work clothes also. "As the surgeon began his work, all realised that this operation was to be done without anaesthetic, hence the retention of the four to hold Tom....Tom groaned a lot, but didn't complain much, though the stitching must have been painful."[70] Pratt survived the war.

There is occasional evidence that medical affairs could be conducted in what was, to the western prisoners, a normal manner. Cmdr. Page recorded one case in which a patient seems to have had exemplary handling, included letters of referral among both POW and Japanese physicians. There exists in the archives a letter from a Capt. Paul S. Roland, MC, USA, to one Dr. Nosu re: a patient named William Larsen, injured at work. Laboratory results were enclosed. Also a letter from Cmdr. Page to Dr. Nosu after Larsen was transferred to Kobe, March 1945, with a detailed history by Page. This seems almost normal in handling,[71] reflecting the willingness of Dr. Nosu to deal with POW doctors as professional colleagues. Few Japanese MOs emulated him.

Quantities of medical equipment, supplies, and drugs were uniformly inadequate in the POW camps maintained by the Japanese in the Home Islands. After the war, large amounts of Red Cross materials were found stockpiled in various locations, supplies that might well have saved prisoners' lives had they been made more readily available. The explanation by the Japanese was that until the use of the atom bombs and the resulting precipitate collapse of Japan, every assumption by the armed forces was that the war would continue into the foreseeable future for years—perhaps many years. Consequently, supplies such as the Red Cross items had to be conserved and doled out gradually to assure long-lasting availability. Not surprisingly, perhaps, many former POWs were and are unimpressed by this argument.

However, a post-war survey by the United States seems to confirm this attitude. The discovery of large stocks of clothing and drugs in the hands of the armed services when the war ended would confirm that there were still substantial supplies in existence, but that they were being conserved.[72]

Another factor was at work here also. There is unequivocal evidence that medical supplies of all kinds were increasingly difficult to obtain in Japan as the war progressed. There were many reasons for this. Importation of all goods from abroad was seriously impeded by the shortage of shipping, a direct consequence of Allied action. Moreover, Allied bombing attacks on occasion were targeted explicitly to interdict Japanese medical materials. A former member of US Medical Intelligence has described how a particular plant in Japan was identified and bombed. The selection was based on the knowledge that most glass containers for injectable drugs in Japan were made there. Destroying the factory would have a significant impact on the supply of medicinals to the armed forces, the civilian population, and incidentally, of course, to POW camps.[73] While the primary aim was to strike at Japan's ability to fight by reducing medical supplies to the Japanese people, particularly the armed forces, inevitably the Allied successes directly affected POWs.

Dr. Tsuneo Muramatsu, assistant director of the Matsuzawa Psychopathic Hospital of Tokyo, reported after the war that by the end of 1943 the shortage of drugs had become critical. Drugstore stocks were depleted by civilians trying to stockpile what supplies they could:

> [S]erums, drugs, and vaccines were very scarce; imported medicinals, such as boric acid, were all but impossible to obtain. An ill-conceived and wholly inadequate system of establishing stockpiles of important medical items throughout Japan was instituted, but with the onset of air attacks the plan broke down, and the situation reached very serious proportions. About one-third of all drug-producing facilities were destroyed by air attacks.[74]

Moreover, many histological laboratories ceased functioning because they could not get dyes and stains for slides; analytical work virtually came to a halt. However, the shortage of doctors was not nearly so serious as had been anticipated. Of an estimated 100,000 physicians in Japan (including those in the armed forces), roughly one-half were serving the civilian population, a ratio of 1 to 1,300.[75]

Most civilians in Japan just before the launching of the large-scale air attacks in March 1945 were in need of many routine, everyday items. Cotton and wool cloth consumption for 1944, based on 1937 consumption as 100, had fallen to 8, leather footwear to 16, and household furnishings to about 25 to 30. Housing was overcrowded. Medicines and drugs were generally in short supply, while food consumption was about 10 percent below the official minimum caloric requirement.[76]

Japan therefore made a sharp distinction among consumers. By 1945 large classes of the population were receiving less and less in favour of those considered essential to continuing the war—the armed forces and war workers.

> The staple ration theoretically guaranteed consumers specified amounts of food according to sex, age, and occupation. The favoured heavy worker class in essential industries received approximately 75 percent of its staple requirements from the ration. General workers, however, received only about 50 percent, while other consumer categories received even less. The staple ration itself was not sufficient at any time during the war to provide the total caloric requirements of consumers, including the favoured heavy workers. This serious defect in the nation's food position compelled all classes of the population to supplement the staple ration by staple and other food purchases outside the ration structure.[77]

Officials of the Mitsubishi Mining Company reported that coal miners on Kyushu in 1945 could obtain only 10 to 15 percent of the amounts they had secured in 1940 of foods such as vegetables, soy sauce, fish, and meat. By the end of the war, these workers were living virtually by the staple ration alone. The average daily per capita availability of food in Japan in 1941 was equivalent to about 2,000 calories. By 1944 the figure had declined to 1,900 and by 1945, to 1,680.[78] A survey conducted by the Welfare Ministry in 1943 on national nutrition attributed the marked wartime increase of tuberculosis, beriberi, disorders of the digestive organs, skin diseases, and evidence of vitamin deficiencies mainly to "malnutrition due to the tight food situation."[79] In May 1945, the medical authorities at the Maizuru Naval College recorded that 30 percent of the 417 students then enrolled suffered from malnutrition.[80]

One former Hong Kong POW categorized the food in Japan as being "very tasty but insufficient and always the same thing—Rice and Soup!"[81] The rice mixture in his camp was usually 60 percent rice,

20 percent barley, and 20 percent beans. They also received a loaf of bread daily, weighing between five and ten ounces. Green tea was issued at every meal, hot water morning and evening. In January 1944, sprats were included in the ration about every fourth day, but beef only twice in the month. Pieces of dried salted herring appeared in most of the evening soups.

On 7 February 1944, the second shipment of Red Cross food arrived at Oeyama POW Camp, and for the rest of that month and most of March, rations were substantially supplemented with bully beef, Spam, and similar foods. The one previous parcel issue was at Christmas 1943.[82] As a POW in Hong Kong and Niigata, Harry Atkinson's weight dropped from 170 to 105.[83]

Work

"We used to have to drill, blast and shovel 20 tons [coal] per night—four of us."[84] Once, when Albert Delbridge was working in a coal mine, he went to pick up a shovel lying on the ground about 30 yards from where he was working. The Japanese foreman asked him what he was doing. Delbridge tried to explain, but the guard accused him of not working. He then began to hit Delbridge with a mine hammer. "I was beaten about the head and the legs, and my arm was broken. I fainted. We put two boards on each side and wrapped it up like a splint. That was all we could do. I went out to work the next day."[85]

Of course, the Japanese laboured also while their military-dominated government drove them towards disaster. One survivor remembered being in grade six in 1945. "We no longer had many classes at school. The main thing we did was dig an antitank ditch in the corner of the schoolyard. 'Dig a hole,' they told us sixth-graders. The older children were no longer around. From April 1945 on, everyone above us was mobilized daily for work in war plants."[86]

As the Allied POWs arrived in Japan they found little beauty outside the often magnificent scenery. What they did find was a pinched country, struggling for survival and determined to obtain maximal input from every member of the working community. Increasingly, that group included women and children; prisoners of war were soon to find that they had arrived not at a pleasant station to wait out the war, but rather at a place of torment and hunger, of misery and disease. The earliest arrivals had almost three years ahead of them, a fact of which they were, fortunately perhaps, quite unaware. But as they spread out to the camps to which they were assigned—Niigata, Oeyama, Kawasaki, Sendai, and a hundred others—they began to realize how unpleasant their situation had become. For all too many, their war would end in these Home Islands.

Chapter 8

POW Camps in the Japanese Home Islands

*A*llied prisoners of war found themselves incarcerated in camps all over the four Home Islands—Honshu, Kyushu, Shikoku, and Hokkaido. POW camps were located wherever heavy work needed doing, near businesses, docks, mines, or manufacturing plants, to provide a nearby, cheap labour force. There were about 160 POW camps in Japan between 1942 and 1945.[1] The camps described in this chapter housed substantial numbers of Canadian POWs. In most camps these men were intermingled variously with POWs from Britain, the USA, Australia, New Zealand, the Dutch East Indies, and other countries.

Detailed accounts follow for seven camps: Oeyama, Niigata 5B, Kawasaki 3D, Omine, Narumi, Sendai 2B, and Omori. The main POW hospitals at Sagamigahara and Shinagawa are discussed also.

Oeyama (Osaka Camp No. 3)

How many died we do not know,
It could be hundreds, long ago
From stark starvation, fear and woe,
In Oeyama prison, long ago.[2]

Oeyama is a village on the northwest coast of the island of Honshu on Wakasa Bay, a few miles north of Miyazu and just east of Iwataki (see outline map). When not looked at through strands of barbed wire, the area is beautiful. Low mountains ring the bay, which leads northwards into the Sea of Japan. Very close to the camp site is a wide canal along which barges carried, among other cargo, nickel ore from the mines in

---

Notes to Chapter 8 are on pp. 360-70.

which the prisoners laboured. Miyazu, the nearest town, had the typical narrow winding streets and wooden buildings of every Japanese town in the 1940s.

The camp, located about a 15-minute walk from the Oeyama railway station, was set in a depression. Almost surrounding the camp area, distant perhaps half a mile, are low hills. The factory was also in the depression. The camp occupied a rectangle three to four acres in area, enclosed by an eight-foot-high fence topped by sharpened bamboo stakes.[3] Behind the camp was a field of five or six acres used as a garden.[4]

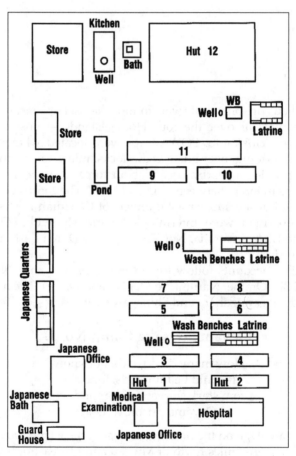

Figure 8.1. Plan of Oeyama POW Camp, Japan.

The camp was first occupied in 1943 by British, Canadian, Australian, Dutch, and Norwegian POWs. The British came first, in early autumn. Then 100 Canadians arrived from Hong Kong in September and a further 48 early in 1944, making a total of 148 Canadians in the camp.[5]

American POWs began to arrive on 5 August 1944. In addition, a group of Allied officers entered Oeyama on 31 March 1945,[6] and a further 161 American POWs came from Yodagowa Camp in May 1945. (Moves such as this were common late in the war as urban camps or the factories where the men worked were damaged or destroyed by Allied bombing.) The total number of prisoners on VJ Day was 645; only 73 were Canadian, the remainder having been transferred elsewhere.

Surg/Lt. S.E.L. Stening was the POW medical officer at Oeyama from October 1943 until June 1944. He thought the camp reasonably well laid out: 12 living huts, all single-storey except one, with Japanese mats and good ventilation, walls of mud over a bamboo base. The hospital was similarly constructed and separate. The kitchen was large, with a concrete floor. Food stores and clothing stores were separate. Wash benches were adequate, latrines adequate but with the usual poor system of sewerage. Unfortunately, the water supply was polluted with larvae from the latrines. At all times ground water was just two feet down.[7]

On average, 32 POWs slept in each hut, so that each man had a space about 2½ by 6 feet to himself—about one-third as much as was prescribed for the ordinary British soldier and, as some of them noted wryly, about the basic dimensions of a coffin. In the winter of 1944-1945, in order to raise the temperature in these huts, the Japanese increased the number living in a hut to 50, so that men were sleeping so closely together that they touched each other.[8]

A few hundred yards from the prison camp was a factory where nickel was refined after being dug by pick and shovel from the adjoining mine. The enlisted men worked either in the mine or the refinery. The officers had moderately heavy camp duties. After Surg/Lt. Stening was moved to another camp, Maj. H.M.S.G. Beadnell, RAMC, arrived and was the medical officer for the British and the Canadians. Capt. LaMoyne C. Bleich, US Army Medical Corps, was the senior officer in the American group and remained in charge of the Americans, administratively and medically, throughout their time at Oeyama—the last 13 months of the war.

The Japanese camp staff was led by Lt. Hazama Kosaku, who was commandant for the entire two-year lifespan of Oeyama, August 1943 to August 1945. (He was tried for war crimes in 1947, found guilty, and sentenced to 15 years in prison.[9])

In Oeyama the winter of 1943-44 was unusually cold. For the Canadians, who had spent the previous two winters in Hong Kong, Japanese winters were a rude shock. One man noted that on his second day there, 8 January 1944, the temperature was -24°C.[10] He had seen, during one day, snow, sleet, rain, hail, and sunshine.

Internal administration of POW camps posed many problems, especially in multinational camps such as Oeyama. Some men believed that life as a POW should be different from the disciplined life in their military units before capture. There was a feeling, fostered by the predictable core of malcontents, that their officers had failed them and that in captivity the duties owed to rank should be diminished or negated.

Within units that remained more or less intact in POW camp, responsible officers or NCOs usually re-established military discipline without major difficulty. The men were influenced by habit, by threats of post-war retribution, and by the pragmatic realization that some form of discipline was necessary for survival. In less cohesive groups the problem became potentially volatile, particularly if officers were separated from their men and a natural leader among the NCOs could not be identified.

Surg/Lt. Stening observed that as hunger increased, the men became more difficult to handle. They stole from each other and from the Japanese; these latter thefts customarily led to beatings and worse. In May 1944, Stening was empowered by the commandant to take control of discipline of the camp and of all punishments. Lt. Hazama forbade the Japanese guards to punish the men without reference to Stening. The Japanese appointed, as camp Sergeant-Major, "the senior warrant officer (WO1 H.L. Deane) and several selected non-commissioned officers were given extra disciplinary powers…serious cases were referred to me for examination and judgment."[11] Deane and three other NCOs became what the POWs labelled, among other epithets, The Big Four.

Stening had occasion to report one of them, Sgt. John Harvey, RAMC, for disobedience and cruelty; Harvey, contrary to Stening's orders, repeatedly struck his fellow prisoners with his fists. "The P.O.W. so struck may have been detected in wrong doing by the Japanese or by Sgt. Harvey. Sgt. Harvey claimed that orders given by the Japanese took precedence of all others and that the Japanese had given him leave or orders to strike and administer punishment to men."[12] Nevertheless, on the whole, Stening thought, this system worked well.[13] But he soon left the camp, after which irregularities characterized the internal operation of Oeyama for many months.

Under Japanese aegis the small group of NCOs assumed complete control. One was a Canadian, CSM Marcus Charles Tugby, Winnipeg Grenadiers; the others were Sgt. John Hugh Harvey, RAMC; WO1 Deane; and MQMS Rogers, the last two both Royal Engineers. Deane apparently was the ranking NCO in camp in the beginning, and both Rogers and Tugby were well up in seniority. Harvey was not, although he was the senior medical orderly in the camp.

Harvey would have been remembered by some of the Hong Kong POWs for his frequent appearances on stage in Sham Shui Po: "Johnny Harvey guitar & vocals." Mark Tugby also performed.[14] After Oeyama the memories were less pleasant.

In 1946, Tugby and Harvey were tried at courts martial in Winnipeg, Manitoba, for alleged illegalities and excesses in the way they reacted with their captors and towards their fellow prisoners.[15] The Big Four met in what was described as the Blue Room, where punishment of wrongdoers was sometimes carried out in the presence of the Camp Commandant and some of his staff.[16] A man who committed a petty crime might be beaten up severely by Tugby and the others.[17] Although some of the POWs considered the men self-appointed, in fact the Japanese commandant, Lt. Hazama, put them in power or openly approved of their activities.

One man recalled that Tugby "was perfectly OK up until about the middle of November, 1944, roughly between the 15th and 20th and then I don't know what happened but he appeared to have buried the hatchet with Sergeant Harvey."[18] Perhaps it was then that he received notice that his wife had been killed.[19] Harvey became "notorious in the Camp for co-operation with the Nipponese." He enforced Japanese penalties against the men, using corporal punishment. Harvey spoke Japanese fluently and he seemed to have been highly regarded by the commandant.[20]

Although the group of four NCOs did not interfere with actual medical treatment, they "controlled the activities at the hospital."[21] When asked if he ever heard any of the medical officers protest, an ex-POW stated that Major Beadnell, RAMC, did. "He was told to mind his business, that this was the way the Camp was run before he came and the way the Camp is going to run as long as he was there. Major Beadnell would have nothing to do with this Sergeant Harvey, who was actually one of his own men."[22]

One complaint against the four men was that they appropriated Red Cross food for their personal use. According to one man, the Japanese gave Harvey boxes of Red Cross food to distribute to underweight men "but what these men got wouldn't make up for the amount of parcels that went into the Blue Room."[23]

Whatever the truth on that question, Red Cross food parcels were used to bribe the men to go to work, a compelling prize for those who were ill but not so sick as to prevent them from shambling out to the mine or the factory each day. At his trial, Tugby asked Maj. Beadnell if he remembered the terms applied by the Japanese for the men to receive the first half-parcel, early in December 1944. "What I understood from Sergeant Harvey was they would issue half a parcel per man provided 85 percent of the men went to work until Xmas."[24] Since it was Japanese policy to cut the rations of sick men, the bribe was a cynical move to keep the working force up to maximum numbers even if some of the men truly were too sick to work.

In April 1945, 30 POW officers, British, Australian, and American, were moved to Oeyama. They found it a depressing place. They also found that the American prisoners, who had arrived shortly before and who were reasonably healthy, had already begun to improve matters by intimidating the British NCOs. The officers immediately set about restoring morale. Their task was not easy.

Many men owed food to a gang of racketeers. A hungry man would obtain an extra half-ration of rice in return for a promise to repay a three-quarter portion at the end of the week. Some men, despite their hunger, would buy cigarettes with a promise to repay in food. Several had sunk deeply into debt. The officers ordered all debts cancelled and arranged for debtors to eat their rations together, under supervision, to protect them from the racketeers.[25]

Often the men found themselves in an ethical or moral dilemma. For example, a POW named Thompson was beaten. The reason was that because he didn't smoke, he saved his cigarettes to trade them for food. Tugby was trying to stop this practice because nobody was getting enough food to sell for cigarettes.[26] But Thompson was punished for attempting to use his own cigarettes to his own advantage. Maj. Beadnell attempted to control the trading of cigarettes for food by forbidding the practice, with limited results.[27] This problem affected every camp to some degree.

Medical Conditions at Oeyama

Surg/Lt. Stening had under treatment at one time in 1944, "209 suffering from beriberi, 156 suffering from pellagra, 120 suffering from defective eye-sight, and eight suffering from nerve deafness."[28] There were about 300 British and Commonwealth prisoners in the camp and in his care at this time.

Among Stening's patients at Oeyama was a Canadian with a severe non-fatal case of "beriberi," hospitalized for many months. He had massive amounts of fluid in his body cavities as well as enormous edematous swelling of his feet and legs. This man had a full range of treatment, including large doses of thiamin, riboflavin, and niacin. His abdominal cavity was drained through tubes more than 40 times, with more than 161 litres of fluid being removed. He also had fluid removed from his chest cavity. In his case a high-protein diet completely cured his edema; the patient had none when Stening last examined him.[29] As with many of the POWs, what was thought to be wet beriberi was, in fact, edema because of inadequate protein in the diet.

Detailed figures on the health conditions in Oeyama exist only for the American POWs. Capt. LaMoyne Bleich kept excellent, terse, sometimes deliberately cryptic notes on his patients, but his responsibility was for the Americans only, 384 men. Medical records exist in his files (loaned to the author by Bleich's widow) for 177 of these US POWs (46%).[30]

Analysis of these data shows major weight losses. Among the other ranks (approximately 150 men), weight fell from an average normal figure of 75 kg (165 lb) to 54.9 kg (121 lb) by July 1945; among the NCOs the numbers were 76.5 kg (169 lb) to 58 kg (128 lb).[31] Larger men generally suffered more and died oftener when sick than did smaller men.[32] The food rations were grossly inadequate: "in the camp it was rice (maggoty at that) daily, with barley mixed and yam leaf stew, very occasionally containing a little meat or fish."[33]

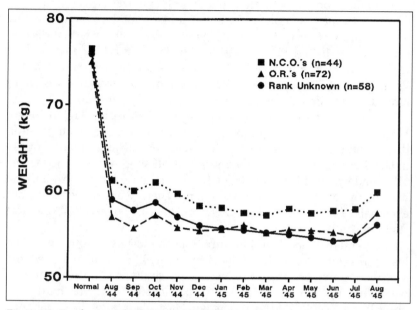

Figure 8.2. Graph of weight changes of POWs held in Oeyama Camp, from records kept by Capt. LaMoyne Bleich, US Army Medical Corps. (Reproduced with permission of C.G. Roland and Harry Shannon, "Patterns of Disease among World War 2 Prisoners of the Japanese: Hunger, Weight Loss, and Deficiency Diseases," *Journal of the History of Medicine and Allied Sciences* 46: 65-85, 1991.)

Bleich's records refer to a wide variety of diseases. The men suffered from malaria, vitamin deficiencies, injuries, undiagnosable fevers, exotic parasites, gastrointestinal diseases, respiratory diseases, skin disorders, neurological diseases, afflictions of the heart and blood vessels, disturbances of the bones and joints, psychiatric problems, diseases of the eyes and ears, and urological afflictions.

Malaria was a major problem among these men before coming to Oeyama; they had been in the Philippines where malaria has been a killer for centuries, or in Hong Kong. But in Japan, though the disease did occur, the attacks were few in number and probably were old disease recurring. On the other hand, although only six of the men had been diagnosed as having vitamin deficiency diseases in the Philippines, these disorders escalated rapidly in Japan. Bleich recorded a diagnosis in this category 545 times among 177 men between July 1944 and August 1945.[34]

With respect to injuries, there were 6 recorded before arriving at Oeyama (i.e., in 28 months of captivity, May 1942 through July 1944), but 128 during the 16 months at Oeyama, where the men were forced to do heavy labour. But it is also instructive to note that the injuries occurred most often between arrival at the camp and the end of February; then incidence fell, suggesting that by this time the men had learned their jobs well enough so that accidents were less frequent.

Three other categories of disease showed marked increases during the captivity served in Japan. These were: gastrointestinal disease (71 instances in the Philippines, or 2.5 per month; 782 instances at Oeyama, or 56 per month); pulmonary disease (6 occurrences in the Philippines; 307 in Oeyama, or 22 per month); and skin diseases of all kinds (3 in the Philippines; 369 in Oeyama, or 26 per month).[35]

Med. 2nd/Lt. Fujii Hiroshi represented IJA medical HQ in Tokyo. He testified at his trial that many medicines, including vitamins, sulfa drugs, and those for respiratory diseases, were lacking in the camps—in fact, he said, the Japanese Army was itself short of those medicines. "We made requisitions for drugs to the Japanese Army hospitals by way of the Main Camp Commandant. There were times when not even half of what we requested was delivered."[36] This, POW medical staff knew all too well.

Several men had their hair turn white almost overnight, and some lost their sight.[37] A man had to be desperately ill to be hospitalized; the men were convinced that once inside, "we could be almost certain that we would not come out alive."[38] The hospital hut was hardly an appealing place, loaded as it was with fleas, bed bugs, lice, maggots, flies, and rats; "all efforts to disinfest the hospital had failed."[39]

When questioned at his trial about abuse of POWs, Lt. Hazama could recall only one instance: he had heard that every day when the prisoners of war went to work at the mine, the children of the Iwataki School threw rocks at them. Aside from this, he did not remember any mistreatment.[40] The men remembered differently.

The Japanese medical officer directly responsible for Oeyama was Lt. Nosu, a subordinate of Lt. Fujii. His duty was to perform physical examinations, distribute medicines, and see that the medical orderly performed his duties. Maj. Beadnell came into fairly close contact with Nosu while Beadnell was a prisoner in the headquarters camp. From discussions with him, Beadnell became convinced that Nosu was not a qualified doctor, but probably a medical orderly with a commission. He was in charge of all medical matters in all POW camps in the Osaka Area. His duty was to visit all camps in the area regularly. "He visited Oeyama only twice while I was there…. It is my opinion that much of the improper medical arrangements in Oeyama camp must be held to be the result of having this man in charge of medical arrangements for the area. He was quite unqualified and incompetent for the post."[41]

According to WO2 Rogers, when he arrived in Oeyama Camp in September 1943 the rations issued by the Japanese to the prisoners were of good quality but too scanty to keep up the strength of the men. Initially the rations consisted of rice, lima beans, soup, vegetables (cabbage, eggplant, squash, and onions), fresh fish fried in oil perhaps twice weekly, and meat about once a month. Even this food, although better than any Rogers had had as a POW previously, proved insufficient to maintain the strength of the men at a working standard.

When work ended in the afternoon, the men frequently were soaked and so chilled that they were numb. On the train to camp the boxcars were very cold; there were no fires in them and they were drafty, so that by the time the men reached camp all of them would be numb with cold and exhaustion.

> On my return to Camp I went sick and was marked for work in the factory the next day. Some of the men, however, who had to return to the mine next day, came down sick two or three days later, and it was about this time that the Canadian and British Prisoners of War who had been working in the mines started to die in considerable numbers from exposure.[42]

This, then, was Oeyama POW Camp. It did not differ significantly from the other camps in Japan except for the unhappy influence of The Big Four.

Niigata Camp 5B and Niigata 15D/15B

Today, the city of Niigata adorns the Shinano River, a modern, clean, pleasant, and pretty place to visit. Half a century ago, few prisoners found Niigata pretty. Exhaustion and gnawing hunger dim one's appreciation of aesthetics. Few of the Canadians and Americans who occupied Niigata Camp 5B, a few hundred yards from the Sea of Japan and the docks where so many of them laboured so painfully, comment on its beauty. Instead, they recall viciously cold winters, heavy snowfalls, the agonies of dysentery and frostbite, brutality, and the deaths of too many friends.

Planning for this camp began in the spring of 1943. Officials of the Niigata Land and Sea Transport Company (Niigata Kairiku Unso Company or NKU) applied to War Minister Tojo Hideki for 300 men to work at the Rinko Coal Company, a branch of NKU. Three firms, NKU, Japan Transport Co. Inc., and Niigata Ironworks Inc. cooperated in building the camp. Wages would be 1 yen per day; working hours were to be 0700 to 1700 (10 hrs) in March, April, September, and October, 0700 to 1800 (11 hrs) from May through August, and 0730 to 1630 (9 hrs) from November through February.[43]

Niigata, then a very small city, was an important port on the north shore of Honshu Island about 150 miles directly north of Tokyo on the Sea of Japan. The POW camp was established in August 1943, when 200 Canadians arrived, the majority of the second large Canadian draft from Hong Kong. A month later, 300 Americans arrived from the Philippines. The Americans believed themselves relatively well off on arrival, because the Canadians looked alarmingly sick and emaciated: "We looked a lot fleshier than they did—they were skin and bones."[44]

The permanent camp covered an area of about 8,000 square metres, on dunes several hundred metres from the sea and from the dockyards.[45] (In the 1990s the dockyards were still in use, but the site of the camp was thick with post-war three-storey apartment buildings.) Because construction was incomplete, the POWs could not occupy the so-called permanent camp immediately. Instead, they were housed in a flimsy temporary camp referred to as the "Rinko Camp."

This initial temporary camp was described by an American POW who arrived there in September 1943. Each barracks was a one-room stable measuring about 10 feet by 12 feet, and divided horizontally by a shelf, giving the room an upper and a lower section. This divided room was occupied by about 20 men. There were 24 of these divided rooms in the stable building, which was about 110 feet long and 30 feet wide. Heating in the wintertime was inadequate because the Niigata Iron Works refused to provide more than 20 small pieces of green pine a day for each of the three stoves in the building. During the winter of 1943-1944 the men had almost no heat and suffered severely from cold and dampness. About one-quarter of the 600 POWs died of exposure or disease that winter, an appalling record.[46]

Lt. Fujii Hiroshi testified at his post-war trial that he had urged Col. Suzuki to move the camp to a better place for the health of the prisoners of war. Suzuki was the senior officer in charge of POWs in the Tokyo area, which included much of central Japan. When Fujii visited the temporary camp in December 1943 he found it to be overcrowded. Even the bathroom had to be used as a barrack; straw was strewn over the concrete floor in the latrine, a blanket was placed on the straw, and the prisoners slept there. They were packed tightly, sleeping side by side and touching one another. If one got a cold or influenza the entire group was infected. "Because they slept on top of the concrete, cold penetrated to them. The latrine water pipes were in very bad condition. I told Colonel Suzuki if they stayed there their health wouldn't improve."[47]

On 24 December 1943 the POWs moved to the permanent location officially known as Niigata Camp 5B. They stayed less than a month; the new camp apparently had been built hurriedly, perhaps on the principle that it was only for prisoners. During the night of 31 December 1943-1 January 1944, one of the buildings collapsed while about 150 men were sleeping inside. Eight were killed and many more injured.

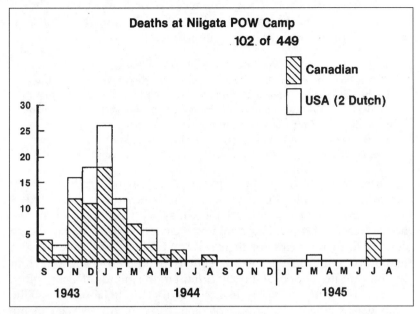

Figure 8.3. Graph of deaths at Niigata POW Camp; figure derived from medical records kept by Maj. William Stewart, RAMC, camp medical officer. (Reproduced with permission C.G. Roland and Harry Shannon, "Patterns of Disease among World War 2 Prisoners of the Japanese: Hunger, Weight Loss, and Deficiency Diseases," *Journal of the History of Medicine & Allied Sciences* 46: 65-85, 1991.)

The accident in the "permanent" camp at Niigata was catastrophic to the morale of men who had already suffered much. The hut was built on sandy ground and no nails had been used—it was pegged. The main beam down the centre of the building was an eighteen-inch log supported by six-inch logs. "That December there was an abnormal amount of snow. If the buildings had been constructed properly it would not have collapsed."[48] On the effect of snowfall, opinion differs. The British medical officer, Maj. Stewart, testified at a war crimes trial that weather conditions were not extreme: winds were not blowing strongly nor was snow falling the night of the accident, though it did snow later in the day on 1 January.[49] In a letter to the author, 50 years later, Stewart commented that the building had been supported by outside struts. Some of these had been removed, in order to permit the passage of the benjo carts removing excrement. The building was thus weakened, leading to the tragic accident.[50] A cynic might suggest that dysentery and diarrhea caused the collapse.

Dr. Fujii was sent from Tokyo to investigate. He arrived on 2 January 1944, bringing Dr. E.S. Kagy, an American POW surgeon, and Shaw (a medical NCO) from Omori Main Camp, as well as medicines, bandages, gauze, and surgical instruments. They found that eight men had died and 20 were injured, five or six very seriously.

After arriving at the camp they helped the POW medical staff treat the injured prisoners. Five or six men had fractures of ribs or pelvis.

> I took them to Shintetsu Clinic and had them x-rayed. After x-ray was taken it was shown to Doctor Kagy and it was discovered two or three men had fractures. I requested Captain Yoshida, the Camp Commandant, to have them hospitalized at the Shintetsu Clinic Hospital and they were hospitalized. Doctor Kagy was left there to treat them. I stayed there for four or five days and then returned to the Omori Main Camp. Doctor Kagy and Shaw stayed there for about one month to treat them.[51]

After the accident, some of the severely injured Canadians were moved to another place for treatment. Ken Cambon, a volunteer orderly, accompanied them: "four of the chaps with pelvic injuries were moved to a small cottage hospital in the city. I was lucky enough to go along with them to care for their needs." In this way Cambon had a temporary reprieve from the inadequate food and housing and from the constant threat of brutality by certain of the guards at Camp 5B.

One consequence of this disaster was that, on 18 January 1944, the camp was divided. One group of men, those who had been in the Shintetsu gang that worked at the steel mill, moved to a separate camp nearer the mill, designated Camp 15D briefly, then 15B.[52] Although the POWs were told that the separation of the Shintetsu group was to be temporary, in fact that group never returned to Niigata Camp 5B.[53]

Routinely, the men came in from work at six-thirty in the evening; they ate and then the sick and injured lined up for sick call. There was nowhere else, so it was held in a corridor, which made sick call a drafty, cold, and highly public affair. For most the publicity was immaterial—they all had more or less the same desperate problems, and the medical officers had no cures. The men filed past and Stewart examined them:

> [A]nd according to the orders which I had from the [Japanese] medical staff I took the numbers of those whom I considered were unfit for work. These numbers I submitted on the completion of sick call to the Japanese medical staff. Sometimes they would see the cases themselves; sometimes they would permit me to admit the first number to be specified, possibly ten cases. On other times they attended the sick calls themselves and saw the cases at the same time as I saw them. Sometimes they showed very little interest either in the lists which I brought to them or in the cases when they examined them.[54]

The senior American officer was LtCol. Francis E. Fellows. When he arrived at Niigata, 18 October 1943, he was 37 years old, the senior

Allied officer, and was designated by the Japanese as Prisoners' Representative.[55]

Lt. Yoshida Masato was camp commandant at 5B from 3 September 1943 until 5 February 1944. He was arraigned for alleged war crimes in the spring of 1948, but never came to trial. He was seriously mentally ill by then and, while the trial was delayed pending his possible recovery, he died in Sugamo Prison, 16 June 1948. Yoshida was not liked by his POW-charges, apparently for good reason.

Yoshida was replaced by Lt. Kato, who had more interest in his prisoners and the general health of the command. "However, Lieut Kato was ruled by an ungovernable temper and when this temper got the better of him, he took it out physically against the prisoners."[56] Nevertheless, this man provided a more humane medical environment than did any other commandant at Niigata 5B.

One medical problem recurred at Niigata as it did in most Japanese POW camps throughout the war. Ill men, attested as being ill by their POW medical officer, were declared well enough to work and were forced to do so. Because the lowliest Japanese soldier believed himself superior to all POWs, a Japanese medical corporal might defy a grey-haired Allied medical officer—and customarily won.

> The reason, when we were sick and unable to work, that we did not stay in camp was that the Jap guards would come around in the A.M. and give you a beating with a stick. The Japs would tell the real sick fellows: "Sukoshi mate chiisai hi hak"'[57] ("in a little while, little box" [referring to the small boxes used to contain the ashes of the dead]). Very cheerful fellows, those guards.[58]

There were five diagnostic categories permitted by Japanese regulations. A man could be hospitalized outside the camp (extremely rare), hospitalized in the camp hospital (rare), permitted to rest in quarters (infrequent), assigned to light duty (grudgingly), or assigned to do ordinary work (the Japanese aimed for at least 90% here).[59] Japanese NCOs, even medical NCOs, were almost invariably medically ignorant and thus failed to understand that men could be genuinely ill without having obvious physical signs such as ulcers, cuts, boils, and deforming fractures.

The same excuse cannot be put forward for IJA medical officers. Yet these physicians often followed the same course, demanding that sick prisoners labour in mine or factory. "Dr. Fujii decreed that many of the men marked 'unfit for duty' by the prisoners' medical officer were fit for duty and ordered them out to work. This order was carried out despite the protests of both the prisoners' doctor and [even] the Japanese medical corporal."[60]

As an example of the consequences, Stewart related the case of POW Wallace, a patient with an abnormally rapid heartbeat; he was examined by Fujii who ordered Wallace to work the next day. Stewart believed that Wallace's high heart rate was caused by previous bouts of diphtheria and beriberi. With prolonged rest his chances of recovery should have been good. But on Fujii's orders, Wallace worked each day until 24 December; then he became incontestably ill, and died on 26 December.[61]

Medical involvement by the Japanese was not always negative. Dr. Fujimake Shigeo testified that in March 1944 there were large numbers of diarrhea patients at the Niigata POW Camp. Dr. Fujii came to the university to ask for cooperation: "as a consequence the university authorities ordered me to conduct the examination of the stool, which I did."[62] Because the result of the test was that amoebae were found in the stools, emetine, which was effective for treating amoebic dysentery, was provided.[63] The POW medical officers agree that this was the case.

The POW hospital was purely a makeshift affair. One man ordered into hospital in 1944 found himself in a room filled with "cripples and beriberi cases." There were 15 patients in a small room, faintly heated by a tiny stove in the centre. "The usual wrangle going on between patients and orderlies, the beriberi are mad for water and mustn't have it, those on restricted diet want more food and can't have it."[64]

Once, Randy Steele looked in the "agony ward" to seek out a friend. He found the man between two POWs who had been dead for some time and were badly swollen: "he was crying and he said he was dying. I started to laugh; I don't know why. I guess it was my nerves or something." The man survived, came home to Canada, and often told Steele that his laughter had made him so mad, it had saved his life by keeping him from giving up—if only to spite Steele.[65]

Fortunately, from about April 1944 the sanitary and medical conditions in the camp improved slowly, "so that by approximately Christmas time of 1944, we had a serviceable and fairly well equipped hospital and dispensary."[66] At times, the camp was visited by doctors and students of the medical school in Niigata, and these rendered much valuable assistance to the camp surgeon in laboratory diagnoses.[67]

The men slept and ate in barnlike huts about 200 feet by 40 feet. A platform ran down each side of the building about a foot off the ground; the POWs slept on this, and sat on it while eating. A tatami or thin straw mat was laid on the platform, then blankets. "We had one good wool American Red Cross blanket and four thin cotton frayed Japanese blankets which were much too short for us. If you pulled them up to your chin your feet stuck out a foot."[68]

The floor was loose sand heavily infested with fleas. It was impossible to keep the fleas out of blankets and clothing. On awakening, the men found fleas dancing around them "like hundreds of young grasshoppers springing up around your feet as you walk through the new grass in the spring."[69] Their bites caused welts and the worst sufferers looked like they had bad cases of hives. The fleas were difficult to catch and equally hard to hold for the death-nip between thumbnail and fingernail.

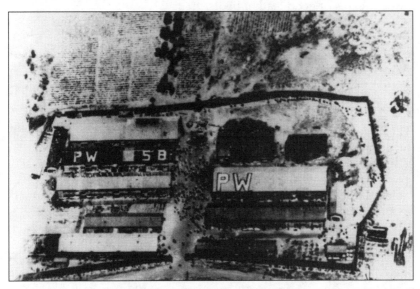

Figure 8.4. Aerial view of Camp 5B, Niigata, taken from a US bomber just after the war. Building top left (white roof) was the cookhouse and warehouse; next below (PW 5B on roof) was a US hut occupied only since spring 1945; next below (white roof) the "daikon hut" occupied by Americans after spring 1945; next down the garden space where the collapsed hut (1 January 1944) had stood; below, smaller hut was Japanese quarters, connected by passageways with bottom hut, the Japanese offices. Top of right group, large dark building, was the bathhouse, and right of it the laundry hut and disinfector hut; below marked PW the hut occupied by POWs working at Rinko coal yard; below that, hut for Marutsu dockyard workers; larger of the huts on the bottom row was the guardhouse. (Photograph loaned and identifications made by Harry Atkinson, 23 October 1989.)

When the men came in from work, they removed their boots and put on a sort of wooden sandal with a strap across the top—"skivies," or "go-aheads" (because you couldn't walk backwards in them). The straps frequently tore away from the sole and many of the men were prone to "borrow" a neighbour's when one of his became unserviceable. This was a constant source of friction. Japanese workers wore a rubber-soled shoe with a cloth top that hooked up the back. The big toe was divided from the other toes. Some POWs tried to wear old worn pairs of these shoes, but they were too small and blistered the men's feet cruelly.

The first winter in Japan, 1943-1944, the POWs were issued with boots woven entirely of straw. If they had had heavy woolen socks to wear, and if the snow had been dry and frozen all winter, the men might have managed. But the straw boots weren't big enough and it was impossible to keep them dry. Once wet, they became a sodden mass. The men couldn't dry them. Night after night they went to bed with cold, wet feet, falling into the sleep of utter exhaustion until wakened, shaking painfully with the cold. "I used to dream at night, fantastic dreams of good leather boots."[70]

Niigata is largely a port town, and therefore much of the prisoners' physical work was on the docks. The POWs worked at the Rinko coal yards, the Marutsu Dockyard, and the Shintetsu iron foundry. Also, some copper was mined nearby.

Rinko Coal Yard

There were two types of jobs in the coal yard: heavy carrying of a difficult but straightforward kind, and the work of the so-called trestle gang, which was especially arduous and often hazardous. The trestle, also referred to—without affection—as "the race track," was an oval of railroad track about three-quarters of a mile in length. The entire track, mounted on trestles, was approximately 25 feet above the ground.[71] Coal, unloaded from freighters, was placed in small open railway cars that the POWs pushed around the track to various dumping points.

CWO Maynard Lee, USN, was permanently in charge of the trestle gang. In his testimony at a trial in 1947, he described this painful and dangerous experience: "Our trestle detail consisted usually of from 60 to 120 men....During the period that I am speaking of now, no man was allowed off the trestle from the time he went up until the time work was over for rest. He would sit on the bench for rest, not lie down—that was forbidden; and if a man would lie down he would get hit with these clubs that all hanchoes had."[72] For the first year in particular, guards used force to spur workers on. One guard was fired because he was too good to the POWs.

This Rinko work detail, regarded with fear and loathing by the POWs, was avoided whenever possible. Lee knew two men whom he believed had deliberately mangled fingers that had to be amputated. They apparently found mutilation preferable to losing their lives at this desperately hard work.[73]

The clothing supplied was lightweight, and the wind seemed much more penetrating to men struggling to balance back-breaking loads 25 feet above the ground. Lee actually saw men blown off the tracks in high winds. Terse diary accounts document the dangers in a grimly matter-of-fact way: "One of the coal gang carried in here with a broken leg. Fell off trestle."[74]

The coal cars, 44 in number, were of varying quality. A few pushed relatively easily, some with great difficulty. On the night shift,

Japanese women pushed the cars, possibly less heavily laden than in the daytime.[75]

An American recalled his time at Niigata on this work detail, carrying coal in baskets. The end result was disastrous:

> I worked there as a stevedore, unloading coal off the ships. We put it on this trestle. We had to put a pole on our shoulder with a basket of coal swinging in front and a basket swinging in back to walk this plank and fill up the railroad car. In January 1944, I fell from the trestle about thirty-five feet. I broke a joint in my back and am paralyzed. The Japanese come every day and kicked me and want me to go to work....I tell you what got me to fall off. About four o'clock in the afternoon, I had to urinate. This boy back behind me didn't see me, you couldn't see over this coal, and he knocked me down.[76]

In the Rinko coal party, approximately 120 men, there were 11 deaths; all 11 men were coal-pushers.[77]

Marutsu Dockyard

By autumn 1943, when the POWs at Niigata began to work, Japanese seaports were in poor condition. Stevedoring capacity was inadequate. Bad summer weather, peculiar to the Japan Sea coast, damaged large quantities of material.[78] It was into these conditions that the Canadian and American prisoners were pushed.

At Marutsu dockyard the men were detailed to load and unload boxcars. A common cargo was pig iron, slabs about 2 feet long, each bar weighing as much as 200 lb (90 kg). Thousands had to be picked up by hand and loaded into boxcars.[79] As soon as a ship docked, the men began unloading its cargo of pig iron. The nets that lifted the rough slabs of pig iron out of the ship's hold were made of steel cable with lengths of thick rope woven into the net. These ropes frayed and tore frequently, and a group of Japanese women repaired these continuously, threading fresh rope into the spare net. The winches and donkey engines were also run by women.

> When a ship was unloading iron, you could hear the dull clash and clank a half mile away, and when we heard the sound and saw the tall masts of a big ship towering up on the far side of Okeedasan's warehouse or Obasan's warehouse, we shivered apprehensively. We could stand it, we said, in summer, but in winter when we had to dig the iron out of the snow with bare hands it was misery pure and unadulterated.[80]

The iron slabs had rough and jagged edges, "like crystals of ice forming along the edge of the horse trough in late fall."[81] Each month the men were issued one pair of mitts woven from rice straw, but often a pair wore out in a day. Later they were issued small square rubber pads and were told to handle the pig iron with these. After a few months the Japanese put a daily quota on the work. Each man was required to load 15 tons of pig iron per day. "This was held over us like a club. If we hadn't completed our quota it was an excuse to cut our rations, or work longer hours."

They handled many other commodities as well. When the freighters unloaded soybeans the bags might be piled as high as a house and two or three times as long. The beans were in large sacks that weighed, when wet, as much as 200 lb (90 kg).

> It took three men to lift, and load one of these on the back (high up, right across the neck) of the man who was going to carry it, through the warehouse and up a plank and into a freight car. To put it mildly it is hard work, particularly the last few yards up a steep plank. When the pile on the docks got a heavy rain the bags weighed 200 lbs, when they were swollen up, some bags would burst.[82]

A common item in the Japanese diet was bean curd. This arrived packed in 50-lb. wooden kegs; the lids were seldom tight, and often the several inches of oily liquid that had risen to the top would leak out and run down a man's back as he carried the keg off the dock, through the warehouse, and up a plank into a freight car. The oil saturated their clothing and irritated their skin, adding another misery to life.

Once, the men realized that they were unloading bales of Japanese money. When a bale broke, the workers loaded themselves with bills that they smuggled into camp. They had no way to buy anything, so they just gambled with it. Then they discovered that some of the more friendly guards were delighted to have the money and would bring the POWs cigarettes and even saké in return.[83]

The POWs were divided into groups, each with a leader. Forsyth recalled that his group lost three leaders. One was Capt. Laurie, Chief Petty Officer of a Dutch submarine. "Laurie was our first leader, he died of pneumonia, from being soaked to the skin while we were working in the rain day after day. Next leader, Staff Sword died in hut crash, third leader, Mac Hawes, a handsome young giant, beloved by all his men, died of poison only a month before the war ended." Of this group of 50 men a few worked in camp but most went to work on the docks. Sickness took a heavy toll; once during the first winter the work party was down to 10 men. The rest were sick in camp. Any man who could walk kept going out as long as he could, because the Marutsu docks provided them with extra nourishment in the form of a soup, often consisting mainly of soy beans, which the men believed helped them more than anything else except, perhaps, the few Red Cross parcels they received.

There were no yard engines to shift cars, so the workers had to push cars up one track, then switch across and down another, for an hour or more before they could begin their real day's work. When a car was heavily loaded and could not be moved, they would have to crash an empty car into it, hoping the impact would jar the stuck car loose. "When a gang of us were on the hawser of a barge towing it along the water front, I will always remember Bobby McLeod striking up on the chant of the Volga boatman. He always did his best to keep our spirits up. I will always regret that he did not live to return with us. He died a month before the war ended, 1 July 1945."[84]

Shintetsu

The Shintetsu Camp (numbered 15D and then 15B) had a separate existence from the spring of 1944 until the end of the war. But it was located in Niigata and its inhabitants frequently crossed paths with those of their old comrades from 5B; these contacts allowed inter-changes of rumour, information, and sometimes supplies between the camps. The Shintetsu Camp served an iron foundry.

Shintetsu acquired a medical officer soon after the camp was established, Maj. John Francis Breslin. He was the MO and also senior officer until USN Commander Callahan arrived early in 1945. At the same time, a second medical officer arrived, Maj. Kenneth Brown, RAMC. In an affidavit Breslin described himself as being "morally responsible for the medical care of about five hundred (500) American POWs, including some Dutch and Canadian POWs."[85] He and Maj. Brown worked cooperatively, "attending in general to the sick, attempts at good sanitation, protests for more and better food, protests against poor working conditions of the men, and in general tried out all kinds of psychological tricks against the Japanese to attain our ends."[86]

Breslin arrived at 15D with only a stethoscope and some clamps for blood vessels. The Japanese provided a thermometer, a few scalpels, and bandage scissors; medicines comprised small amounts of Mercurochrome, aspirin, a vitamin B1 product made of rice husks, and "a very poor Japanese brand sulfanilamide tablets," plus bandages and adhesive tape.[87] Later, the supply improved slightly and included sulfathiazole ampules for injection, iodine, alcohol, creosote tablets, and various samples of drugs whose intended use was cryptic since directions were in Japanese.

Breslin and Stewart, in Niigata 5B, were able to cooperate in some clandestine ways, the contacts beginning at the end of April 1944 when the men of 15D began to be allowed to go to 5B for baths. This occurred two to four times monthly. One consequence was that Stewart and Breslin exchanged information, discussed various medical problems, and made arrangements for men of 15D who had dental problems to go to 5B to see the American POW dentist confined there. Other con-tact between the two camps was maintained by surreptitiously pass-ing notes at various worksites.

In his affidavit, Breslin also mentions a helpful Japanese doctor. This civilian, Dr. Yoshida, was hired by Shintetsu officials; he was a professor of medicine in the Niigata medical school, and "turned out to be the only Jap who befriended us." Through Yoshida's efforts they were able to get a microscope, English-language medical texts, cigarettes, eggs and bread for the sickest patients, as well as instruments and laboratory reagents. This was done surreptitiously and on Yoshida's own initiative.[88]

Another Japanese physician with whom Breslin had contact was a Dr. Shirai, head surgeon of the Shintetsu foundry hospital. The two MOs met roughly monthly; Shirai operated on several POWs, apparently satisfactorily. He was also present when various medical procedures were carried out. For example, the entire camp was tuberculin-tested once; on another occasion all POWs had chest x-rays. Breslin visited him to request drugs, which they usually received, though only in small quantities.[89]

Contacts with the Japanese Population

One Japanese worker at Niigata was notably kind to the prisoners. All his fingers had been cut off by the Chinese while he was their prisoner, some time before. One of the POWs would be sent out with this man to gather greens for the camp kitchen. They would visit his home, a tiny one-room dwelling where the man lived with his mother. There they would have a modest meal, sitting cross-legged on the floor.

But many of the inhabitants of Niigata became hostile towards the POWs as the war situation worsened. Some took to waylaying the columns of POWs marching to work, throwing rocks at them and spitting on them. Steele remembers that, more than once, mobs of Japanese gathered at the camp in the evening, shouting at them menacingly.[90] Fortunately, the guards were businesslike in their duty of protecting the POWs. Things improved significantly as the summer of 1945 drew near and, obviously to most of the Japanese, the end of the war as well. A new camp commandant proved to be an old man who was "quite gentle."

Even in hostile foreign cities, the POWs frequently were reminded that another gender existed. In the camps in Hong Kong there was little opportunity to see women except from a distance, though workers at Kai Tak airport seem occasionally to have made contact, as has been mentioned. In Japan, the POWs often found themselves working alongside or near women and girls. The number of women in the workforce increased dramatically as the armed forces absorbed more and more men.

When we first went to work on the docks the Japanese women were frankly afraid of us. We may have been the first white men they had ever seen. The first day they ran and hid. After that they stared at us from a distance, and finally they decided to ignore us, and pretend we never existed. The last summer they were beginning to be interested, and would have been friendly if we had given them any encouragement. Particularly one of the girls who handled one of the "boshas" (carts) and learned to giggle and roll her eyes.[91]

That there was sexual interest was inevitable. Communal bathing was still the norm in Japan in the 1940s, so men and women were accustomed to seeing each other nude. This was routine. What was not routine were these large, hairy strangers. Seeing them bathe became a fascinating exercise for some Japanese women, who, during the occasional communal baths (at which the POWs routinely bathed as a group, last, in dirty water) "looked at us and pointed to the fellows with the big ones and made quite a fuss."[92] Apparently the women fantasized about the size of the occidental penis. It seemed logical that such giant-sized men should sport giant-sized penises. "Avid curiosity drove them into the benjos to find out. Time and again while I was standing, penis in hand, I would find a leering face nosing around my elbow with the hope of beholding a deliciously, shockingly monstrous organ, only to find their grandiose visions dashed."[93]

Bathroom facilities tended to be rudimentary and unisex. As did many others, Will Allister noticed how different—for westerners—the relations were between the sexes. Japanese society seemed full of restrictions, yet there was

[A] refreshing openness and freedom about the human body. No His and Hers toilets, we were all one happy evacuating family. Each stall had a hole in the floor and a narrow swinging door with ample space above and below to see the occupant. It was common to see a man lean over the door to greet a lady squatting inside and remain for a nice little chat.[94]

Some of the Allied POWs, unused to this custom, had difficulty urinating in front of Japanese girls at work: "I'd turn my back and I'd start right away. Then the girls would come around me to see what I was hiding and say to me: 'Nanda?'—what's the matter?—and I would shut off right away."[95]

The shortage and poor quality of food in Niigata Camp 5B was Problem Number One. Knowing how far the amount of food actually delivered fell short of what should have arrived, the Japanese falsified the records. Sgt. Ross, RRC, was forced, under threats of physical punishment to himself and reduced rations for the entire camp, to sign receipts for a complete shipment regardless of the quantity received.[96]

The day-to-day ration was painfully limited. Lugow (a sort of barley porridge) was a common item on the menu and often constituted the entire menu. Dr. Fujii believed that all of the POWs' illnesses originated from the inadequate diet. Moreover, he testified explicitly that the diet at Niigata 5B was insufficient. Excerpts from his testimony are revealing. He claimed to have told his superiors that the Allied prisoners of war in general needed more food, especially in Niigata. However, there had been a substantial reduction in the amount of food given to the prisoners in the Tokyo area, which included Niigata. Fujii testified:

> Major General Yamaji of the Military Affairs Department of the Eastern Army at that time began a movement to conserve rice. Major General Yamaji was a classmate of Colonel Suzuki at the Military Academy and they discussed the matter and they decided that there was no need in feeding the prisoners of war more than the Japanese personnel, and furthermore the prisoners of war did not care for rice anyway. They instituted the policy of feeding the prisoners of war substitutes like cereals, potatoes, etc.[97]

Red Cross parcels were an infrequent bonanza for the POWs. How many each man received depended on what camps he was in, a matter of luck. Individual memories differ. One prisoner remembers receiving 2½ parcels in Hong Kong and 2½ in Japan.[98] Another, in the same camps—Sham Shui Po and Niigata 5B—noted that he received two Red Cross parcels while in Hong Kong in 1942. From the British Red Cross, they "were like Manna from heaven.…While in Japan ('43-'45) we received four and one seventh American Red Cross parcels. They were very good and a wonderful help to us. We often wondered what the Canadian parcels must be like."[99]

Discrepancies in numbers are understandable after all these years. The important fact was that while their fellow POWs in Europe were receiving a package each, every week or every second week (except in the early months of 1945), the Far East POWs had a package about once a year, and often that had to be shared with other men.

Sgt. Lance Ross recorded, on 29 April 1944, that they had a day off because it was the Emperor's birthday. The Japanese were all drunk. They gave the POWs a can of bully beef and a can of vegetables between two men. These, it proved, were Red Cross supplies. The Japanese also gave the men an egg, an orange, and a bottle of beer between four men; "not much chance of getting tight on that."[100]

Culinary delights were rare indeed. Once they were given shrimp, and one might be excused for thinking that this was sumptuous fare. However, Ross was not enthusiastic: "Had shrimp for dinner. They are so rotten they just smell like dead Chinamen. We must be tough."[101] Fastidious tastes had to be abandoned: "a fish head for breakfast, I ate it all, even the eyes, I am very hungry."[102]

A major problem affecting not only the individuals involved, but also camp morale, was the trading of food as speculation. In order to eat heavily now, some of the prisoners would trade their meals for

weeks ahead. Eventually they were so deeply in debt they had everything going out and nothing coming in. Maj. Fellows made the men
turn in a statement of their indebtedness and laid down a schedule
whereby they could pay off their debts. They were forbidden to do any
more trading. This didn't work. They continued trading, so Dr. Stewart
took a hand: "he ordered them to report to hospital, he had their meals
served there and watched them eat so they could not carry anything
out to trade. They were known as the 8 ball club."[103]

Enormous importance surrounded the process of serving out the
daily ration. Men were loathed or praised depending upon the general perception of their fairness in serving out the meagre supplies:

> The Japs had a small brown bowl made of some plastic material and it
> was a standard measure for dishing out our rations....The server out
> would get the wooden bucket on the ground between his knees, and
> using a wooden paddle would pack the steaming mixture into the small
> brown bowl, and level it off. There might be a small dipper of stew to go
> with it or a piece of salty yellow daikon pickle, or two spoonfuls of
> grasshoppers. If the server saw he was going to be short the cry would
> go forth, "Hold onto your rice," and the server would go around with a
> spoon and collect a spoonful from each, or more, till he had made up the
> ration he was short.[104]

Most of the men stole food whenever the opportunity arose; most
of the time—though not invariably—they stole only from their captors. When discovered by the guards, punishment was prompt and
painful. Harry Atkinson was beaten twice. He and some buddies stole
soybeans to smuggle back into camp and they were caught. Stood at
attention, they were beaten in the face, groin, and stomach using fists,
then this was improved upon with a wooden sword.[105]

Dysentery, a debilitating and sometimes lethal disease, had a devastating effect on malnourished, overworked men. There were almost
always a few cases, but in the early part of 1944 a serious epidemic ravaged Niigata Camp 5B. By mid-March even the Japanese became concerned at this threat to their labour force.

Later, Lt. Kato cooperated with Maj. Stewart in stopping what
could have been a devastating outbreak of bacillary dysentery: "On
the 19th of December 1944, at which time Lt. Kato was the camp commandant, I reported there were cases of dysentery in the camp, and I
expected to find on survey that there would be many more. Lt. Kato
immediately stopped all work."[106] None of the men went to work for
two weeks. This prevented the spread of the dysentery, and Stewart
could treat those men who were already sick. In all, about 40 cases
were diagnosed, with no deaths.

For any patient, the impact of dysentery was profound and, all
too often, lethal. Gabriel Guitard, of the Royal Rifles of Canada, kept a

terse diary. On 11 October 1943 he wrote that he felt weak and still had beriberi and a cold. Three weeks later, on a beautiful day, Guitard noted that the ration was small—he was, as usual, hungry and under-nourished. "My back and stomach aches all the time a dull tiresome ache which leaves me weak and dizzy. Have Beri Beri in chest and stomach."[107] Three months later, still ill and hospitalized continuously, Guitard at last surrendered to his final enemy. He died of dysentery, malnutrition, and associated disorders.

Dr. Fujii testified about some of the medical procedures used to combat pneumonia. He had the POW medical orderly make up a gargle solution with potassium permanganate. Before roll call, morning and evening, bottles containing this deep purple solution were distributed to each barrack. The POWs would bring their teacups and the section leader poured a measure of the gargle for each man. Asked about effectiveness, Fujii commented: "After the policy of gargling was instituted there were some pneumonia patients the first year, however, there were no pneumonia patients during the winter of the second year and so I think that it had beneficial effects."[108] Possibly it did help.

The senior American officer in Niigata 5B—not a medical officer—was appalled at the treatment given one of his men by the Japanese. The unfortunate patient had advanced pneumonia. Here is his outraged account:

> The first medical treatment which I saw administered to any prisoner was given by a Shinto priest to a man who was ill with pneumonia. The priest with his assistants went through a ritual covering a period of about four hours, during which time he kept the entire hospital in a turmoil from the beating of the gongs and a weird chant and during the same time placed some type of powder upon the chest of the patient. This powder was then ignited and large raw burns were received by the patient. When I attempted to protest this treatment, I was forcibly ejected from the room and placed under guard until the ceremony was completed. Of course, the patient died.[109]

This is a classic example of the clash of cultures. The impact reverberated all over Asia whenever Japanese captors and western prisoners collided. The treatment given sounds like cruel torture. The major thought that it was, and wrote his account in appropriate language. But to a Japanese, the officer's outrage seemed genuinely mysterious. The prisoner was not being tortured, he was receiving a standard Japanese folk remedy called moxibustion.

The rationale for moxibustion relates to acupuncture, where fine needles are inserted at prescribed points on the body. Long experience has indicated to the healer that stimulating certain places on the body produces effects in related (though often widely separated) organs or areas. In moxibustion the points are stimulated not by a needle but by the heat produced by igniting the moxa, which is dried mugwort, *Artemisia vulgaris*.

As is true of many folk remedies, western as well as eastern, effectiveness often depends on having faith in the efficacy of the method. In Asia, where moxibustion was and is used in Chinese, Japanese and other cultures, people are used to the procedure and often get at least symptomatic relief. Westerners knew nothing of this—to them—bizarre practice, so they interpreted what they saw as torture. Moxibustion did not cure this POW's pneumonia. Neither would most western remedies of that era.

Despite desperate conditions, major psychiatric disease was infrequent, though several men have suggested that perhaps they were all a little mad. Occasionally there were significant problems. Rarely could these be handled in any appropriate manner medically. There was no proper, humane way to segregate mental patients.

Unhappily, there was even less likelihood that the Japanese would permit this sort of treatment anyway. In general, only men with obvious physical lesions would be spared from work. Those with conditions that showed nothing obvious to uninformed Japanese soldiers—whether the patient had heart disease or schizophrenia—usually would be forced to the mines or the docks. An exception was the patient with mental disease who exhibited unquestionably bizarre behaviour. "The Japanese were scared of him. He just went totally mental and we had to guard his door day and night just to keep him alive."[110]

At Niigata, at least one man came to a tragic end because of mental disease. Pte. Frank Spears, US Army, was mentally unbalanced. When Maj. Fellows requested his transfer to a hospital so that he could be adequately safeguarded and treated, this recommendation was not approved. Spears was placed in the custody of the camp doctor. After about six weeks, the Japanese pronounced him cured and insisted that he return to duty.[111] Shortly afterwards, Spears escaped, was recaptured, and escaped again. On the testimony of Maj. Fellows, Spears was manifestly unbalanced mentally. He never was seen again; the morning after his second escape the camp commandant ordered a casket made, which was taken out of camp by the Japanese. After the war, the POWs were told that Spears had died of a heart attack while attempting to swim a river. Fellows was convinced Spears was recaptured and executed.[112]

Disease Statistics

Maj. William Stewart, the medical officer at Niigata, arrived shortly after the camp's construction (September 1943) and remained there until his release, after the surrender of the Japanese, in September 1945.

He was in charge of over 500 POWs. Medical records exist for 407 of these prisoners.

As in all Japanese POW camps, the men at Niigata suffered from malnutrition and avitaminosis. The more common manifestations in these camps were beriberi and edema. No significant peaks or trends are seen in the number of occurrences except for a sudden increase in August 1945, which may represent a final closing-the-record diagnosis made by Dr. Stewart at the end of the war. Or many of the prisoners may have avoided reporting illnesses until then for fear of being denied food. The incidence of vitamin deficiency was extremely high. There were 349 diagnoses in this category, an average of 12.5 each month. But the cases did not occur equally often over the two years. Of the total of 349, 199 (a monthly average of 50) occurred between December 1943 and March 1944[113]—the time labelled by Stewart and by many of the POWs as the worst period at Niigata 5B.

NCOs seemed to suffer less from vitamin deficiencies than did Other Ranks. Both the malnutrition and the vitamin deficiencies suffered by most of the prisoners were aggravated by disease, poor living conditions, and heavy physical labour. Usually, these factors weighed more heavily on Other Ranks than upon NCOs.

The number of occurrences of diarrhea or dysentery demonstrated no specific peaks except for that peculiar rise in August 1945. But the number of occurrences was impressive: 685, or 24.5 per month. Even after Red Cross supplies were received, it was difficult to treat these diseases satisfactorily due to the highly inadequate and monotonous diet of polished rice, and not enough of that.[114]

Respiratory and skin diseases were also prevalent at Niigata. There were 227 recorded diagnoses of respiratory diseases (about 8 per month), and 196 (7 per month) of skin diseases. No significant rise or fall was noted for any month or year. However, Maj. Stewart stated that for respiratory diseases, the first winter there (1943-1944) was the worst period in the camp,[115] and the number of occurrences was generally higher than in the winter of 1944-1945.

The number of injuries that occurred in Niigata varied from month to month. The men were exposed to harsh physical labour and long work days. One report indicates that the peak period for accidents was similar to that for diarrhea and other diseases. The generally weakened condition of the men and the nature of the work performed combined to make them subject to accidents. Lack of proper attire, such as warm clothing and boots, also contributed to the number of accidents on the work site.[116]

In some instances crude surgery was carried out under unpleasant and painful circumstances. Randy Steele was working at the coal yard when he got a sharp piece of coal in his foot. Unable to get it out, he kept on working. After a week his foot became infected. "I was limping about when a Jap guard asked me what was the matter and I told him. That night, two guards came and they made me lay on the floor and they took a knife and cut a hole in the bottom of my foot and took a piece of wire and dug the piece of coal out, then took a piece of rag and pushed it in the hole....After a few days, they changed the rag and my foot healed up after a few changes."[117]

What are the caveats to be kept in mind in assessing the significance of Maj. Stewart's data? There are several. The figures for the amount of sickness are lower than would have been the case for the same group of men had they not been under severe pressures not to report ill. Rations were reduced for the sick, so many men who were unquestionably ill and who would, under more normal conditions, have been excused from work and possibly hospitalized, continued working. In most camps—perhaps all—the internal POW administration found ways to avoid cutting the rations of the sick directly; that is, they arranged for the total ration intake to be divided equally among the total number of POWs. Thus everyone went short because the intake for the sick was decreased. This provided another reason to be reluctant to go ill, since by doing so they shrank not only their own diet but also that of everyone in the camp.

Moreover, the sick who remained in camp were cut off from two sources of extra nourishment, sources that could be crucial to survival. POWs working outside were sometimes paid—trifling amounts, it is true, but nevertheless some additional food could be purchased. Also, those working outside often were able to steal food, or materials that could be bartered for food. These facts further increased the pressure on men to work even when unwell.

Despite the often desperate conditions, the men nevertheless did find the energy to put on a few "entertainments" at Niigata. Two Americans, Bill Barbour and George Francis, were largely responsible for the concerts.

> Anyone at 5B will not soon forget the two plays "Eadie was a Lady" nor "Romeo and Juliet." The bard of Avon might have been profoundly shocked if he could have heard Romeo borrowing Hamlet's speeches but an audience of POWs was not critical. The Jap camp staff enjoyed the third act of "Eadie was a Lady" so well they ordered it repeated a second time. Was it only a rumour that the commandant was disappointed when he discovered that Eadie was no lady but only Sgt. Neal masquerading as one? What would the commandant have thought if he could have seen Sonny Castro, in the "Biaderes," at Shamshuipo.[118]

Tom Forsyth remembered one splendid concert. "Red" Barlow played Little Red Riding Hood. He brought down the house when he cried in a shrill falsetto, "But Grandma, you've got a nose just like Huhmicky's."[119] Huhmicky, obviously, was "Grandma."

Christmas

Christmas 1944 turned out to be a great improvement over Christmas 1943. The day was declared a holiday and each man received an American Red Cross parcel. The kitchen staff had hoarded a few extras to give the men good meals on Christmas Day. "[A]long with the parcel I am sure everyone was full for once."120

Moreover, rarest of rare, mail had come in. One man received a letter from his brother, and it was only a year old. There was a photo enclosed, "the only photo I received while a prisoner, of Kay and the two little boys, Donald and Graeme, sitting beside the decorated Christmas tree. I really got a lump in my throat. Everyone around wanted to see the picture; if one man looked at it, I bet fifty did."121

Death and Burial

Death was a common and eventually almost banal event among the prisoners of war at Niigata. Few camps had a higher death rate. There were some fatalities in the sick period immediately after the Canadians arrived in September 1943, but the catastrophe that shocked the camp thoroughly was the collapse of the roof on 1 January 1944. Eight men died. "Next day I was one of three men detailed to put the dead men in their coffins. It was a cold day, snowing and blowing. We were shivering. The men lay stark naked in a row and cold as ice. The coffins, cheap, flimsy affairs roughly and crudely made, were too short for the bodies."122 The coffins had been designed for the smaller Japanese.

When the first deaths occurred in the autumn of 1943, the bodies were put beside a shed containing the water pump. Each morning and evening on the way to and from work, the POWs had to step over them. Soon the bodies were swollen and turning dark. The Japanese said they were waiting word from Tokyo to know what to do with the corpses. Ultimately, they took them out, on a three-wheel motorbike with a box on the back, to a local crematorium. A POW witness accompanied them and, after the cremation, they gave the witness chopsticks, instructing him to pick out a few bones. These were put in a box about eight inches square, labelled with the dead man's name and army number, and the box was put in a shrine.123

Similar ceremonies were observed at other Japanese camps, puzzling the POWs at this apparently sudden respect for men whom the Japanese had treated abominably for years. For example, at Hanawa Camp in October 1944:

> Our first death. He had been ill a couple weeks, diarrhea, malaria, and edema. Nips did nothing for him except a mouthwash. Though after death they gave him a hypo and put him in a room, set a bowl of apples at his feet, laid a couple of small bouquets of flowers by him and burned punk sticks all the time.

The following day this diarist, a medical officer, added: "They brought the ashes back from our boy. They are in a small crockery jar. They put them on the floor where the body lay. Still burning incense."[124]

At Niigata, the Japanese brought motorcycles and put the bodies in the sidecars, covered with blankets, to be transported downtown to the crematorium.[125] One dead Canadian was extra tall. "They said the legs were too long for them, too long for the motorcycle, so they made us cut the legs off at the knees, so it would make it easier for them to work with, once they left the POW camp."[126] On another occasion legs were broken to make them fit:

> I remember a couple of men dying who were tall men. One day I had to put one of these men in the bike. Rigor mortis had set in and you know anyone that's cold lying in bed is all curled up with their knees up under their chin. That's the way we slept there because we were always freezing. They had no heat in the buildings. They deliberately made us jump on the legs to break them and straighten them out. You could hear the bones cracking just like so much dry kindling as you stomped on them.[127]

When a Canadian sergeant died, he was put in a crude wooden coffin too small for his body. To to fit him in, a fellow prisoner had to break his legs and arms. The POWs made a coffin out of rough boards. The Japanese ordered a fellow POW to accompany the body. On the way to the crematory, he bumped around inside his coffin so much that it came apart, "and his limbs gradually slid out of the end of the coffin and dragged along on the road, but the drunken soldier who was driving the motorcycle didn't stop to repair the coffin, so the corpse was half dragged through the city streets to the amusement of the civilians and the Japanese driving the motorcycle."[128]

Tokyo Camp 3D, Kawasaki

To most westerners, the Japanese word Kawasaki conjures up images of motorcycles or electronic gear. But to the survivors among some 400-plus Allied ex-POWs, Kawasaki has a completely different meaning. These men were imprisoned in a camp in Kawasaki for more than two years from early 1943. To them, Kawasaki—then and now a western suburb of Tokyo—forcefully conjures up memories of painfully hard labour in the nearby shipyards, of biting winter cold from which there was no respite, and of gnawing, endless hunger.

Yet in many ways Kawasaki was one of the better camps. Or to put it differently, there were worse camps: Niigata with its horrendous death rate, or Oeyama where the men struggled with the psychological burden of finding that not only the Japanese but also some of their supposed allies were acting against them. There were many reasons why Kawasaki was different. One positive factor was the medical officer, Capt. John Reid, RCAMC, the only Canadian officer to leave Hong Kong with a labour draft to Japan. In Reid the Kawasaki POWs had a man of integrity and vigour who worked tirelessly to benefit his men. I have not heard any former inmate of the camp speak other than positively of him. Many camps, including Niigata and Oeyama, had energetic, devoted medical officers, but for the Canadian prisoners it was a special benefit to have a Canadian medical officer, a man they had known for years, as their MO.

Originally (and throughout this book) known as Kawasaki 3D, on 6 August 1943 the camp name was changed to Tokyo POW Camp 3D. The letter "D" was used to indicate camps that were detached from the army and instead were under industrial management, though all such camps had army commandants.[129]

Mostly, the men worked at the Nihon Kokan Shipbuilding Yard. Kawasaki was a new camp, not quite finished when the prisoners arrived in early 1943. It consisted of two large huts, each accommodating 250 men.[130]

There were almost 500 Canadians at Kawasaki 3D. One characteristic they noticed immediately was the remarkable authority given to Japanese junior officers and NCOs. NCOs did jobs officers would do in any western army. Typically, Japanese POW camps were commanded by a 2nd/Lt. or 1st/Lt., with a sergeant or corporal in day-to-day control in camp, and two or three privates.[131]

One of the greatest differences between Kawasaki 3D and other camps was the fact that at Kawasaki they had the good fortune to have a few helpful and humane Japanese in charge. Dr. Reid's Japanese counterpart, Dr. Inoue, was most helpful. He never interfered with Reid's assessment of sickness and, even more remarkably, became "a good personal friend whose conversation, books, flowers and general tolerance and education do honour to our profession and make a bright spot in my routine here."[132] Moreover, Reid characterized Lt. Uwamori, the camp commandant, as a gentleman whose regime was most understanding. One important consequence was that instances of physical punishment were few and soon became negligible.[133]

The men had left Hong Kong after enduring numerous inoculations and isolation for a week. Besides Reid, the two other accompanying officers were Maj. Robertson, RAMC; and Surg/Cmdr. Page, Royal Navy. The draft of 650 left on 19 January 1943 on the *Tatuta Maru*, a large luxury ship that provided an atypically fast, safe voyage.[134]

They landed at Kobe and from there went by train to Kawasaki, between Tokyo and Yokohama. On the train the men sat packed in rows, forbidden to move. In the memory of one of them, that trip took a part of a day and a night and into the next day,[135] a distance of about 300 miles (450 km). Arriving at Kawasaki with 499 Canadian POWs, having left 150 at Kobe, Reid made the disconcerting discovery that 17 percent of the men had malaria.

Capt. Reid described the camp at some length. It looked a bad camp, bare and squalid. Typically, the huts were one-storey, with sleeping areas on a raised shelf, each individual place marked off by a strip of lath. There was no heating system or arrangement, and the roofs leaked.[136]

In all camps, the serving of food became a source of worry, paranoia, and—all too often—theft. Servers were changed often, sometimes because of hanky-panky. Promise of a cigarette could cause a server to pack one bowl more firmly than the rest, thus squeezing in more food. The nourishing value of the soup depended on how deep a man dipped the ladle, since the few vegetables settled at the bottom. "In our section, [Lionel] Speller lasted longest and somehow managed to rise above the clouds of hostile suspicion and twisted paranoia."[137]

Capt. Reid was assigned the combined tasks of being commanding officer and medical officer. He found this draining.[138] Nevertheless, he continued to hold both jobs for many trying months. Details of one problem that can epitomize Reid's non-medical responsibilities are those involving the alleged beatings and torture of Ernest M. West, James Reuben Pattingale, and Mitchell Soroka, Canadian Army.[139] This matter became the chief charge against the interpreter, Kondo Kanechi, at his 1946 trial.

West, caught trading clothing to a civilian for food and cigarettes, was beaten severely by several Japanese NCOs, including Kondo. Pattingale became implicated and was beaten. These beatings lasted for an hour or more daily for several days, the fury of the Japanese increasing when it was found that a pair of Japanese army boots had also been traded. West initially refused to say where he got the boots but, when he had been held on half rations for 10 or 11 days, he weakened. Then there are two stories: one, that Soroka came forward and confessed that the boots were his, the other that West named Soroka. The violence now was turned on Soroka.

Ultimately, a Japanese court martial was held in Tokyo. West and Soroka had no lawyers (Pattingale was not tried). Kondo appeared as a witness and, according to his statement, he was able to sway the court to give reduced sentences: "for an offense which would have brought a Japanese soldier at least five years, West received only eight months and Sirocca [sic] about two months."[140] West and Soroka served their time in the state penitentiary in Tokyo, where they said they were fairly treated, and then returned to Kawasaki.[141] At his own trial, Kondo was found guilty and sentenced to one year at hard labour.

This is the kind of situation that must have confirmed Capt. Reid's preference for limiting his duties to the medical side. As the SBO, Reid would have been heavily involved in protesting the beatings to the Japanese, in trying to find out from his men exactly what had happened, and in trying to work out a strategy to resolve the mess with minimal damage. Meanwhile the bulk of the men went about their daily lives, working in the shipyards, queuing for food, reporting for sick call, all with the backdrop of their colleagues being beaten noisily at various locations around the camp, sprayed with cold water, and then locked in the crude jail.

The dispute shows clearly the inevitability of clashes between POWs and camp administration. The men were hungry and wanted cigarettes. They had brought extra clothing with them from Hong Kong. Japanese civilians by 1944 were short of clothing. Yet it was a crime to trade away or sell your equipment in the Japanese army. When someone was known to be involved in an offence it was routine Japanese military practice to beat the accused to get him to confess. (The *Kempeitai* had subtler but infinitely crueller methods for persuading compliance—fortunately these butchers were not involved in this case.) Given the ingredients, conflict was inevitable.

Reid had attempted to use trading within the camp as a means of occupying the POWs' minds. About trading, a former Winnipeg Grenadier recalled:

> Now, some people always get stung. There always has to be, there always has to be a winner somewhere, eh? Some guy might end up, from half a parcel, he could end up with one and a half; somebody else could lose all his parcel. This, Dr. Reid wouldn't stop. As a matter of fact he put a board up, just outside where his little room was, on a post there. This was the daily market: a square of chocolate was worth one package of cigarettes. In some parcels you got prunes, and in other ones you got raisins; well, raisins are worth a package of prunes plus something else....Dr. Reid felt that even though that guy was losing the parcel, what he was going to get out of it wasn't going to do that much for him anyway, because you only get a little bit. So he was getting more out of this parcel in trading, to keep his mind off all the other things. And it's true.[142]

One Canadian medical orderly, Pat Poirier, exercised—not entirely willingly—with his MO. They had a medicine ball that weighed 12 pounds. The other medical orderlies refused to take part, claiming they hadn't the strength, so Reid would "pick on the Frenchman—on me—'Now, Poirier, you come and play with the medicine ball.' Every time he threw that ball I used to be backed up about three or four feet."[143]

One day Reid had asked an orderly to check the temperature of a patient with a high fever. The orderly returned to report and the doctor turned his head just as Poirier threw the ball; it hit Reid in the stomach, and he went down. "I went over, to give him aid to bring him back up, and he said, 'Go away, God damn you, you almost killed me! Wait until I get back here; you are going to get it!' Anyway he used to call me 'Poirier-for-the-medicine-ball.' I used to hate that because it took part of my strength."[144]

Occasionally there was some communication with home and loved ones. Once a batch of about 300 letters arrived in camp, divided among about 100 of the men. Most got none. In June 1943 they had the experience of recording messages from 40 men, plus a musical program, for rebroadcast to Canada.[145] "Some of the boys had written some music, we had the instruments, ukeles [sic], and this orchestra broadcast some numbers on this first broadcast. They actually broadcast a number one of the boys wrote and here it was copyrighted and it has been played some, and he is going to get some money I suppose."[146]

The Japanese Army medical college established a special group to investigate the health problems of POWs. One of the conclusions combines nicely the attributes of Japanese xenophobia, humaneness, and empiricism:

> When our people are going through hardship and deprivations there is no need to satisfy to the full the desires of the prisoners of war whose countries have been satiated with natural wealth. It would be enough to guarantee for them the lowest standard of living allowable from the humane standpoint. On the other hand, however, when we face the question from the point of view of the utilization of their labour it proves necessary to preserve their health and ensure their working ability by creating good living conditions which will improve their labour efficiency.[147]

At the shipyards of Nihon Kokan, Will Allister laboured as a ship's painter. He decided that he would move like an old man. That would be his personal battle: both a kind of sabotage and an aid to his own survival. "The Japanese painters gossiped about us and I was nicknamed *suromoshon*, slow motion. I found a tortoise painted on my locker to confirm the success of my campaign."[148] (Allister's book catches as well as anyone has the psychological workings of prisoner-of-war life and its impact.)

Pat Poirier also became a painter at Nihon Kokan, in a paint gang of about 15 men. With brushes about a foot wide and an inch thick they slathered on five gallons of paint in the morning and five gallons in the afternoon. Other men did different jobs, some working with an oxygen tank, others becoming iron markers, some learning a trade working with chisels and other tools.[149] Lionel Speller also laboured for months in the shipyard, but the Japanese learned that he was a shoemaker and set him up in camp with a shop, to repair the men's shoes and keep them on the job.[150]

The company supplied a few medicines. In April 1943 a contribution came from Nihon Kokan of about 250,000 fish-liver-extract tablets.[151] Three months later, the POWs received two batches of medicine paid for by the company. But by late 1943 supplies of many kinds were short all over Japan. Dr. Reid observed that even the Japanese were lousy, in spite of not living in the same filthy conditions. They bathed more frequently and could get some soap, though much less than in peacetime.[152]

The shortages quickly impacted on POW life. In October 1943 Nihon Kokan told the men they could no longer meet their requirements for medicines, though they still supplied Mercurochrome and some bandages. Aspirin was unobtainable. Reid was able to buy at some nearby drug stores a thousand aspirin, plus some trianon, sulfanilamide, and quinine.[153] Work became the ultimate necessity for all POWs. Dr. Reid had to saw wood in order to be assigned food. "Medical work did not count, you had to be producing in Japan, so I sawed wood."[154]

At great personal risk, many of the men found ways to sabotage the Japanese war effort. At shipyard launchings, for example, some ships, when they hit the water, were unseaworthy.[155] The saws used to cut steel girders were made in England and Scotland, and the Japanese had only a limited supply. So Harold Englehart broke saws.

> It wasn't difficult to break them—if you twisted the steel girder, the saws would break. But you had to do it when they weren't watching because they were working there too. And it was pretty dangerous, because when this saw broke there was pieces flying everywhere. They were unaware what I was doing. I told them the saws were made in England and were no good compared with Japanese saws.[156]

It is, of course, impossible to document this activity with certainty or to quantify it.

In December 1943 Nihon Kokan formed a special group of POWs called the slow-walking group, beriberi patients who were required to work but were able to proceed to the shipyard only at a slow pace.[157] The problem of keeping the sick in camp rather than working became worse in February 1944. A new IJA sergeant took over a section of POWs; Sgt. Ino, according to Reid, was a hypocritical, cruel individual. "He has taken over full medical responsibility for his section and has stated that I am no longer to take his men off work."[158] Consequently, Reid began to see men who were literally totally exhausted. This was not the physical exhaustion of home, but that of POW days "in which a man is unable to stand any longer."[159]

A remarkable event took place during this painful winter: Reid, under pressure to send more men, and with Uwamori beginning to switch his support away, "more or less handed in my resignation....[Uwamori] thought it over for twenty-four hours and then said okay, you go back."[160] Neither action nor reaction was customary.

The medical college study referred to (on page 257) contains a revealing paragraph that makes clear a major reason for this investigation: "We also fear that those prisoners of war who have lived under unhealthy conditions in the fighting zone and have contracted various diseases might carry epidemics to our people on their being transported to our homeland and put to work in all areas as labour material. It is not only for their health but also for the safety of our own people that we should give thorough consideration to maintaining them in good health."[161]

The investigating medical team noted that many POWs were down 20 to 30 percent in body weight. The report alerted its recipients to the necessity to prepare for much sickness in the POW camps and hospitals, and noted the potential need for special foods suiting the prisoners' taste; they seemed not to like rice-gruel.[162] Some statistics showed that dysentery and diphtheria carriers were included in the men brought to Japan. Although these Japanese physicians were observant and prescient, their findings evidently fell on deaf ears, a fate common to all armies.

Because their warnings went unheeded, the medical situation among POWs became much worse than it might have been. We can easily feel both pity and empathy for the POW patients. But we should also remember the intense frustration that burdened the lives of their medical officers who, despite the best of training and of intentions, could do so little for their men. After the war, Reid explained his strategy in dealing with the Japanese medical staff:

> I always tried to get these Nips to the place where we were fairly friendly—they thought so anyway—and my request would carry some weight and they would do what we wanted them to do. If they didn't like you and you wanted a man off work, it didn't go. If they did and you wanted a man off work, it did and that's about the size of it.[163]

Reid commended several medical orderlies who were at Kawasaki, including Mel McKnight, Morgan ("the best nursing orderly I ever had"), Matheson, Sgt. Veale, and Sgt. Mulcahy.[164] Reid, when he was the only medical officer in camp, had a personal medical nightmare: "One night I thought I had appendicitis and thought I would have to operate on myself but it passed off during the morning and there was no recurrence."[165] On one occasion, two Canadian POWs were taken into the company hospital and each operated on, with no anesthetic. One went in after the other. "The first one didn't scream because the other one was following him. But, the second one did. Can you imagine having an operation without that?"[166] Once, Ken Gaudin had a bad accident, injuring his back and leg. He had a bone in his leg scraped "without benefit of anesthetic."[167] Dr. Reid was told by the Japanese doctor that his inability to transfer cases to outside hospitals was because there was only one military hospital for all the POW camps in the Tokyo-Yokohama area and the maximum number of patients allowed at any one time was 30. But acute surgical cases could be sent to the civilian hospital connected with the shipyard where the men worked.

At one point in 1943, Reid had excused from work about 160 men daily, of whom 110 had beriberi of such severity that they were excused without argument by the Japanese. Each working man received a full ration of rice and barley daily, the men who are off work but not in hospital get two-thirds of a ration, and only one-half for the hospitalized men. They pooled all rations received and each man drew an equal share. The consequence was that everyone in camp was on shorter rations, "giving rise to a downhill course for those doing heavy physical labour and a downhill course for the beriberis and other nutritional diseases."[168] The camp collectively lost 3,000 pounds in August 1943 and 1,000 pounds in September, an average of six pounds per man one month and two pounds per man the other.[169] The Japanese doctors continually tried to send sick men to work, but Lt. Uwamori continued to back Reid's judgment and let him keep in those he felt needed the rest urgently.[170] Reid outlined his medical strategy for the men under his care:

> The policy I've always held as the final criterion in this episode is to consider the main factor is not illness nor even disability that may be more or less permanent, but to consider as the main factor the danger to life in the reasonably near future. I think all the Canadian medical officers have held this criterion before them. Thus my endeavour here is to take back as many men as possible to Canada whether well or ill and not to concentrate on complete health. I would rather return with five hundred men in various stages of beriberi, which perhaps in the future could be cured, than to return three hundred men in good health and leave two hundred dead behind.[171]

In the spring of 1943, for the first time, patients travelled to an outside hospital—three men with severe beriberi.[172] Eventually, all the men who had beriberi improved. The disease eventually vanished from the camp over a period of a year and a half.[173]

On 1 August 1943, 22 isolated infectious cases (20 patients with amoebic dysentery, 1 diphtheria carrier, 1 case of tuberculosis) and four general hospital cases were sent to the new POW hospital at Shinagawa.[174] Several of the amoebic carriers returned from Shinagawa in October 1943; they had been given 10 injections of emetine but some still had enteritis. They had lost an average of another 16-17 lbs. "After much argument I prevented a further three patients from being sent to the hospital as I felt they had a much better chance of getting well in camp than in Shinagawa."[175]

After tests showed that 49 percent of the men had positive tests for tuberculosis, Reid was offered BCG vaccine for them and declined. But one night the Japanese medical staff suddenly appeared in camp; all POWs previously negative to the tuberculosis test were injected with BCG vaccine. "This was done after considerable argument—I argued—I was very much against giving any of the men BCG."[176] The use of this vaccine remained a controversial subject until long after the war.

Reid had to buy whatever medicines he could outside the camp. Once he noted that he had spent 70 yen for drugs and supplies the previous night (the value of the yen before the war was about $0.25 Canadian), including Trianon, sulphur ointment for scabies, bismuth, thermometers, and yeast.[177] "I am beginning to collect 5% of the men's wages to keep a reserve of medicine. Previously I spent my own money."[178]

Supplies of all kinds were grossly inadequate: "we only had three needles, and they had to do; that's what they had to use all along. So these things were so blunt that they had to throw them. Lots of times you'd walk away with the needle in you still, and they'd call you back and pull it out."[179] The men found that there was essentially no paper in Japan—certainly nothing that could substitute for toilet paper. The men had to use their hands to clean themselves, wiping them on the wall when they were finished. "They had no soap and only cold water. We had an antiseptic solution around and so on, but it was pretty terrific from our viewpoint."[180]

Sometimes the system worked. In June 1943, Pte. Zytaruk, WG, had an accident at work: "He was removed to the Company hospital, the hospital operated in connection with the Company; the fracture was fixed with silver wire and a brass plate, the leg splinted with hip abduction, extension of the knee and full extension of the foot. I saw the patient on the morning of June 12th and his general condition was excellent. The Japanese had operated. They took him right off from where it occurred to the hospital."[181] Certainly this patient had prompt and apparently appropriate treatment.

On 30 December 1943, an American medical officer, Lt/Cmdr. E.V. Dockweiler, USN, and Ensign Pollak, USN, arrived in camp.[182] Later, another American medical officer, Maj. Kagy, arrived also, coming in with a group of American POWs. According to some of the men, they much preferred Reid. Kagy had come from Niigata 5B, where the roof had fallen in; after that tragedy it seemed that he had little empathy for the Kawasaki POWs. "After what he had seen, this was nothing."[183]

At Kawasaki, the disease that became especially troublesome during the winter of 1943-44 was an unusual type of pneumonia associated with pleurisy.[184] Reid had no opportunity in camp to do any laboratory work.[185] Medical supplies became less and less available. On 11 March 1944, Reid was told by the Asano company doctor that they had no sulfapyridine in their hospital. Reid was advised to use quinine, "which was just as good," and that there was no prospect of getting Trianon or any form of sulfapyridine or sulfathiazole in the future. Moreover, white blood counts had become too inconvenient for them to do for the camp.[186] Conditions were worsening rapidly.

As was common for most camps, the men interviewed after the war could remember little or no homosexuality being evident. Yet, as Roy Robinson pointed out:

> You bunked together. It didn't happen in North Point and not in Sham Shui Po, there it was pretty hot; but when you got to 3-D, to Kawasaki, and when we went up north to the mine, it got cold, and you bunked together. Each man had three or four blankets and there were several ingenious methods of making a bed so that you couldn't kick it out, double folded over. And two fellows bunked together. It was everybody, just about. There was the odd fellow that was just maybe a little too dirty so that no one would have anything to do with him. But 90 percent of the people at least bunked together. And then no. Whether I was naive or what, I don't know, but I can honestly say that it wasn't there.[187]

Probably he was mistaken, though such tendencies were hidden as carefully as possible six decades ago.

Food, Malnutrition, and Sickness

One "medicine" that Reid guarded closely had come with them from Hong Kong. In preparation for the trip, the Japanese had issued bully beef. Surplus cans—about 150—were turned over to Reid on arrival in Japan. "I lugged it into camp with me and that was the basis for treating some of the sick people for a long time."[188]

Eating rice three times a day for three and a half years proved a depressingly monotonous diet for the POWs, who became ingenious in finding ways to alter the flavour. They used anything, including highly questionable items, to season their rice. A favourite was Japanese-issue tooth powder. Once, the Japanese gave them a tub of grease intended for shoes; it was found to improve rice.[189]

About February or March of 1944, the officials from Nihon Kokan began supplying one meal of unpolished rice daily and thiamine pills to all beriberi patients sick enough to be excused from work.[190] About the same time, some dried pears and breakfast food, plus 1,200 cans of corned beef, arrived in camp from the Red Cross.[191] "We are told that the Japanese intend to continue to cut food until they find the least amount we can live on....They kept on cutting these rations now for the next six months."[192] Dr. Reid protested, to no avail.

Weight losses were always impressive and sometimes profound. Reid noted that late in the war he was at his lowest weight since he was 11 years of age (143 pounds).[193] Less protected than a medical officer, at war's end Colin Standish, at Narumi, found that he weighed 71 pounds, having gone into the camp at 175.[194]

At Kawasaki, some of the men received the Japanese traditional medical treatment known as moxibustion, which was discussed earlier in this chapter. Moxibustion is further examined in a separate section at the end of this chapter, dealing with the collective experience of prisoners of war.

The Japanese apparently expected giants when their POW labourers arrived from the south. The clothing supplied was so large that "we looked like walking tents. We rolled up the pant legs and sleeves. This was no fashion show, we gathered, but it was certainly a circus. The small men disappeared in a sea of cotton. Marching to work, four abreast, we were a wonderful sight to behold—straggling, bumbling, clumping along as though in time to some dissonant arrhythmic music."[195]

The barrack huts in the camp were poorly heated, so Dr. Reid made a bargain. He offered the official army interpreter an exchange. Reid would shave his head if the private would get them some stoves. Happily, the private was a sporting man who thought this was amusing; if Reid followed through, he would get the stoves, four for each hut.[196] Reid shaved. The stoves arrived. The men warmed up a little.

But stoves are useless without fuel. In mid-January 1944, shipments of coal ceased. For several weeks, the POWs tore out most of the insides of the huts, under Japanese supervision, to get enough wood for fuel so that they could cook their food. The Japanese had proven quite unable to obtain fuel elsewhere.[197]

In his debriefing in 1945, John Reid revealed how clearly he saw the complex situation within which they had lived for almost four years. It was emphatically not a black-and-white subject:

> That's one thing you have to remember—whatever they gave us they were looking at from their angle...there were times in Japan when we got as much as the civilians, never as much as the Army—the only thing the civilians had over us, they had a tremendous black market and they could get some things which we could not get. Houses and clothing were the same thing; according to our standards atrocious, according to their standards very much the same thing from the time they were born until they die.[198]

And Will Allister pointed out that they saw clearly how badly it was going for Japan. There was little meat or fish, as the prisoners could see every day at lunchtime; often the Japanese labourers had only a few pickled vegetables with rice in their lunch boxes. "Some told us that rice was scarce at home, sometimes non-existent. And of course when rations grew tight, the *furyos* [POWs] were the first to feel it."199

On one occasion, a combined parcel arrived from the Red Cross and the YMCA. Included were some second-hand phonographs and records (but no needles), carpenter tools, baseball mitts, checkers and chess, ping-pong nets and bats, a mandolin, a ukelele, and three harmonicas.200

Sometimes Red Cross parcels arrived, but the POWs had to wait for Japanese permission to use them, perhaps as long as six months.201 In trials after the war, many Japanese defendants claimed local supplies of food were so scanty that they felt it necessary to save the packages against possible starvation in the camps, if the war continued indefinitely—as Japanese warlords assured the people that it would. And because of the sinking of the *Awa Maru* on 1 April 1945 by the American submarine USS *Queenfish*, the likelihood that any further supplies of Red Cross materials would be allowed into Japan was slight indeed.

Deaths

In addition to his responsibilities as senior POW officer and as medical officer, Reid also assumed the duties of chaplain when there were deaths. It was the rule that a Buddhist ceremony must take place with a Buddhist priest. The camp Commandant would then say a few words and then "I may say what I please."202 For example, on 22 December 1943, Sgt. Goodnough, RRC, died of pneumonia. This was the fourth death among these men in Japan. First there was a Buddhist service conducted by a priest, who was paid by the company. Then the POWs had their service. Six sergeants served as pall-bearers, hymns were sung by the chorus, and "The Last Post" and reveille were blown.203 No other dignified handling of funeral rites in any Japanese camp has come to light. In general, dignity did not exist.

Dr. Reid found no evidence of religious conversion as conditions worsened. A man's convictions didn't change when he was about to die and he didn't speak about them when he thought he was going to die. No POW, Reid believed, suddenly became a Christian if he had not been a Christian before, and nobody seemed particularly interested in any religion at the end, "they just went out without any comments."204

In the spring of 1945 many of the men were sent to Suwa POW Camp, where they laboured at open-pit iron ore mining. Suwa was considered (by the Japanese) a camp for troublemakers.205 W/C Leonard Birchall, RCAF, was senior officer there; POWs could not speak too highly of him as a man and as a leader.

Omine

Omine Camp, also known as Fukuoka POW Camp 5B and as Omine Camp 8D, was located near the little town of Kawasaki on Kyushu

Island in Japan, in a small community located at Omine.[206] This camp must be distinguished from the POW camp in the Tokyo suburb of Kawasaki that was known by that name, and which also contained a large complement of Canadian prisoners.

Kyushu is the southernmost and third largest of the main islands, separated from Shikoku by Bungo Strait and from Honshu by Shimonoseki Strait. Kyushu has a subtropical climate marked, as the POWs readily testify, by torrential rainfalls. The island's heavy industry has always been located in the north part of Kyushu because of proximity to Japan's oldest coal fields; the POWs were sent to Omine to mine coal.

The Japanese commandant from 23 January to July 1943 was Lt. Yanaru Tetsutoshi.[207] Yanaru established codes of conduct on daily activities such as saluting: "If you had a hat on you would be required to salute in the Japanese style with your index and second finger touching the right brim of your cap, or if you had no hat on, you would have to come to attention and bow."[208]

The drill at the time of leaving Hong Kong is a familiar one: "About the 10th of January we were called out on parade on the main road of the camp leading down in front of our huts. We were all put on one side of the road and an interpreter told all the men who could walk properly to walk across the road to the other side." This selection process did not produce enough men, so the Japanese guards went down the other side of the road, where the "unfit" were, and simply picked out men here and there arbitrarily. In this way the required 1,200 were chosen.[209]

They sailed from Hong Kong on 19 January 1943 on the *Tatsuo Maru*, landed at Nagasaki on 22 January 1943—an unusually rapid and comfortable trip—and travelled by train from there to Omine. Maj. Robertson took charge of the draft from Nagasaki to Omine. Sgts. Roberts and Churchman, both RAMC, acted as medical orderlies.[210] The men arrived at the camp on 23 January 1943, 163 Canadian and 37 British POWs.[211]

At Omine, Maj. H.G.G. Robertson, RAMC, was the senior POW officer, a position he held until the war ended two and a half years later. Though a medical officer, he was forbidden to practise his profession by the Japanese except in a limited way under direct orders from the mine physician. Robertson knew of no explanation for this curious and harmful order. For more than a year, until Maj. J. Smith, MC, USA, arrived, there was no functioning medical officer in the camp. Smith was then put in charge of the medical arrangements of the camp until the surrender of Japan. About a year later several Dutch and British medical officers arrived.[212]

On arrival at Omine the POWs' physical condition was examined under the direction of 2nd Lt. Kaneko. Many men had imported illnesses from Hong Kong. The chief complaints were beriberi and skin diseases, and the majority were suffering from bad eyes; they assumed that the causes were lack of Vitamin B and other vitamins.[213]

In May they had their first planned recreation. "I played Volley Ball with *San Shonti* against *Ni Shonti*" [No. 3 Shift vs No. 2 Shift].[214] Later that month the Japanese ordered that all notebooks and pencils were to be handed in. No reason was given, of course, but many clandestine diaries ended at about this time.

The Allied prisoners of war imprisoned in the Omine Camp were employed by the Furakawa Mining Company in their Omine Mine No. 2. This work continued from the opening of the camp on 23 January 1943 until Japan's surrender in August 1945.[215]

When the men arrived they found two inclined shafts leading underground, one of which was in operation, one blocked by a cave-in. On the surface were mine offices, winch houses, a blacksmith shop, and a site for making concrete blocks. No coal was being mined from this section of the mine. "We later worked our way down into the coal and it began coming up from the point we started working."[216]

On 28 January 1943 the men were issued their work clothing: "One pr Rubber boots with split toe, 1 pr. black shorts & coat cotton, Rubber Belt. Handkerchief for the lunch. Miners hat & water bottle."[217] By 14 February 1943, the men had started to trade their clothes for cigarettes.[218]

One hundred and seventy-six men went to the mines when work began on 2 February 1943. They were first trained in the use of picks, scraping boards, and name tags. In addition, they learned the Japanese symbols needed to identify such items as mine-pillars and stone-hauling cars.[219] Instruction ended after one day and work began in the mine on 3 February 1943. The first Canadian to enter the mine was Sgt. Lance Ross. It was, they quickly found, very hot below the surface.[220]

Directions for the mine workers were preserved in the papers of F.W. Ebdon. Some excerpts give insight into how the Japanese viewed their hapless labourers:

> Part 1: 1. When going to work inside mines you must have medical examination. 3. When medical examination is held, let the doctor examine you without your saying anything. Part 9: 2. Never touch power lines. When people are sweating or have a weak heart it takes only 50 Voltage of electricity to cause one's death. Part 13: 5. As much as possible regulate bowel movements and do your business before leaving, or on arrival back in camp. Part 14: 7. One who has been accidentally hurt must be treated like a brother. By ones kindness wounded people will keep courage and strength.[221]

By 8 March 1943, the reality of enforced labour was evident. Eighteen men reported sick, complaining of cramps and diarrhea; they were ordered back down into the mine. A month later Sgt. Ross lamented: "I have dysentery, passing blood but I have to go to work just the same. There are about 15 with it, one poor fellow fainted and we had to carry him."[222] Nevertheless, some were ill enough so that even the Japanese realized they could not work. Thus on 17 April 1943, only 49 men out of a working party of 64 were at work. The remainder were sick with fever and diarrhea.[223]

The state of the mines was frightful and frightening, the work dangerous and exhausting. Shafts were constructed to accommodate the much smaller Japanese bodies. Therefore, the POWs had to stoop constantly and painfully. One survivor remembered it like this:

> The timbering was stuff that had been in there for years and was kind of rotting, breaking through in spots due to the fact that the mine had been out of operation, the shaft had been out of operation for sometime. There was a lot of loose rock on the walls and ceiling that dropped down every now and then. The ventilation was exceptionally bad with no air-line in there for ventilation purposes. With the cave-in, the position of the cave-in was above where we were working, and therefore no air could come down from the surface to us. What air was in the shaft was that air which circulated down underground and was on its way back up again. This caused us considerable discomfort, the dust from the drills and the dynamite smoke. It was also very damp down in there, the water running down the shaft, and later on we ran a pipeline down for concreting purposes. The pipes were leaking very badly and caused a lot of discomfort with wet feet and so on.[224]

At Omine they mined soft coal. Men well enough to do heavy labour made up a party that worked in the mine itself, while a group of men not physically fit for underground work laboured on the surface, loading sand, gravel, and cement, and making cement blocks used for retaining walls in the mine. The Japanese called the latter group the *Aows*, and the Canadians translated this into The Blues.[225] Once, a prisoner saw men taken on stretchers to work. They might only perform some small tasks on the surface or in the vegetable garden, "but you had to work."[226]

A Japanese army medical officer was stationed at Fukuoka Headquarters. He visited the camp once a week. Maj. Robertson testified: "He was in official charge and I was allowed to do certain medical work by his permission, but I was not allowed to run the MI room or look after the sick on my own authority."[227]

There was a recreation room available to prisoners at first, from after work until roll call. But after one month it was converted into a hospital and no one was allowed in but patients and the medical staff. A man could visit his friends for about an hour each evening. This recreation room/hospital had steam heating, and was the only building in camp with a permanent heating installation.[228]

By mid-February 1943, the men had been given at least seven inoculations or vaccinations, some of them in the skin of the back near the shoulder blades. So some attention was being given to keeping them healthy. Unfortunately, what they needed was good food, warm clothing, and rest. These were not forthcoming. "I wonder when it is going to end?...TIME MARCHES ON. 1 year 5 w. 3 days: 403 days."229

As with all camps, Omine was guided by official regulations. One of these, in typically garbled English translation, refers to food. It was a rule the POWs found no difficulty adhering to: "Endeavour not to make remnant."230 The British medical officer at Omine believed that the amount and quality of food supplied was extremely poor. But, he added, "in fairness it must be admitted that it was not much worse than the Japanese Army personnel in the camp were getting and it was also greater in quantity than the civilian mine workers were getting." Maj. Robertson believed that most prisoners who ate their full rations managed to survive the war. The men could do their work "though with considerable discomfort and with some loss in weight."231

On 26 February 1943, F.W. Ebdon noted that his weight was down to 103 lb. He and his fellow POWs had lost three or four pounds in recent weeks. "Hope now they will give us some more food."232 One component of the food was unappreciated despite its protein content: maggots. Some men sought dark corners to eat their food so that they wouldn't have to see the maggots as they spooned them in.233

Many men had trouble with culturally forbidden foods: "If a stray dog came in the camp, somebody would kill it. You would hear a yelp and so forth. But I tasted broth, just a spoonful of broth, from soup made from a dog one time, and one spoonful of broth that some guy had made from a snake. Other than that, I didn't try to find... I'd just starve to death. I couldn't bring myself to do that."234 Most men were less squeamish—or found ways to make themselves less so.

Nor did the arrival of Red Cross parcels necessarily improve the food shortage. On at least one occasion, parcels were received but not distributed. The Japanese camp commander refused to let the men have them, reasoning that if the Allies invaded Japan, Red Cross food might be their only food.235

Compared with most camps, Omine apparently had well-con-structed quarters. Opinions differ as to the pre-war use of the struc-ture, one source identifying it as the Omine Hotel,236 while another claimed it was an old sanitarium.237

> We get to Omine, we found that there was a two story building enclosed by a twelve foot wooden fence. The building was of the usual Japanese construction of wood with the sliding doors and windows. It was very poor construction. The windows didn't fit properly and there were plen-ty of gaps where the window sashes were put onto the actual building. The place was infested with fleas which didn't make themselves appar-

ent until the warm weather came along. There was no heating system in the prisoners' rooms. There were mats on the floor, but no other furniture.[238]

The prisoners' living quarters consisted of about 25 rooms, each about 10 by 20 feet and divided in half by sliding doors. Eight men lived in each room. There was no furniture in the western sense. A charcoal pot was used as an ashtray. There were mats on the floors. At each end of the room was a large cupboard for clothing and other personal effects. Another small cupboard was used to keep mining clothing in, to keep it separated from the men's other belongings so that they wouldn't get dirty. Bedding was a thin mattress and five Japanese army blankets.[239]

The quarters may have been better than most camps, but work conditions remained grim. The usual diseases became prevalent. Food was inadequate in quality and quantity. The men who died first, according to one POW, were "the big heavy fat guys that had enormous appetites....I was considered a very light eater, and that may have saved my life."[240]

Narumi Camp (Fukuoka Camp No. 2), Nagoya

As usual, the changing Japanese designations for this camp are a source of ongoing confusion. Osaka POW Camp No. 11 Branch Camp (Narumi), or Narumi 11B, was established 28 December 1943; on 6 April 1945 it was transferred to Nagoya District and was known as Nagoya POW Camp No. 2 Branch Camp (Narumi), or Narumi 2B, until September 1945.[241]

Narumi was located 10 km south and east of the city centre of Nagoya, just north of the Meitetsu Nagoya main railway line. Nagoya is on Honshu Island, in the prefecture of Aichi, and is a port on the Pacific Ocean about 200 km west of Tokyo.

One Canadian POW thought that the Narumi Camp looked like a Hollywood-style Indian fort. It was built of wooden posts and staves, with wooden gates cut into the wooden fences. There was one main gate and a couple of smaller gates, with the main gate facing the mountain. The camp had been constructed for POWs.

There were four barracks for Canadian and British POWs and four more for Americans, plus a cookhouse and the Japanese quarters. Each barrack building held about 200 men. The barracks had double-decker bunks, each bed about five feet by two feet, covered by a straw mat. Any tall man necessarily overlapped his bed. At the head of each bed a shelf held shaving equipment and other belongings. The men had little.[242] "I kept two or three lizards. I'd give them a little bit of rice and they would keep the bed bugs down."[243]

The Commandants were Lt. Tanaka Hiroshi (28 December 1943 to 6 April 1945)[244] and Okada Miyoroku (6 April 1945 till war's end).[245] Later, war crimes courts sentenced Tanaka to 16 years and Okada to 50 years at hard labour, both having been found guilty on many counts of brutality at Narumi.

Following the Japanese surrender in August 1945, the Narumi commandant, Okada, argued that since he and his personnel were now prisoners of war they should be entitled under the Geneva Convention to food and shelter. That, the POWs observed ironically, was the first indication he had given that he knew the terms of the Geneva Convention.[246]

On 13 December 1943 a draft of POWs left Hong Kong. The fifth draft, it included 204 members of the Hong Kong Volunteer Defence Corps (HKVDC), 200 British regulars, and 97 Canadians. On 18 December they entered the harbour at Takao, Formosa, and three days later the men were transferred to the 8,000-ton *Toyama Maru*. On 5 January 1944 they reached Moji and on the 7th they arrived at Narumi Camp, Nagoya.[247]

Seven months later the camp population swelled with the addition of 199 Americans from the Philippines.[248] There were also crews of two Dutch and two Free French submarines. The French all died; they died, Colin Standish believed, because they gave up. They suffered severely from pneumonia and pleurisy.[249]

One major complaint voiced by the prisoners, during the war and at the war crimes trial afterwards, was the alleged ban on the wearing of overcoats in the cold Japanese winter. A member of the Winnipeg Grenadiers stated that early in 1945, some prisoners of war who were sick and confined to the camp area broke this regulation and wore their greatcoats in camp during the day. The weather was below freezing at the time, and all prisoners who were not working were suffering from the cold. Some of these men were caught by the Japanese.

> As I left my hut I saw Rodgers and the three other Englishmen being forced by one of the Japanese camp guards to stand to attention in front of the guard room. Rodgers and two others were clad only in pajamas. All of them had some protection on their feet. I believe it was wooden clogs. The fourth man had on a greatcoat. The weather was severely cold on the day in question. There was no snow on the ground but there had been a considerable amount of frost and there was some wind. I could see the Japanese guard who was supervising this punishment, in the guard room immediately next to the prisoners, keeping warm by the fire which the Japanese kept going continuously in the guard room. These four prisoners of war were forced to stand at attention for some hours.[250]

Writing after the war, one American concluded that the British had been courteous to them, "but we did not reciprocate too well. The

Americans were made generally uncomfortable by the 'Limeys.' To put it another way, the well-spoken and unflappable British made us Yanks feel a little inferior."[251]

Some POWs complained that Canadian NCO Colin Standish was a "favourite" of Lt. Tanaka, camp commandant, who had him to tea.[252] Certainly, Standish was selected by Tanaka, the commandant, to be the permanent day duty officer for the British and Canadian POWs when he arrived in camp in January 1944.[253] It is not surprising that a few men criticized Standish's activities, though most praised him. Any man forced to be the liaison between captors and captives ran that risk. Some things he did displeased a portion of his charges: he was too tough, or not tough enough, and so on. But most of the men interviewed have nothing but praise for Standish, who did a difficult job as well as one could. Standish set standards:

> One thing I made sure that every Canadian was identified as a Canadian with CANADA badges. You wore them, and they were priceless to get hold of because you needed one. The Japanese respected the Canadians much more than anybody else. Canada was their plan to hope and glory. A lot had been to Canada on ships and landed in Vancouver and they thought this was the place to go. So as Canadians we got along better with the Japs than the British or the Americans did. I always made sure the word "Canadian" came in.[254]

Dr. Riley noted, at the end of his post-war summary letter, his "high regard" for Sgt. Standish, RRC, "who was of great assistance to me in many ways and who did much to maintain the high morale of the Canadian POWs in Narumi Camp."[255]

The men worked at a factory, or *kaisha*, manufacturing locomotive engines. It was located in the middle of Nagoya, the third largest city in Japan. The Narumi POW Camp was situated on the outskirts of the city, about 20 minutes from the factory.[256]

In addition to locomotive construction, the POWs were pressed into work in other related areas. Most tasks, ignoring the Geneva Conventions, directly aided Japan's war effort. Among others factories in the area was one building Mitsubishi Zero fighter planes. Allied prisoners also helped to build landing craft, and motors for the biggest battleship ever laid down for the Japanese navy, the *Yamata*, in the Mitsubishi factory where there were 25,000 workers, including 5,000 prisoners.

The daily timetable was crowded and started early. Reveille at 5 a.m.; depart for dockyard 7 a.m.; start working 7:30 a.m.; stop working 5:00 p.m.; arrive at camp 5:40 p.m.; bath 6:00-7:30 p.m.; evening muster 8:30 p.m.; taps 9:00.[257]

The medical officer, Capt. Riley, visited the locomotive engine factory once. He had been invited by the Japanese medical orderly,

Sgt. Haiashi. In the middle of the morning the men had a break of 10 minutes, repeated in the afternoon. Work was demanded every day including Sunday. Although they arrived in Japan early in 1944, their first half-holiday took place only on 4 July.[258] That this was Independence Day in the USA must surely have been coincidental.

The type of work at the factory varied; the men were divided into seven working parties, the personnel in each changing from day to day. The largest group, Party No. 1, was engaged in the moulding shop doing very heavy work; No. 7 was composed of men who, under normal circumstances, would never have been allowed to do any work at all. Most of the men on No. 7 Party suffered from malnutrition diseases such as beriberi. The party was first formed by the camp commandant as a way of reducing the camp's official sick figures. Their work consisted of sweeping, carrying pieces of scrap metal, making string, sorting nails, and similar tasks.

The factory was run by civilians. Each workshop had its own leader, or hancho. "I understand that the civilian personnel at the factory treated the men fairly well on the whole."[259] Unfortunately, there were also semi-military escorts who conducted the men to and from the factory. These men, called *gunzukos*, were recruited from ex-soldiers who had received some war injury of an incapacitating nature. The *gunzuko* in charge of No. 7 Party was named Tanaka (no relation of the camp commandant). This man was particularly cruel to the men in No. 7 party. He refused to allow them to sit down and kept them on the move the whole time.

Before the men left camp for the factory they had to parade for *tenko*, or roll call, and afterwards to march down to the railway station. They would often have to wait half an hour for the train and, while waiting, they were obliged to stand in ranks and were not allowed to move about to keep warm. One POW recalled an incident: an American asked permission to leave the ranks to void urine, and this was refused. He was in agony, so eventually he broke ranks and urinated against a wall. The *gunzuko*, Tanaka, made the American lick his urine off the ground.[260] At the factory, sabotage was attempted whenever possible:

> We probably did some of the worst sabotage because we were building locomotive engines and stuff, so it would show up, whereas a lot of sabotage never would show up....We sabotaged a lot of motors and we burned all their template plans for anything. We burned the template shed. Left a candle going and it fell over and it started under a bench at night....To sabotage engines we'd groove the pistons, and then we'd smooth the grooves out with grindings, and we'd put it in and then put some oil over it. As soon as heat got to those she'd open right up. Or we'd fill blow holes in the pistons with a soft core rod, our main way, and they never caught us.[261]

The first medical officer, Dr. Norman Riley, RAF,[262] was SMO at Narumi from 15 January 1944 to 10 May 1945. Riley had one good IJA medical orderly to work with, Sgt. Haiashi; the others were unsatisfactory.[263] Riley had been captured in Java and was in four camps there, one at Singapore, and three in Japan. Riley's main complaint against camp commandant Tanaka had to do with his attitude towards sick personnel. He always insisted that full working parties were sent out, irrespective of the number of men who were unfit for work.[264] An American doctor was in the camp from 7 August 1944 to September 1945, Dr. Elack Schultz.[265] An American POW wrote:

We had but one American and one British doctor for the entire camp. We lost several men from starvation and pneumonia, but would have lost a great many more had it not been for Dr. E.A. Schultz of Toledo, Ohio.[266] He worked hard. Every time a man died "Doc" wept, knowing he could probably have saved the man with the proper medicine. Unfortunately, the Japanese rarely gave him authority to excuse us from the factory work.[267]

At the hospital, Standish recalled, they had no medical equipment or supplies. But they all apparently agreed that they had a good American doctor—Schultz.[268] Because of the distance between Nagoya and the prisoner-of-war hospital in Osaka, it was never possible to transfer serious cases there.[269]

Bathing facilities at Narumi were good. This was fortunate, because in the summer, and to a less extent during winter, the camp was grossly infested with fleas.[270] The latrines were adjacent to the barracks: the stench was almost unbearable throughout the summer, and the camp swarmed with large flies that bred in the latrines. Late in 1944 and early the next year they experienced earthquake tremors of varying intensity.[271] Dr. Riley noted that during an earthquake the fluid in the tanks used to spill over in large quantities, flooding into the barrack rooms.[272]

As has been mentioned more than once, a common source of frustration and bitterness was the perceived inequities in the way precious food supplies were doled out. At Narumi, an American thought that the British did this job well:

The distribution of food by the POW administration was fairer and more efficient than in the Philippine camps because of the virtual absence of corruption. That was so for two principal reasons. First, the British managed and operated the Nagoya camp's central kitchen without American participation or intervention. The British personnel appeared to be so equitable and capable that the American POWs came to consider them more trustworthy than their American counterparts.[273]

According to Hubbard, most of those who died at Narumi did so because they failed to consume their daily ration regularly. The POWs who manipulated food rations put themselves at great risk. "Rabbits," who deferred current rations to the future, and "gorgers," who mortgaged future rations to increase current consumption, were flirting with death. At even greater risk were those who gave nicotine a higher priority than food. Most of the men who traded food for cigarettes did not return home. A special group was formed to deal with the bankruptcy problem, the so-called Rabbit Commission. They received a "rabbit's" daily rations and gave him only that amount the Commission deemed necessary to sustain life. The Commission restructured his debt on a long-term basis, set up a precise schedule of repayment, and saw to it that creditors received payment on a prorata basis. "Notices of 'rabbitcy' were posted, and the Rabbit Commission prohibited everyone from trading with the rabbit."[274]

One Canadian apparently "let himself go," became lousy and filthy, and sold all his clothing and food for cigarettes. The senior British officer had to appoint a personal guardian for him.[275] As detailed elsewhere, the nicotine habit became a serious problem for a few of the men. One, an American navy warrant officer, died in camp. "One of the cadavers I helped to haul to the crematorium was a friend of mine, a Navy chief, who literally traded his life for cigarettes. Despite pleas from his friends and his promises to reform, he continued to trade a good part of his food ration for tobacco. In short, he chose starvation for a few more drags of his precious cigarettes."[276]

Once, the camp received a barrel of pickled grasshoppers as part of the ration.[277] Red Cross parcels containing more mundane food arrived at least twice. Again more fortunate than other POWs, those at Narumi received these parcels quite promptly. Those arriving on 9 April were distributed on 18 April, while those arriving 26 November were saved to make Christmas cheerier, being issued 24 December.[278]

On 22 March 1944, Capt. Riley reported to the commandant on the medical situation at Narumi Camp. At this date there were 13 POWs with beriberi, 17 with "happy feet," 34 with edema, and four with optic neuritis.[279] He mentions that the men from Hong Kong lived for several months on a diet of rice and vegetables only, and many of them had had diphtheria.[280] He comments on his attached list of weights as being a "selected" list of 55 men. Their average weight at time of capture was 77.8 kg (171.5 lb); weight on arriving in Japan averaged 60.7 kg (133.8 lb); "present weight" was 57.2 kg (126 lb).[281] Ronnie Edwards recorded his own weights during captivity, and his figures support Riley's. When captured he weighed 70 kg (168 lb); when he left Sham Shui Po for Japan this figure had fallen to 56 kg (121 lb), and he kept within a few pounds of this weight until war ended.[282]

The prisoners who were in Japan for only the last 18 months of the war could see that food for the Japanese civilians was scarce and getting scarcer. Though their rations were still superior to those of the POWs, there was plenty of evidence suggesting serious hunger among the Japanese workers.[283]

Japanese civilians in the factories were watched, as were the POWs, so the men couldn't communicate with them. The main foreman at the shipyard was called "Blue Coat," and he was fair. But some of the women, and the 15- or 16-year-old military cadets, were indoctrinated to hate westerners, and "they were a bad bunch. They hurt you. The old Jap, say a guy of 45-50, he was all right. Very seldom would you run into trouble with him, except you may run in one that just got notice that his son has died or something. But fundamentally the old Japs were OK, but the young ones were bastards."[284] The Koreans were often brutal as well. Many Koreans were treated as semi-prisoners by the Japanese and they were in no way sympathetic to the POWs.

One of a POW NCO's worst troubles was making sure that his men didn't steal from the Japanese, particularly the civilians' food. "I was death on any of my people stealing the Japanese food. Because they had no food either."[285] One thing the POWs did steal was newspapers. A few men could read Japanese, so they had some idea, reading between the lines of the propaganda, of what was going on outside.

In May and again in July 1944, Narumi Camp was visited by representatives of the International Red Cross. A special show was put on for their benefit. This included the temporary stocking of the canteen, which had hitherto been empty for some time. A truck arrived laden with goods including canned milk, bottled beer, biscuits, and tinned fruit. "Within ten minutes of the departure of the Visiting Party the lorry returned and took all the supplies away."[286]

Narumi POW Camp 2B, being so close to heavily bombed Nagoya, was substantially reduced in numbers in the spring of 1945. On 10 May one group including most of the Canadians, left Narumi and was transferred to Toyama.[287]

Sendai Camp 2B

The city of Sendai is located on the Pacific Ocean, in the prefecture of Miyagi, ca. 300 km (180 miles) northeast of Tokyo. This camp was known as Tokyo 14D when established in March 1944, but it later became Sendai Camp 2B after the general reorganization by the Japanese Prisoner of War Bureau. This camp was located at nearby Yoshima to supply labour for the Furukawa coal-mining company.[288]

Camp Sendai 2B consisted of two large one-storey huts for living quarters, a kitchen, a guard house, an office, three storehouses, and a hut used as quarters for the staff. The POW barracks had two levels of sleeping platforms on each side, the upper about five feet above the ground-level sleeping platforms. The camp was enclosed by a high board fence. Sendai 2B was located in the mountains and the men had to work in an underground coal mine with seven shafts about 500 yards from the camp.[289]

This draft of POWs was transported by boat to Moji, Japan, by ferry to Shimonoseki, and then by train via Tokyo to Tairi, on the east coast of Japan north of Tokyo. From Tairi they were trucked to Camp Sendai No. 2, which is about four miles west.[290]

The first 200 prisoners arrived in May 1944. These men had been captured at Hong Kong—roughly 100 British, 60 Canadians, and 40 Portuguese members of the HKVDC. The senior officer was Capt. Robinson, RAMC.[291]

At his trial, Ninomiya Yutaka, the commandant, was questioned about Japanese treatment of POWs. During the war he had attended a training course at the Tokyo Main Camp. There, he studied the Japanese Rules and Regulations for the handling of prisoner-of-war camps, including a translation of the Geneva provisions for the treatment of prisoners of war.[292] Ninomiya's trial provides an opportunity to examine how camp commandants, with their life-and-death powers, were prepared for this work.

Ninomiya was an instructor in English in a boys' school when called to army duty in June 1944. In July he received 10 days' training and was then ordered to duty as commandant of Sendai 2B. Col. Sakaba taught him that the first aim was to make prisoners work. Although Ninomiya understood the Geneva Conventions, Sakaba told him to use Japanese Army regulations to govern prisoners, not the conventions.[293]

In many camps in the Far East, including all in Japan proper, the captors insisted that commands be made and responded to in the Japanese language. At Sendai 2B, for example, the men were told they had 48 hours to learn the numbering system so that they could count by the numbers in Japanese on parade every morning. Many men found it difficult to learn in 48 hours.

> One particular fellow in our camp called Novak simply could not learn the Japanese language. The Japanese Sgt Major knew this fellow had a problem and if we tried to hide him in the middle rank or somewhere other than the front rank, he would pull him out and stick him in the front rank just to make sure he would have to give his number. We decided to help him out by putting him in the same spot every time. Novak seemed to be able to remember the Japanese word for the number six. So we would always put him in a spot where he was number six. Invariably [before this], this Sgt Major would pull him out and he would be beaten. This went on and on, beating after beating with a club. After

the Sgt. Major was through with him we had to hold him up—it was awful.[294]

Later, this POW recalled, Novak tried to commit suicide, but failed.

The prisoners of war were contracted out to work in the coal mines of the Furukawa Company by the Japanese War Ministry. The POWs were under IJA camp staff until the work parties were organized. They were then turned over to the guards for dispatch to work details. While inside the mine the POWs were under the control of company personnel. The camp staff received control again upon the return of the prisoners to the camp. At Sendai there was evidence that the mine had been closed until the POWs arrived, at which point it was reopened. "The reason it had been closed was because it was deemed unsafe for operation previously. However, it was good enough for the prisoners of war to work in."[295]

One prisoner reported that, before the earthquake of 1923, the mine had concrete and steel galleries, the remains of which could still be detected. But the 1923 quake broke up these galleries and the mine flooded. Collapses occurred daily in the mine. Quite a number of POWs were badly injured. Pte. Fernandez had his back broken, producing paralysis and, within a month, death. Few days passed without men being cut and bruised after being caught in a collapse.[296]

During the first months, the POWs had to march down an inclined shaft, work hard for eight hours or more, and then march up the shaft again. Exhausted men often were carried out by their comrades. In some shafts, the men had to work with water and mud up to their knees; sometimes they were enveloped in foul gas that induced intense headaches and fainting. Tools were inadequate and safety precautions were essentially non-existent.[297]

One ex-POW complained about the harmful activities of a Canadian NCO. This man was healthier than most and thus was able to work harder mining coal. The problem was that the Japanese reasoned: if he can do that much, then all the others can also. He was setting the quota. The Japanese rewarded him for extra production with rice and fish and cigarettes.

> And everybody was on him to stop doing that because we couldn't keep up. In fact, there's no way I could do the work. There's a chap, Isadore Perrault his name was, and he was a big husky, strong guy and hadn't been too sick, and he used to do a lot of my work, because I just couldn't put my quota of coal out.[298]

Occasionally, a bit of humour relieved the pressure. One man recalled being instructed before they entered the mine. A Japanese miner told them not to be scared or nervous. "'Look at me, I worked in the mines 30 years and look at me.' I bet you he didn't weight 110 pounds. He had a small little neck. We nicknamed him 'The Picture of Health!'"[299]

Capt. Robinson, RAMC, was the medical officer at Sendai 2B until September 1944. Then he was replaced by Capt. Patrick Cmeyla, US Medical Corps. Capt. Tinkler, RN medical service, arrived in May 1945.[300]

Cmeyla recorded the daily routine. Each morning he examined the POWs, accompanied by a Japanese medical orderly. The men whom he considered too ill to go to the mines were excused, on Cmeyla's advice, by the medical orderly. Then a Japanese sergeant, Ozawa, held a parade of the POWs "excused," and decided who among them would in fact go to work, and who would stay behind. Ozawa frequently slapped those in formation. Many POWs certified by the POW MOs as being ill were forced by Ozawa to work in the mines. This destroyed the authority of the POW medical officer and made the position of sick POWs hopeless. Therefore "the sick-calls were a farce, insofar as helping sick POWs."[301]

> It was awfully difficult to be excused. In the shipyards, for instance, the doctor used to have a sick parade every morning before work. I got very run down and developed a series of boils in my armpits. I used to go every morning on sick parade and the doctor would tell me he couldn't put me on sick today because he had too many men sick, so he would lance the boils and then I would go to work. This happened about fifteen times.[302]

The camp hospital was just a plain, unequipped building. It provided nothing more than a relief from work, plus whatever extra food the staff were able to give the patients out of the limited rations. It was difficult to have a POW admitted to the hospital. Cmeyla had minimal equipment to work with, nor drugs, medicine, or bandages. The few bandages were used, and reused after washing. But when inspectors visited, it was the regular practice of the Japanese camp staff to place medical supplies in the POW aid station for inspection, and pick them up again immediately after the inspection ended.[303]

When the POWs arrived at Sendai a Japanese physician examined the prisoners. About 140 of them were sick men: 60 had beriberi, 40 contracted diarrhea, and about 10 had skin disease. Fifty or 60 of the prisoners of war had avitaminoses from lack of vitamins, and many had "weak eyes."[304]

The work was hard in the coal mines and the food inadequate. For breakfast the Japanese provided only a bowl of watery soup with no meat, just a few vegetables. Each man had a small box of rice to eat for lunch. Usually they were so hungry that they would eat that on the way down to the mine, and then have nothing for eight hours. Then there was another bowl of thin soup when they came up from the mines.[305] In the coal mine the POWs wore only a G-string—the Japanese *fundoshi*—and so-called hard hats. These were actually cotton hats with pieces of felt inside.[306]

Apparently only one Canadian died at Sendai 2B; he died from malnutrition and pneumonia. The ration was supposed to be 750 grams of grain per day for workers, 560 grams for those who were working but not in the mine, and 350 grams for the sick. However, the prisoners divided all rations equally among themselves despite these orders, and an honest effort was made to do so without letting the Japanese know.[307] William Overton recalled that they once received, as part of the ration, a horse's head and the four legs from the knees down. The cooks cleaned it and cooked the whole thing in soup. "It certainly provided a lot of the grease that we needed, but I can remember one man going hysterical because he found a horse's tooth in his little bowl of soup."[308] Overton's weight fell from 151 to under 100 pounds.

One morning in April 1945, the prisoners were ordered to do physical training. The American doctor, Capt. Cymela, asked Ozawa to excuse the men suffering from beriberi from this physical training. Ozawa then ordered the men who had beriberi to fall out and line up to the side of the main group. About 30 men fell out. Ozawa then made these sick men take off their shoes and walk barefooted around a cement embankment on the edge of the camp. It was extremely cold, and Ozawa said the cold would do their beriberi good. He forced these sick POWs to do this until the others had finished physical training— 20 minutes to half an hour. On succeeding mornings Ozawa continued this practice until all the men elected to do physical training rather than continue the excruciating punishment of walking barefooted on the cold cement.[309]

Dr. Hironaka, the company doctor, testified that he believed there was an adequate supply of medicine. But "[a]s for treatment, I would not say that treatment was adequate because adequate treatment could not be given due to lack of adequate tools and equipment."[310]

Omori Camp

In this camp, there were about 100 American GIs, 300 British and Canadians captured at Hong Kong, about 40 American, British, and Australian officers, and a handful of Norwegian sailors who had been picked up by German raiders in the Indian Ocean and landed in Tokyo.[311]

Omori POW Camp was partly built by POWs. It occupied a small island of sand in Tokyo Bay, about 200 metres long, 100 metres wide, and located about 50 metres from the shore. It was a disciplinary camp to which "bad actors" were sent.[312]

The camp was in a quadrangle, with a short central street flanked by double-decker wooden barracks, each housing about 100 men. At the far end was the kitchen. Behind the barracks were the latrines, "the nature of whose construction," Dr. Weinstein wrote later, "I was to learn more intimately in the very near future."[313]

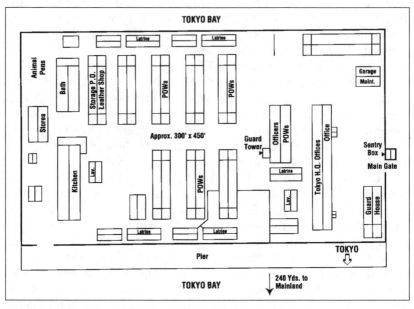

Figure 8.5 Plan of Omori POW Camp, Tokyo Bay, Japan.

On 8 September 1944, a group of 100 American POWs, including two MOs, arrived at Omori POW Camp.[314] They found the camp hierarchy gathered to greet them. Lt. Kato, a wizened, dark-faced man "with thick glasses, closely set, shifty eyes, pudgy nose, and loose slobbering lips" was camp commandant. With him was Watanabe Mutsuhiro, an NCO, well-built, about five foot seven, with sturdy shoulders and what was described as a well-modelled head with features that seemed almost occidental in type. His face was marred only by a cast to the eyes which became intensified when he flew into a rage—this was The Bird of camp notoriety. "Dressed in a white jacket and trousers like an ice-cream salesman, he gazed at us, a wry, sardonic smile on his handsome face." Dr. Weinstein decided that he didn't look as bad as his reputation. Weinstein would be proven unequivocally wrong.

Watanabe was in entire control of the Omori Camp of about 600 POWs and had almost full powers of life and death. "I never knew him actually to kill anyone. But the displeasure of Watanabe might easily mean death to us, poised as we were on the brink of disease and starvation. He hated Officers and above all Doctors."[315]

The obsequious interpreter, Nishino, looked to Weinstein like the pre-war Hollywood version of a westernized Japanese. "Slim, slant-eyes, thin-lipped, with long hair well pomaded, he started off the proceedings by interpreting Lieutenant Kato's speech."[316] The POWs were informed by the interpreter that every prisoner, no matter what his rank, must salute every Japanese, even if he were a coolie. If they did not salute they would be punished accordingly. Because of this regulation, for several months the POWs at Omori went through a reign of terror.[317]

Capt. J.J. Woodward was an Australian in the Indian Medical Service whose name will be remembered from Hong Kong. He thought that the camp, as he marched into it in September 1944, looked much cleaner than had the noisome Shinagawa hospital. Omori was also built on a reclaimed island, but one made of sand instead of black mud, and the huts were larger, cleaner, and lighter than those at Shinagawa.[318]

Lewis Bush testified that on one evening in June 1944, at Omori Camp, he was brutally beaten by Watanabe, who knocked him down, threw water on him, hit him with a fire bucket and was about to finish off by hitting him over the head with a 40-pound fire extinguisher. Then someone struck Watanabe and dragged him away, thus preventing the blow with the fire extinguisher. Bush was later told that it was the Japanese medical officer, Lt. Fujii Hiroshi, who interfered and stopped Watanabe. Bush was convinced that Fujii had saved his life. He considered Fujii to be "a better type Japanese, high strung and rather enthusiastic."[319]

The *Manryu Maru* took Bush and 450 Canadians to Japan, leaving Hong Kong on 25 August 1943. Remarkably, interpreter "Cardiff Joe" Matsuda gave up his cabin to Bush and other POWs.[320] They were not to receive similarly considerate treatment again until after the Japanese were defeated two years later.

Omori Camp was the headquarters for all POW camps in the Tokyo-Yokohama area. Constant theft of POWs' possessions, and various cruelties carried out by The Bird and his minions took place within 100 yards of the offices of the colonel in charge of all these camps, and his large staff of officers. Yet The Bird apparently never restrained his ferocity in any way. He was specially active after air raids, which began at the end of 1944.

Allied officers were beaten, slapped, and stood at attention for 12 or 24 hours at the slightest provocation. The chief purpose apparently was to instill fear among the remaining prisoners, and to permit the Japanese to satisfy their egos as conquerors of the occidental races. For saluting in a slovenly manner, an officer might be made to work for days emptying latrines. Maj. Kaufmann, one of the American MOs at Omori, observed cynically that if only one officer had recently started on this regime, it was soon found convenient for the Japanese to punish a second officer in a like manner so the two men could work together. The Japanese method of emptying latrines required two men, one at each end of a long, springy pole supporting a large odorous bucket.[321]

Conditions improved dramatically after Watanabe left the camp early in 1945. A Japanese sergeant by the name of Oguri, and Kano, an interpreter, took over the administration of the camp. For the rest of the time there were no beatings by camp staff, who did what they could to make working and living conditions decent.[322]

Capt. Woodward was the only surgeon in this camp. He saw a number of cases, but only secretly and at the special request of the official MOs, two Americans. This clandestine approach was necessary, since the Japanese doctor, Lt. Fujii, "would have delivered a general bashing to patient, MO, and consultant had we been detected."[323]

Yet Woodward was responsible for the treatment of 200 men. Of the 200, the only ones against whose names he had no entries for treatment administered were, he found, dead.[324] Woodward has left an ironic description of the way the Medical Inspection Room functioned under the Japanese medical staff at Omori:

> The MI Room was in the charge of Matsusaki San, a benign and courteous old Jap who insisted on an involved ceremony of arrival and departure and enforced the use of conventional polite phrases by us on all occasions. He never objected however to the greetings "Snar ka backera" accompanied by a deep and I hope graceful bow. This bowing was an accomplishment which I had quickly mastered in Omori under the personal tuition of the "Bird." It was bow or croak and I bowed. The bland smile of the dignified Matsusaki as he refused to waste even a 1 mgm ampoule of Vitamin B on a prisoner pale, weak and panting with beriberi heart was the essence of the fine old world spirit of Japan and the unction with which he pronounced the sentence "Shigoto" (work) on early pneumonia cases for whom I was pleading for admission to the "Hospital" hut, was reminiscent of a satisfied Bishop. I believe he caused many deaths. His assistant Higochi was less impressive but just as Japanese.[325]

Fujii has been mentioned in these pages many times. As we have seen, he had both supporters and detractors.

Discipline at Omori was harsh. Often, too, it seemed to be senseless, gratuitous brutality for its own sake. There was, for example, one POW who was sick during the winter and couldn't go to work. Someone had a violin, and the POW could play. "He was playing it in bed, and as a punishment he had to go outside the gate of the camp and play the violin for 24 hours. It was winter time and he was sick."[326]

Happily, at least one Japanese guard showed decency and compassion. If his attitude wasn't contagious to the other guards, at least it offered occasional reminders of humanity to the men. This man, Edomoto, was a student of European art and literature. He made no secret of his opposition to the war—to the POWs at any rate—and in hundreds of unobtrusive ways did his best to improve their lot.[327]

The prisoners at Omori got their share of punishment but one observer thought that they seemed to take it in their stride. Bertram wondered if this was because they numbered so many old sweats, or because the British enlisted man was customarily toughened in a harder school than most other troops. Whatever the explanation, Omori presented "the amazing spectacle of a prison camp under the strictest discipline...in which the prisoners as a matter of course cheerfully condescended to their captors, and never for a moment left them in any doubt as to who were the better men....As a demonstration of morale I have never seen anything like it."[328]

Squadron-Leader L.J. Birchall, Royal Canadian Air Force, arrived at Omori to be disciplined. This fine, courageous officer had been flying the Catalina that first spotted the Japanese fleet in the Indian Ocean as it approached Ceylon in 1942. It was their warning, which they were just able to radio before being shot down by Japanese fighters, that probably saved the island from disaster. Birchall was invariably an outstanding leader in whatever camp he was in. He came to Omori after a long stretch in Ofuna, the cruel interrogation camp operated by the Imperial Japanese Navy.

Birchall had struck a Japanese orderly who had ill-treated a sick prisoner, so he was sent to Omori.[329] As a disciplinary measure, Birchall worked all day in the Omori fur factory, then all night in the kitchens. "I slept in five minute bits whenever I could and any disobedience was punished by having to stand barefoot on the hot ovens holding two buckets of water. Believe me, with our sensitive feet this hurt."[330]

The contrast between POW life and the fondly remembered normal life was, of course, something all the men knew intimately; it was a common source of flagging morale. For some, the contrast was especially poignant. When the Winnipeg Grenadiers were stationed in Jamaica in 1941, one of their duties was to guard German POWs held there. "Those fellows lived the life of Riley."[331] The comparison generated bitter feelings. Many hearkened back to those days with nostalgic yearning.

The Britishers and Canadians from Hong Kong had their musical instruments. There was a tall, sad-faced warrant officer who directed a small jazz band under the starlit sky. Hot trumpets blew, guitars strummed, and violins took up the melody while weary prisoners relaxed and dreamed of home and freedom. The Red Cross sent in a good electric phonograph with a fine collection of records, both jazz and classical. "If The Bird was in a good humour, we got permission to play it. Some of the records that I heard for the first time in October, 1944, were 'Queenie, the Strip-Tease,' 'Don't Sit Under the Apple Tree,' and some harmony by the Andrew Sisters and Bing Crosby."[332]

The enlisted POWs went outside the camp to their jobs every day. The officers, whose number varied from 50 to 75, were not given outside work except for a small group who gardened. Except for the garden detail, all had to labour in the fur shop sewing pieces of rabbit fur together to make waterproof covers for Japanese military knapsacks, or to work as clerks to help the Japanese administratively.[333]

The enlisted men were divided into groups of 100. They left at 8 a.m. for work and returned at 5 p.m. Most of them worked as stevedores at freight terminals and shipyards in Tokyo and Yokohama. "They were a rugged, hard-boiled group of men, survivors of two years of Japanese confinement and cruelty. The physically and mentally unfit among them had been weeded out by privation and disease."[334]

Some gangs worked at the Mitsubishi warehouses, where they were able to steal sugar. Others, in areas of the railway yards unloading tobacco, could break open a drum and snatch a few handfuls to smuggle into camp. Some men smuggled rice. At Omori, to his disgust, Angus McRitchie worked at the railway yard unloading pig iron and lumber: "I couldn't [smuggle]—pig iron and lumber didn't help me any."[335]

The ration run was an especially backbreaking job. Trucks brought sacks of vegetables, rice, barley, and coal weighing from one hundred to two hundred pounds, to the shore of the bay. A narrow road connected the mainland to the small man-made island of Omori, but the road wasn't wide enough for a truck. Thus, heavy sacks of supplies piled on their backs, the POWs staggered into camp, a distance of perhaps 300 yards over the humpbacked rickety bridge, across the island, and through the prison compound into the galley. "Neck, back, feet, and heart took a pounding in this occupation. At the end of it, we were so nauseatingly exhausted we couldn't eat."[336]

For the prisoners, the most important people at Shiodome, the railway yards, were the *sencho* (the senior foreman) and the hanchoes, or Japanese gang bosses. Less important but often possessing power were the ordinary Japanese railwaymen. At the bottom of this heap were the Korean railwaymen, whose status was not so far removed from that of the POWs.[337]

Stealing food from the docks and warehouses was a risky but essential activity. Much ingenuity was displayed. The commonest tool was what they called a "pipe" or a "fiddle and flute," a section of brass or bamboo tubing sharpened at one end, which could be thrust into a sugar sack; sugar siphoned into a bag quickly. When withdrawn, there was no visible hole or telltale droppings. A "flute" was a dangerous object to be caught with, for it was invariably seen as damning evidence of intent if not execution.[338]

Japanese truck drivers were cut in on the smuggling racket. They deliberately came a half-hour late to pick up the POWs; while waiting, the prisoners would obtain permission from the company guards to return to the rest rooms until the trucks arrived. With the help of various "Rube Goldberg" contraptions, they suspended socks of sugar in their sleeves and trouser legs, under their armpits and crotches. They slipped smaller sacks into oversized shoes. They tied socks filled with sugar to the backs of their necks under their turtle-neck sweaters. Sometimes they strapped flat containers to their abdomens, giving them the spurious look of being well fed. When the trucks arrived, the camp guards shooed away the company guards and hurried to load their POW charges onto the truck—without their being searched by the company guards. "Back to camp they went to conceal their precious hoards. Sugar was currency in camp. They traded it for cigarettes from the Nip guards. They traded with prisoners on other work details for food. A half-canteen sugar was standard price of an evening's entertainment with the few homosexuals in camp."[339]

Most of the men had ample opportunity to steal food, and so the general health in the camp was better than in many others. These benefits did not extend to the officers, who were kept in camp for various duties. One of these was the grossly unpleasant task of emptying out the contents of the latrines to serve as fertilizer for the camp garden. This human waste was slopped into buckets and poured on the ground outside the camp fence, a distance of only 20 yards from the POW kitchen. Collecting wood on the beach was also among the officers' duties. These outdoor exercises they considered a welcome diversion from the task of leather-working.

Early in 1945, after a raid by B29s near the camp, the prisoners were taken out to cut fire lanes through still-standing houses in mainland Tokyo. The fire damage was horrific. Many Japanese had dug shallow pits as air raid shelters, covered them with woven bamboo sheets, then covered this with the dirt from the pit. The fire literally cooked those inside, then the roof collapsed to cover the bodies.[340]

At Omori the medical and dental arrangements were adequate, though barely. Capt. Lloyd H. Goad, "a pale-faced, long-suffering, much-beaten American," had been the camp MO from July 1943.[341] He took orders from a sadistic Japanese medical orderly and from The Bird, who passed judgment on all patients whom Goad thought should be rested in quarters or "hospitalized." By a judicious combination of cunning and adroitness, Goad usually was able to wheedle the necessary permission. If the proportions were wrong, he and his patients were whipped. On alternate days, Maj. Berry ran sick call while Goad laboured on the farm. In the winter of 1944-1945 there were a large number of men with pneumonia, and Berry and Goad requested that they be excused from garden duties to care for the sick. Lt. Fujii refused to permit this.[342]

The experience of Capt. Patrick M. Cmeyla, MC, USA, paralleled that of many other Allied MOs. Because of his continuous efforts on behalf of his men at Sendai 2B, as described earlier, he became a nuisance to the Japanese. He was sent to Omori for punishment because of so-called "disobedience."[343] Typically, he could not do medical work—he laboured alongside the other officers at their various jobs.

One problem faced almost routinely was the difficulty in getting a seriously ill patient admitted to a proper hospital. According to Fujii, the final authority to permit a patient to enter a hospital outside the POW camp was the superintendent of the hospital and the officials of the Prisoner of War Information Bureau of the Army Ministry. If permission in principle had been decided upon, then the camp commander could approach the hospital superintendent directly to request the hospitalization of a particular prisoner of war.[344] The system could, and did, break down at several levels.

Except for those men who were on punishment rations, the food issue at Omori seemed to be better than elsewhere; certainly Dr. Weinstein found it a marked improvement over Shinagawa Hospital. Each man received a heaping mess-tin of grain three times a day, plus a fairly thick vegetable soup. Perhaps three times a week there might be a piece of dried salted fish, and occasionally a dish of boiled soybeans. Boring, but enough to support life and replace burned-out muscle.

As Bertram noted, the basic ration at Omori was always called "rice," but seems to have been a cereal base comprising millet, barley, and a small percentage of white rice. It was harsh on western stomachs but probably better balanced in terms of nutrition than the customary Japanese fare of white rice and barley. Bertram believed that the comparative rarity of beriberi and the deficiency diseases among prisoners in the Tokyo camps testified to the vitamin B content of this food.[345]

Dr. Fujii stated in his testimony that a Japanese person had an average basal metabolism of 1,200 calories. The average basal metabolism of a POW was 1,600. He claimed to have written a pamphlet about nutrition and POWs:

> [P]risoners of war…had to have more calories than the Japanese and I also studied the table of menu that was provided for the prisoners of war and calculated the number of calories in that menu; that is, how many grams of proteins there were in the prisoner of war menu, how many grams of fats and how many grams of carbohydrates or the calories in each menu were calculated and this menu was compared with the number of patients in that camp and after this investigation, I wrote in the

pamphlet that each prisoner of war must receive 120 grams of protein per day and that it was absolutely necessary for a prisoner of war to receive more than fifty grams of fat per day. In the Japanese Army there is a regulation stating that one person should have only 5 to 10 grams of fat per day. In the pamphlet I recommended that the prisoners of war be given a lot of soya beans because soya beans contained a lot of protein and fat.[346]

After this was published, Fujii believed that the food situation improved. Officials requested soy beans from the army and these were given to POWs; he also negotiated with the company employing prisoners of war to furnish soy beans.

Periodically the Japanese proclaimed a "weigh day." All the POWs went to the dispensary and were weighed. The Japanese seemed to delight in collecting figures and drawing brightly coloured charts to show weight loss or gain. Actually, what this usually meant was that the POW medical officers collected the figures and drew the charts for them: "the interpretation of data and conclusions drawn from the charts never, in my experience, modified or increased the food handout."[347] When there was an announcement that the food ration was to be increased, the prisoners knew that they needed to buckle their belts—usually the ration would be cut. If the vegetable issue was increased, the rice, barley, or millet would be cut. If potatoes came into camp, they would be issued instead of rice.

According to Lewis Bush, when rations were short at Omori, Dr. Fujii put forward his plan to make miso beer—beer brewed from fermented soybean paste. This he believed would prevent and even cure beriberi. Bush, a Japanese-speaker who knew Fujii as well as any POW, reported that he had a lengthy argument with the supply staff, but eventually they provided him with the supplies necessary for making this brew for the men engaged in heavy labour. It was made in the cookhouse under his supervision from miso, sugar, and fermented barley. Not only did it not taste bad, but it soon had the desired effect. "This was only one of the very excellent deeds of this young cadet doctor, but even so, he was tried as a war criminal. Today he is married and has his own practice in Tokyo. Many of my comrades did not, I am sure, realize all that he did, or tried to do, in order to uphold the medical code."[348] Others who had confrontations with Fujii disagreed.

Each working POW was to receive 250 cc of yeast solution a day. Double that amount was given to the sick. The yeast for each barracks was put in a mess bucket and the barracks section leader divided the yeast equally. The men brought their mess utensils and drank the liquid yeast:

During the first part of this process, that is when the yeast was first given to the prisoners of war I went up to the prisoners of war when they were drinking it and asked how the yeast tasted. There were some prisoners who could not sleep because of their leg condition due to beriberi. Such prisoners of war mentioned that after drinking the yeast solution they were able to sleep and the fact they were able to sleep I think was a sign of improvement in their health.[349]

Norquist observed several questionable though ingenious cooking methods used by those POWs who had successfully stolen raw rice or beans. Of course, these had to be cooked on the sly. One method was to lower canteens of the raw food into the delousing steam vat in the bathhouse, under clothes being treated. Or they might cook their loot in the smouldering trash pile, or on clandestine hot plates.[350]

By April 1945 the Japanese offered the POWs dog meat to add to their increasingly meagre diet. But the food was turned down, apparently on the advice of the medical officers, who were afraid that the meat would not pass public health inspection. By this stage, nutrition was far less than adequate and men with distended bellies because of beriberi were commonly seen in the hospital.[351]

At Omori, as in many other camps, the POWs came to expect the familiar order: "Prepare to gargle. *Gargle!*" When they ordered men to gargle the Japanese were deadly serious. In October 1944, men were stood at attention for an hour after *tenko* because some of them had forgotten to gargle, as ordered, twice a day.[352]

The men were issued an overcoat and long underwear, though these were only cotton. They also received a green coat and pants that were tight-fitting around the ankles. Naturally, these were made for the Japanese body, and the pants tended to extend no lower than the calves or knees; these couldn't be worn to the mines but were used when the men were back in camp and had cleaned up, their "Sunday suit."[353]

Omori was a headquarters camp, and the buildings had been newly built when the camp was opened. They were regulation Japanese barracks, built to accommodate a maximum of 100 men, sleeping in double tiers. During the last 18 months of the war, however, so many fresh drafts of prisoners were moved through Omori Camp that for months at a time the POWs were seriously overcrowded, even by Japanese standards. One barrack accommodated 150 men, which meant that each man had less than 18 inches for his sleeping space, increasing the danger of infection during the winter months. Though there were other buildings not being used at the time for living accommodations, nothing was done to improve these crowded conditions. In the last year the barracks were infested with bedbugs in addition to the ubiquitous fleas and lice. The bedbugs were so common that their bites made sleep impossible for many.

Clothing should have been in good supply since Omori, as a headquarters camp, had large quantities of captured military clothing actually in store:

In fact, however, we fared worse than many other camps in view of the irregularity of issue and the stringent conditions in force before clothing could be drawn. In particular boots and heavy clothing were almost impossible to obtain and during the last winter of the war many prisoners working in Tokyo had no boots and could not get none. They were obliged to work in worn canvas shoes and as a result many men suffered from colds caught in this way and sometimes this turned suddenly into pneumonia, causing several deaths.[354]

One day a handsome, tall Japanese, dressed impeccably in clothes which might have been cut in Savile Row—according to Lewis Bush, they had been—visited Omori and came to the room occupied by Bush and other officers. The man was Tokugawa Yoshitomo, son of Marquis Tokugawa Yoshichika, and brother-in-law of Prince Chichibu. Bush knew of Tokugawa, and he had heard of Bush, and they found that they had many friends in common. Tokugawa was visiting the POW camps representing the Japan Red Cross. Naturally, the POWs told him all their complaints and he promised to do whatever he could to assist. Immediately, he was able to have released to the men boxes of books sent by the American Red Cross, but which the POWs hadn't seen because of the characteristically lengthy delays until books could be censored. "After Yoshitomo's first visit, 'Brown' gave me another bashing and accused me of telling tales, and said that I was not, in future, to speak to Tokugawa."[355]

When asked about the Red Cross and the Swiss representatives (Switzerland was the Protecting Power for the US in the Far East), Dr. Weinstein commented that they didn't come around. "There's one bloke named Prince Tokagawa [*sic*], a member of the royal family connected with Red Cross work, who visits here occasionally. We've complained to him on more than one occasion. He says it is impossible for anybody to interfere with the military in their treatment of prisoners—even if they wanted to!"[356]

A few Red Cross parcels arrived, but often the Japanese camp commander wouldn't let the men have them. His stated reason was that if the Americans invaded Japan, those parcels might become their only food.[357] This occurred so commonly at all camps that the retention of parcels must reflect central edict.

In camp the POWs were warned that the civilians outside were homicidally furious at Allied prisoners, especially Americans. The prison administration announced that they were the "guardians" of the POWs. Yet the latter seemed never to encounter an enraged citizen. "On the other hand, I met several who went out of their way to make my lot more bearable at the risk of their own safety. The civilians I met merely went through the motions of expediting the war effort. They had a bellyful of war."[358]

One American recalled a Japanese woman, wife of a workman (they called her "Ma") who gave each of his group a little parched rice that tasted like popcorn.[359] Also, civilians would hide handfuls of roasted soybeans where the men might find them. Once a guard caught a man doing this and brutally whipped him in the face with a pair of pliers. "Only then did we realize the full depth of the civilians' kindness and their hate for the military."[360]

POW Hospitals, Tokyo Area

There seem to have been two places used expressly as hospitals for POWs in the large Tokyo area. The first was at the Sagamigahara Japanese military hospital, the second—which superseded Sagamigahara—was Shinagawa Hospital.

Sagamigahara Hospital

Sagamigahara military hospital was a regular Japanese Army establishment. Its POW division was grafted on, out of necessity, sometime in 1942. This was coincident with the transfer of POWs from other parts of the Pacific Theatre to the Home Islands for purposes of labour. The POWs were housed in a wooden building originally used to house insane Japanese soldiers. During its existence of about a year, this so-called POW hospital, consisting of four rooms, was still used intermittently for its original function, one room being occupied by the insane.[361] Though one POW who had access to the main hospital, used for Japanese soldiers, found it adequate,[362] the POWs were not admitted there. Instead, they found themselves in the mental ward.

Inevitably, because they are affidavits collected in anticipation of proceeding to a trial for war crimes, the available records paint a bleak picture of patients' existence at Sagamigahara. The records are explicit enough to make it seem unlikely that any former inmate would come forward to praise the place or contest the evidence.

The Japanese soldiers had beds, the prisoners slept on tatamis on the floor. So crowded were the quarters (two rooms each about 20' by 12' and two about half that size) that the tatamis touched and, according to one survivor, no patient had a tatami exclusively to himself.[363] Tatamis are woven sleeping mats about 6' by 2.5'. Though a steam-heat system existed and there were pipes and radiators to prove it, no prisoner could remember ever feeling heat in those radiators, not even in the depths of winter. The large rooms housed 20 or more patients at times, the smaller, up to a dozen. Exiting a room for any reason meant stepping over or on fellow-patients. Since many of the men had dysentery, the need to go to the latrine was urgent and frequent, an exhausting routine for seriously ill patients. Bedpans were not provided. When distressed patients were unable to reach the latrines and soiled their bed space, their neighbours or the orderlies had to clean up after them. Hot water was unavailable as were all types of cleaning materials.

The toilet to which the men flocked out of necessity was a single-hole latrine opening into a cement tank without drainage. The smell was usually grossly offensive and pervasive. The tank was emptied when full or overflowing, by the patients themselves under Japanese orders. If custom was followed, the contents would have been used as fertilizer in the nearby fields.

Essentially no medical care was provided by the Japanese. There was no medical officer present regularly in the POW hospital, either Japanese or Allied. A Japanese MO came over from the main hospital periodically, sometimes every few days, at other times only monthly. Rarely did he actually examine a patient, instead being informed about the patients by Japanese medical orderlies.[364] Whatever he was told seemed to have no impact on treatment. Occasionally unidentified powders would be given to a patient but these effected no cures. Otherwise medical supplies were non-existent. When patients had open wounds, the POW orderly had to steal dressings from the main hospital, and these dressings had to be used and reused.

The unsatisfactory nature of Sagamigahara hospital, even for those rare cases that could be admitted, has been outlined by an Allied medical officer located at Kawasaki Camp. He sent three men with severe beriberi to Sagamigahara. The orderlies who went with them described the experience on their return: "one mile to the tram station, four changes of tram, a stretcher carry of two miles at the other end, to the hospital which consists of fifty buildings on forty-five acres of countryside, thirty minutes outside Tokyo by tram. This is the Japanese Military Hospital and in the area is one building divided into six rooms for prisoners of war staffed by one RAMC orderly and Japanese doctors."[365] Patently, these were not good conditions.

The main preoccupation of the Japanese orderlies appears to have been brutalizing the patients. There was one exception, one well-intentioned individual. Otherwise the ex-POWs unanimously criticized these men. They functioned as guards far more than as orderlies. But as bullies they were assiduous and, in some instances, imaginative. Many of the patients had swollen, excoriated testicles, a consequence of severe avitaminoses. One Japanese orderly insisted on painting these raw weeping surfaces with a painful burning liquid; he continued to do this despite protests and evident agony until it became obvious that the procedure was positively harmful.[366] Aside from this allegedly therapeutic refinement, the usual approach by the orderlies was crude brutality. Patients were regularly slapped and often beaten up. Those whose feet were swollen and painful from beriberi or other causes of edema discovered that their feet attracted vicious attention.[367]

The sole POW medical orderly at Sagamigahara was present only because he was a patient. As his condition improved, he began to assist his fellow patients as best he could.[368] Another man volunteered as orderly when he became more mobile.[369]

Only one activity by the Japanese medical staff can tentatively be classified as therapeutic. A number of patients suffering from severe beriberi received injections of what they were told was a vitamin B-containing liquid. This may have helped some of the men. The injection was made into the spinal canal; according to his patients, the medical officer administering it did his job roughly and caused much pain.[370]

Moreover, the prisoners of war became unwitting guinea pigs used for instructing Japanese medical students from a nearby school. After the Japanese MO made his injection while instructing the students, they then carried out the same procedure, on the same patient or patients, using the same unsterilized needle and syringe. One POW patient reported having this traumatic procedure carried out by a dozen students, one after the other.[371] Nor was this the only training for these students. On other occasions they learned to take blood samples, withdrew stomach contents via a tube, and did other procedures.[372] It seems evident that these activities benefitted only the students; certainly no treatment eventuated for the POWs.

There were many deaths recorded among the patients. One man's passing was succinctly described as caused by "the piling up of mistreatment, malnutrition and imprisonment."[373] Usually the survivors attributed these deaths to a combination of neglect and brutality exacerbating medical conditions. This conclusion seems valid. Here is one case history, which gives the flavour of the place:

> Another British soldier named William Pinnock, of the Middlesex Regiment, died about one month after I was admitted to the hospital. He was suffering from dry beriberi, severe malnutrition and dysentery. He had been there for some time when I arrived and when I saw him he was just skin and bones. He was very weak and a great part of the time he was delirious. When he was delirious he would stagger over the prisoners and out into the hall. Many times when he did this the Japanese medical orderlies beat him with their web belts and rifle butts and continued this until he crawled back into his room. On one occasion I saw him struck on the back of the head with a rifle butt which knocked him unconscious for some time. As near as I can recollect it was two days after he received this blow on the head from the rifle butt that he died. It is my opinion that his death was caused by a lack of proper food and medical attention and the frequent beatings he received from the Japanese medical orderlies.[374]

The impact of vitamin deficiencies on these men, as on so many POWs, was devastating. One of the symptoms attributed to beriberi was the so-called "happy feet" or "electric feet." At Sagamigahara the men suffering with this painful and exhausting disorder received advice on how to alleviate their discomfort. Thomas Marr recorded that when he arrived at Sagamigahara he was examined by a Japanese doctor, who informed Marr that if he wanted to alleviate the pains in his feet, he should put them in a tub of cold water.[375] Marr followed this advice. His feet became swollen and began to turn black. He had been given the worst possible advice: gangrene, followed by the loss of toes, feet, even legs, would have been the inevitable result. After three weeks the regular MO told Marr to stop this treatment. He did and his feet improved. Sgt. Albert Cox, a patient helping change dressings for one of his compatriots, one day removed the bandage and found three toes lying loose there.[376]

All in all, there is little positive one can say about Sagamigahara POW Hospital. But it may have been palpably bad enough to persuade the Japanese that something better was needed. And something better did come—not a western-style modern hospital to be sure, but Shinagawa was initially much better than the hospital it replaced at Sagamigahara.

Shinagawa POW Hospital

Shinagawa is a district in the southwestern part of Tokyo, as that city spreads along the edge of Tokyo Bay towards Yokohama. During 1943, it became apparent to Japanese POW officials, as it was painfully clear to the prisoners, that some new arrangement for handling ill POWs was required. A Red Cross delegation to Tokyo-area camps noted that while technically the sick were admitted to the Red Cross hospital in Tokyo, in practice this hospital was overfilled as a military hospital for the IJA. Consequently, it had become impossible to get POW patients, even those with major injuries, admitted. The POWs were without proper hospital care and had to be looked after, whatever the medical problem, in the quite inadequate sick bays, some even lacking medical officers, in individual camps.[377] It was to correct this problem that Shinagawa was transformed into a hospital exclusively for POWs, who therefore did not have to compete for accommodation with Japanese soldiers.

The Shinagawa facility had a chameleon existence in the world of Japanese POW camps. It began as an ordinary work camp, but after a few months was transformed into the chief POW hospital in the Tokyo area, and remained so until war's end. But the hospital itself saw two distinct phases, before and after the March 1945 assumption of total power by Lt. Tokuda Hisakichi, Japanese Army medical corps.[378]

The work-camp phase need not detain us, since it was unrelated to both the hospital activity and the vivisection that was charged at war's end.

A: "Good" Shinagawa

From September 1943, when it became a hospital, until March 1945, Shinagawa functioned in a straightforward way. The medical staff consisted of Allied POW medical officers and orderlies, with a Japanese administrative staff. A few days after the hospital opened, an RCAMC officer visited it with a seriously ill patient; the hospital, he observed, was just the old Shinagawa Camp, with no new buildings, a camp originally built to house Japanese unemployed in the depression years. S/LtCmdr. Whitfield, RN, was the medical officer in the beginning. There seemed to be no equipment or medicine, but better food than in Tokyo 3D.[379]

The Japanese never intended Shinagawa to be a model hospital. Dr. Fujii pointed out that in the IJA hospital system, Shinagawa Hospital was classified as Class III, the lowest grade hospital. Therefore it would not be supplied with special instruments for neurosurgery or for other specialized operations. Such surgery would have to be done at a Class I hospital such as the Army Medical College.[380]

Although September 1943 is the official date cited as the beginning of Shinagawa Hospital, patients were being sent there a month earlier, according to Capt. John Reid, Canadian medical officer then at Tokyo Camp 3D. "On 1 August 1943, 22 isolated cases (20 amoebic, 1 DIP carrier, 1 suspect TB) and four hospital cases were sent to the new POW hospital at Shinagawa."[381]

Many Allied POWs were shocked to find that beds were rarely provided in hospitals in Japan. However, this was true in many civilian hospitals, not just those used by POWs. Not everyone found these arrangements unsanitary. S/Cmdr. J.A. Page, RN, had this to say: "Patients were nursed on mattresses on the floor, or on platforms covered with a thin straw matting, Japanese fashion. In spite of this it was possible to keep the wards comparatively clean and surgical cases did well and secondary sepsis was rare."[382]

Maj. Alfred Weinstein, MC, US, spent part of his POW existence at Shinagawa. He found much to criticize. A surgeon, he noted that the same gloves, gowns, and homemade operating table were also used for autopsies. This practice raised the spectre of cross-infection. The small operating room had only a single low-wattage bulb. The only source of heat was a small coal-burning stove. Linen was sterilized in a home-made steam apparatus. There were only a few of the usual surgical instruments:

> To supplement these, we made many instruments ourselves out of scrap iron and wood that we picked up in the compound, such as resectors, bone chisels, Steinman pins for bone work, Gigli saws, splints, walking calipers, traction beds, suspension frames, and the like. After Red Cross

supplies came in, we had more surgical tools, and got Dr. Tokuda's consent to separate the autopsies from the surgical work, and shortly before my departure, with Red Cross funds, many surgical instruments and lights were purchased and made available.[383]

Capt. A.J.N. Warrack was at Shinagawa from May 1944 until August 1945. He described the physical setup of the camp in an article published just after the war ended. The hospital was located on an island about half a mile square. It contained several wooden barracks apparently built for Korean labourers. The walls were two layers of thin boards about four inches apart. Each barrack contained two small rooms accommodating three or four officers or orderlies and four wards each housing up to 20 patients. The floors were raised about a foot from the ground and were covered with the standard Japanese straw mats or tatamis. At the end of each barrack was a latrine—a urinal plus four compartments built over a two-foot-deep concrete tank.[384]

Drugs were available in generous supplies from the Red Cross.[385] Abdominal surgery carried out by Allied POW MOs produced excellent results.[386] Spinal anesthesia and intravenous pentothal were used. And sulfa drugs were available and used extensively. "We also resorted to the smuggling of drugs to other camps by secreting them on the persons of patients who would be discharged from our hospital to their respective camps."[387]

Although the results of surgery by POW MOs were considered satisfactory, the surgical skills of Lt. Tokuda were slight. An American medical officer experienced this problem as a patient. Capt. Lloyd Goad, POW MO at Omori Camp, developed appendicitis, and was sent to Shinagawa, where Tokuda did the necessary surgery. After three days Dr. Goad still had much pain. The POW MOs operated again, during Tokuda's absence from the camp. Blood clots were removed and the wound resutured, after which convalescence was uneventful.[388]

The latrines were emptied onto the camp gardens and farm. The POW medical officers protested against this practice on sanitary grounds, but without avail, since this was common practice in Japan. "A concession was made, however, with regard to faeces from the dysentery barracks. These were emptied into a pit dug adjacent to the Naval School."[389] Hot baths were allowed twice a week. These took place in a wooden tub capable of accommodating six men, under which a fire was lit and the water kept continuously hot.[390]

The Japanese supplied few drugs. Only the generous supplies sent by the Red Cross permitted the work of the hospital to be carried on efficiently.[391] Japanese officers would periodically inspect the charts of the patients and recommend or delete certain drugs. These decisions were usually arbitrary and seldom based in science. "For these reasons they invariably forgot what they had said on a previous occasion and the Allied Medical Officers continued to prescribe drugs as they thought fit."[392]

No operation could be done without the permission of the senior Japanese officer. It was usually given but, if the Japanese commandant was in camp, he would insist on either performing or assisting at the operation himself. The commandant's knowledge of surgery was considered abysmal and, as a consequence, the task of the senior POW surgeon, SurgCmdr. Cleave, was made much more difficult.[393]

After a visit by the International Committee of the Red Cross, their report commended the excellent treatment given in this hospital. They pointed to the fact that 174 operations had been done with only four deaths. Overall, there had been 53 deaths since the hospital was opened almost eight months before; mostly the causes were tuberculosis, amoebic dysentery, pneumonia, and beriberi.[394] A year later, Gottlieb reported that approximately 1,100 prisoners had been treated between July 1943 and March 1945, with a mortality of only 66 patients.[395] In February 1945, Shinagawa POW Hospital held 259 patients. The POW medical staff comprised three British officers and seven Other Ranks, and five American officers and 16 ORs.[396]

Pneumonia was a major cause of mortality in work camps and at the Shinagawa Hospital. Patients sent there seldom arrived before the third day of illness. They were treated with sulfa drugs and usually did well if caught early enough. "The Japanese practice of making patients walk part of the way to hospital and of moving cases on the third and fourth day of illness did not improve the recovery rate."[397]

Food and its preparation excited anger here as elsewhere. The cooks, mainly British Other Ranks, reputedly sold and traded food. They were favourites of the Japanese, so that they could and did defy orders from their own officers in regard to matters of food. "We could do nothing about it as they invoked the Japs....One could always tell a cook or a friend of a cook by his size and shape."[398]

One of the many hazards of POW life in Japan was moxibustion. In many instances the Japanese made its use compulsory, inflicting it by force if necessary, on prisoners suffering from such diverse ailments as beriberi and amoebic hepatitis.[399]

All convalescent patients and medical staff were required to work, the latter in addition to their medical duties. This work included emptying latrines, farming, and digging. Two groups were sent out each day to the adjacent shipyards.[400] If they did not work, the officers' ration was only 390 gm grain, whereas for a working man it was 705 gm, and bed patients received 570 gm.[401]

B: "Bad" Shinagawa

The internal-medicine side of the hospital was generally less a problem than the surgical, there being less interference by the Japanese. Then, in March 1945, the Japanese commandant—Med/Lt. Tokuda Hisakichi—decided to take over complete control of all patients with tuberculosis and other serious medical conditions. These 53 men were isolated in one barrack which was out of bounds to all prisoners except for two medical orderlies retained as nursing orderlies.[402] These segregated Allied prisoners remained in Barracks No. 5 until about 15 August 1945.

Warrack mentions Tokuda using such therapy as intravenous soya bean milk and intraspinal Vitamin B, Vitamin C, and riboflavin. Tokuda also gave intramuscular injections of sulphur and of castor oil, and performed (unskillfully) artificial pneumothorax on inappropriate patients.[403]

In May 1945, SurgCmdr. Cleave was relieved of his responsibilities as senior POW medical officer. Someone had stolen beans from the warehouse; therefore, the Japanese concluded, Cleave did not have control of his men. After Tokuda took over all the serious cases, and until the day of liberation, all medical personnel in the Shinagawa POW Hospital laboured with pick and shovel from 7:30 a.m. until 7:00 p.m.[404]

Lt/Cmdr. J.R. Davis, USN, was at Shinagawa for one-and-a-half years. In a deposition he recalled some details of the chief Japanese medical officer:

> Tokuda is repulsive in his appearance. He is slender, about five feet in height, slightly stooped, and very bow-legged. His weight may be about 100 pounds. His vision is bad, and at Shinagawa he wore heavy spectacles without which he was helpless....He was quite studious, and he would spend hours and hours, day after day, in his room with piles of books all about him. When a shipment of books from the International YMCA came for Christmas of 1944 and again in 1945, he appropriated the very excellent medical books included therein and kept them for his own use.[405]

Davis also mentioned a systematic study Tokuda did of body weights and calories. This study did, in fact, result in increased food supplies for the prisoners.[406]

Tokuda's surgical ineptitude and the resulting dangers of operative disaster and post-operative infection caused much worry. The operating room was small. Tokuda invariably managed to touch some unsterile object while putting on his gown or during the operation. Thus the whole aseptic procedure became a farce. There were flies in the operating room in the summer and, if it was an interesting case, Japanese soldiers would crowd in (none wearing masks) until the doctors scarcely had elbow room. Davis therefore thought it wise to leave inside the abdomen several grams of powdered sulphanilamide. "I got almost no sepsis as a result."[407]

Davis records a total of 784 patients with 75 deaths—11 Americans, 18 British, one Indian, 6 Australians, 24 Dutch, 12 Canadians, 2 Norwegians and one Royal Italian Navy. And many more patients were treated before Davis arrived in the camp. Many patients arrived almost dead.[408]

Maj. Saldivar witnessed Drs. Fujii and Tokuda perform an appendectomy. It lasted almost three hours; they appeared to know little about surgical technique "and were actually butchering the patient." Eventually they left the operating room and ordered Col. Edwin Kagy, US Army Medical Corps, to complete the operation.[409]

Dr. Tokuda escaped retribution for these activities. Trial was interrupted frequently because of his poor health, and he died in prison.

Moxibustion

Allied interrogators took statements and, when appropriate, affidavits of evidence from thousands of prisoners of war in the immediate aftermath of the Second World War. They heard allegations of appalling conduct against POWs by some Japanese, several hundred of whom were tried and a high proportion convicted of war crimes in trials during the last half of the 1940s.

One complaint expressed by a few of these POWs was that the Japanese had tortured them, burning their bodies by lighting some sort of combustible substance piled up on various places on the skin. For example, here is an excerpt from a post-war deposition, made by Lt. Norman Eugene Churchill, who was assigned to Adjutant General, GHQ, as officer in charge of recovered personnel. He described his immediate post-war visit to the sites of Kamioka and Funatsu, 4 September 1945, giving some indication of the use of moxa as torture or punishment:

> Riggs was burned on the arms, approximately that far (indicating) on both arms. A fellow by the name of Thomas was burned on the ears and neck, behind the ear and on the back of the neck (indicating). Swisher was burned on the stomach and arms in the same manner (indicating an area about a foot long)....The scars were large, red, ugly looking things. I have never seen anything quite like it. It was very apparent that there was a lack of proper equipment for them to treat the wounds properly.[410]

What was done to these men? Some Allied prisoners were subjected to torture, but the vast majority of such cases refer to the use of torture to obtain evidence, carried out by the *Kempeitai* (the Japanese Army's special police division). The picture in such cases was unequivocally if unimaginatively torture, with ample evidence by hundreds of victims of barbaric procedures such as the water torture, hideous beatings, and burning various body parts, particularly the most sensitive. Most western POWs escaped such malevolent treatment; theirs was generally a more banal kind of brutality.

The quote above bears scant resemblance to typical *Kempeitai* activities. And setting aside the nefarious activities of the *Kempei*, torture per se was used relatively infrequently against Allied POWs. The explanation of Churchill's deposition seems to be very simple, yet tantalizingly complex. Distressing and painful as the burning was to startled, resentful POWs, in fact the procedure was medical therapy of a type having a history extending back more than two millennia: namely, moxibustion.

The procedure has several names, and the variety is increased by a creative approach to the terminology and its spelling by interpreters at war crimes trials, by the legal typists who prepared the official transcripts, and by those who typed depositions and affidavits throughout the world. Thus moxibustion also appears as moxybustion, moxa as moksa and Maksen, and the Japanese *okyu* also as *kyu* and *oque*.

A British POW officer who had lived in Japan for many years and married a Japanese woman, Lewis Bush was more culturally attuned to moxibustion than most:

> The captain of the "Morioka Maru" was passionately fond of moxa treatment. He used to burn himself all over every day. One night he persuaded me to be his victim when I complained that my stomach was upset. The doctor was disgusted with my meek acquiescence. All the officers and engineers not on watch were present. I lay on the saloon settee and the captain burnt me just below my navel. All present thought this most humorous and, I must confess, that I too, saw the funny side of it, especially as the captain took it all so seriously. But the climax came when as I got up from the sofa I passed an enormous blast of wind. Yes, it did relieve my stomach condition.[411]

The Japanese were unwilling to hear debate about their orders to have moxibustion administered. At Taisho POW Camp, the medical officer discovered painfully the futility of arguing with Nipponese Medical staff over this treatment. For "Beri Beri Pellagra & diarrhoea the treatment consisted of burning some sort of fusee on various parts of the body and to be done every day for 10 days." Because he protested against this procedure he was beaten for an hour and a half. And, of course, "[t]he treatment was that day & subsequent days carried out by the Nipponese."[412]

Other Allied prisoners of the Japanese recognized what their captors were trying to do to them, at least after a period of post-war reflection. Smith wrote in 1991:

Moxa, an age-old panacea prepared from the leaves of certain Chinese plants, was used on POWs in an attempt to eradicate the various diseases resulting from malnutrition. A Japanese doctor would designate primary locations on the anatomy of the poor ailing victim, where little cones of the dried material were to be placed, lighted, and allowed to burn themselves out. It was administered as a treatment for beriberi, pellagra, and painful feet, so prevalent among POWs. Although brutally uncomfortable, the patients submitting to this ridiculousness would survive, but for the rest of their lives, as a reminder of the practice, they would carry moxa scars on their bodies as a result of the questionable procedure.[413]

But many, perhaps most, saw the burning as either a kind of cruel experimentation or as deliberate torture. Lancelot Ross, a Canadian sergeant, was sure the burning was a type of experimentation having something to do with beriberi:

One time they took four or five of us, stripped us completely of our clothes and made us lie flat on our backs with arms and legs out. They came along with this cotton rope, about a half-inch. They would cut a half-inch length off of that rope and set them on their ends, at, I think, about six points. I had one on each side of my chest, one on each hip, on the side of my stomach, one on each wrist, one on each ankle and one on the centre of my forehead. Before they put them on they would light them with a match, and you know how slow cotton burns. They put them on a nerve center. And they would let them burn right down to nothing.

My God, it was awful the pain with it, when the fire came close to your skin. If you showed any tendency of moving they would holler at you and raise the rifle butts, and you had to stay there until all the rope had burned away, and then they would let you up. I had open ulcers and sores for months after.[414]

But another Canadian, Randy Steele, who had severe wet beriberi while at Niigata 5B, believed that moxibustion saved his life. One evening two Japanese, a woman and a man, came into the camp. They made several of the POWs lie on the floor, applied what appeared to be little sulphur wicks to their stomach and legs, and then set fire to them. "They burned right through the skin and the water came out the holes, big pans of it. They drained the fluid and I felt much better. I fainted during the burning but I guess that saved my life. Many of the boys who had it as bad as I did died before that treatment was given them. My swelling came down and I felt better."[415]

The medical records from Niigata make no mention of this unorthodox—by the standards of western medicine—treatment. But these records do make it clear that Steele was seriously affected by beriberi. He was confined to quarters for this disease from 22 December 1943 until 25 July 1944, and then again from 7 January 1945 apparently until the war ended. Thus beriberi was sufficiently severe to incapacitate him for work for 15 of the 23 months he was in Japan. On 18 August 1945, Maj. Stewart, the MO at Niigata 5B, noted Steele's condition then: "Still has swelling of legs otherwise feels & appears healthy."[416] So it seems obvious that moxibustion did not cure Steele, even though he believed that it had helped him.

Kondo Shoogo testified about giving moxa to various POWs, including a man named Rubia. This prisoner saw Kondo giving himself a moxa treatment and requested one for a headache he was suffering from.[417] Kondo had no connection with the medical department in the camp; his responsibilities encompassed finance and supply. He was asked how many men it took to hold a Japanese patient while he was being treated. "Usually when we receive these moxa treatments we go of our own accord so we try to take the pain as much as possible so usually we don't have anybody holding us."[418]

When asked if he was a licensed practitioner of moxa, Kondo testified that he was not. His understanding of the procedure stemmed from his previous war injuries:

> I did have a little trouble with my injuries sustained, so I went to a moxa teacher and had it done and returned to the prisoner of war camp and gave myself these treatments. A soldier whose father used to be a moxa teacher was here at the camp and worked for awhile and used to apply these moxa treatments to me practically daily.[419]

Kondo denied that he had treated a POW, McEwen, who subsequently died. Capt. Samuel A. Newman, MO in McEwen's camp, also testified about his treatment. Before his arrival at Kawasaki, the Japanese had been using "some kind of oriental therapy" to treat beriberi, appendicitis, gallstones, and other disorders. The POWs were burned on various nerve centres. McEwen had been burned on both ankles and on the tops of his feet. Like McEwen, Capt. Newman thought the treatment had helped.

> I got on the thing after the burn got so bad that it became infected, and it got so sore that I was able to get McEwen off work and eventually this burn worked its way through the skin and within a twenty-four hour period this liquid within McEwen drained out of him so that I could not recognize him the morning after this had drained out. He had gotten down so thin that he looked like skin stretched over a skeleton.[420]

As for the "oriental treatment," Newman was able to get it stopped when he arrived. To accomplish this he recruited the camp interpeter, Numano.[421] Why, one wonders, was he so eager to have moxibustion stopped when, despite the burns, it seemed to help the sick prisoners? Maj. Milton L. Kramer appeared as an expert medical witness for the prosecution. Counsel asked him a hypothetical question of some complexity:

Assuming that a person were afflicted with beri-beri and had been subjected to the treatment known as "moxa" by the burning of a punk-like
substance upon one of his legs in numerous places and that the resultant
burns became infected to the extent that large blisters of a reddish color
formed and finally a dark discoloration progressed from the toes of the
leg burned to the hip, would the failure to render medical attention to the
infected burns contribute to the death of the person so afflicted?[422]

Not surprisingly, Kramer answered yes. Equally unsurprisingly,
he stated that moxibustion had no place in the modern treatment of
disease. He went on to make an analogy between moxibustion and
cupping, a procedure that was a fundamental part of medical therapy
in the west for centuries, though ending in the nineteenth century.[423]

Numerous further examples could be cited. Burning by Artemisia
vulgaris, the mugwort species most commonly used, was performed
on Allied POWs by the Japanese. But the evidence strongly suggests
that in most instances—perhaps all—the procedure was intended to be
medical therapy. Some of the Japanese observers may well have rather
enjoyed watching the prisoners squirm with pain, but they knew that
the "torture" was incidental, a discomfort routinely experienced by
Japanese of both sexes and all ages.

The War Ends

Yet despite the sickness, the hunger, often despair, most of the men
endured. The months and years rolled by. Finally it was August 1945.
Suddenly, and for some almost unbelievably, the war ended. The survivors had seen their predictions of "next month" finally come true.

> Where the *Kempei* post used to be, now there was a U.S. road halt with a
> white-helmeted M.P. yawning as he slapped the pockets of pedestrians.
> One night I saw a bored American guard doing just what the Nips had
> done so often to us—ordering a man to stand to attention, beating him
> when he did not respond smartly enough. *Plus ca change.*[424]

Eventually the former POWs travelled by train to Yokohama and
were put on a hospital ship. "And that's where we lost everything. All
the souvenirs we had and everything that we had in our possession,
the pictures, or souvenirs like swords and things like that, they took it
all."[425] They stripped and passed through a disinfectant bath, after
which they all were issued with shorts, sailor's white pants, a tee-shirt,
and a white sailor's hat. From Yokohama they were taken to Guam
and then, after all those weary, desperate years, back to their homes.

Chapter 9

Less Than Perfect Soldiers

To obey Imperial commands, to be brave as well as just, to be humane as well as brave, and to realize the grand harmony of the world—such is the spirit of the Emperor Jimmu [first Emperor of Japan]. Bravery must be stern and charity must be far-reaching. If there is any enemy resisting the Imperial troops, we must destroy him with our tempestuous military power. Even if we succeed in subduing our enemy with our unrelenting power, if we lack the grace of refraining from attacking those who have laid down their arms and of treating kindly those who obey us, we can hardly be called perfect [soldiers].[1]

*T*his was the official position, referred to by Tojo Hideki at his trial. Those at the receiving end of the gun barrel, such as internee Agnes Newton Keith, had a pithy assessment of how well Japanese in the field adhered to such standards: "They were not sadistic, or masochistic; they were not Oriental, or Occidental; they were just a gang of lowdown young hoodlums who had complete power over a hundred people who could not strike back."[2]

Instances of maltreatment, cruelty, and brutality can be duplicated many times over, in examining the experiences of Allied POWs in the hands of the Japanese during World War Two. But it is not enough to recapitulate such stories as evidence of maltreatment. Why did such events occur? How widespread were they? What do we know about the motives of the perpetrators? The conduct of members of the Imperial Japanese Army towards their prisoners of war needs to be examined.

Notes to Chapter 9 are on pp. 370-73.

I do not suggest that the Japanese Army was incapable of atrocities; the evidence was produced in Manila. But brutality, not torture, was the army's besetting vice, and accident and callousness played a larger part in their misbehavior than calculation.[3]

The words "Japanese brutality" require definition. "Japanese," in this World War Two context, usually means citizens of Imperial Japan, but in particular situations the word may encompass Koreans, Formosans, East Indians, Burmese, and others who had volunteered or been suborned to join the Imperial Japanese or ancillary armed forces. Korea and Formosa were under Japanese domination before and during World War Two, and many men joined or were impressed into the service of the Imperial Japanese Army. For example, several thousand Koreans were rounded up and made POW camp guards. Rarely was this a voluntary action. See, for example, the account of Korean I Gill, better known to POWs at Haruku as Kasayama Yoshikichi, his adopted Japanese name. He stated that even though "it might look like you'd volunteered, force was behind it."[4] India and Burma were to be part of the Greater East Asia Co-Prosperity Sphere, and many men of these two countries were seduced or coerced into Japanese service; and, of course, some joined willingly and even gladly.

"Brutality" bends to definition less easily. It is used here as shorthand to include a wide array of insults to body and mind, both those resulting from direct physical violence and those consequent on indirect effects of starvation, overwork, humiliation, and despair. Brutality encompasses a wide spectrum, from the Japanese or Korean third-class private casually smashing a POW's bare toes with his rifle butt, to the implementation, as policy, of the equation that no work means no food; from the packing of hundreds of dysenteric POWs into the holds of slow, fetid cargo ships, to the refusal to permit local populations to aid prisoners; from "disciplining" POWs by making them stand, bareheaded, in the tropical sun for hours, holding heavy stones at arm's length, to withholding or refusing to supply medical supplies and equipment.

Insofar as that is possible, "brutality" will be used without bias and without inherent value judgment. But it is important to examine motives and reasons. Much of the brutality was deliberate, but even in these instances the motivation was often complicated and contradictory. Simple cruelty or sheer barbarity explains only a portion of the brutality. And at least some of the brutality to which Allied POWs were subjected in the Far East was unintended and sometimes even undesired by their captors. Brutality, therefore, will be used to refer to the effect on POWs without necessarily reflecting intent on the part of the Japanese.

Nor is there any suggestion here that only the Japanese, or only the Axis Powers behaved brutally during World War Two. Brutality of one kind or another is coeval with humankind, and will remain so. Large-scale brutality has occurred with depressing regularity throughout history, ancient and modern. We are all uncomfortably familiar with the barbaric brutality occurring today in many parts of the world as the new millennium dawns.

Inhumane and brutal treatment occurred in Far Eastern POW camps: that statement needs no further documentation. That its causes are complex and multifaceted seems evident. In addition to physical brutality, several factors contributed to the discomfort of POWs: lack of political concern for prisoners, lack of sympathy for them because of *bushido*, unexpectedly swift defeat of the Allies exposing logistical inadequacies, and almost total lack of qualified camp staff.

Bushido

This word appears in many accounts of the war in the Pacific, both in the Japanese and in the English-language memoirs. By the 1930s, *bushido*[5] was a languishing cultural hangover from centuries earlier, until the military establishment promoted it as providing guidelines to appropriate Japanese behaviour on the battlefield.

It might seem as if *bushido* and chivalry are similar, but that is not the case. One student of the concept has pointed out some of the differences:

> Chivalry not only laid down the correct conduct between knight and knight, but between knights and their enemies, civilians, women, and children. *Bushido* on the other hand was solely concerned with relations between *samurai* and their conduct in battle. The *samurai* could have no relation with his enemy, for one would be the victor and the other would be dead. Women and children were not protected either, and could be slaughtered as thought fit. A *samurai* had complete power over the women of his own household, and his interests were paramount; if it were necessary for his daughters to become prostitutes to pay his debts, then the code laid down that they should do so without hesitation. This facet of *bushido* explains the wide divergence of treatment given to prisoners of war by Japanese troops, from civilised to bestial.[6]

Bushido began during an age of great poverty. Life was cheap, and only by offering his life could the samurai eat and, later, if he survived, obtain a grant of land and other privileges. These pressures were something like those that might have forced his sister into prostitution. "With technological advance and the advent of a complex industrial society, one might have expected it to decay, as the medieval orders of chivalry decayed in Europe. But, in fact, no such process happened, and even in 1942 Renya Mutaguchi could write in an Order of the Day, when his campaign was heading for disaster: 'If there is no breath left in your body, fight with your spirit.'"[7]

When a Japanese soldier left his family to join his regiment at the front, his departure was punctuated by a ceremony to which family and friends were invited. This ceremony resembled funeral rites. A lock of the soldier's hair and a piece of fingernail were kept by his relatives. "From that moment, the man was dead, so far as his family was concerned, and was regarded by them as having returned to his ancestors. He could only come back alive as a conqueror. In the meantime, his relations experienced no wish to receive news of him."[8]

> Twice a year elaborate rituals were observed at the *Yasakuni* shrine (the Army shrine in Tokyo) and in these the names of the fallen were placed in an ark and carried up to the altar where, in the rites of the Shinto faith, they were deified. Sedulously the idea was propagated that any one man dying in battle would join the Gods if any part of his body, his nail parings even, could be brought back for the ceremony.[9]

The principle that no Japanese fighting man should permit himself to be taken captive, and that he should commit suicide should he be captured after being wounded,[10] was a fixed part of the Japanese attitudes in the 1930s and 1940s. Tojo Hideki testified to this point during his trial:

> The Japanese idea about being taken prisoner is different from that in Europe and America. In Japan, it is regarded as a disgrace. Under Japanese criminal law, anyone who becomes a prisoner while still able to resist has committed a criminal offense, the maximum punishment for which is the death penalty.[11]

If the Minister of War held this opinion, it seems safe to conclude that it was one that permeated the armed forces. The effect was profound, and impacted on both the Japanese soldier and the Allied POW. This attitude was seen as being part of the spirit of *bushido*. The corollary was that if a Japanese was taken prisoner, he was considered to be dishonoured, and his relatives were expected to look upon him as being dishonourably dead. Given that, the likelihood that opposing POWs would be seen with sympathy was slight.

A former US ambassador to Japan has discussed this topic, recalling that a year before war began he received from the Chinese government the name of a Japanese soldier who had been taken prisoner in China and who wished to notify his family that he was alive and well. Communicating this information to the government in Tokyo, he ultimately received the official reply. The Japanese government was not interested in receiving or transmitting such information. "So far as they, the Government, were concerned, and also so far as his own family was concerned, that man was officially dead. Were he to be recognized as a prisoner of war, shame would be brought upon not only his own family, but also his Government and his nation."[12] Purportedly,

Tojo ordered that if any Japanese serviceman should let himself be taken prisoner, his regiment was to execute him, if re-taken and, more-over, his crime should be visited on his entire family.[13]

In 1932, during the siege of Shanghai, a Japanese officer was taken prisoner and sent to Nanking (Nanjing). When World War Two ended, this man returned to Shanghai, found the spot where he had been cap-tured, and killed himself.[14]

Japanese soldiers knew that they were not to become prisoners; throughout the war this attitude became all too evident to the Allies. At Okinawa a survivor recalled seeing a Japanese soldier climb down the cliff. "A Japanese soldier raising his hands in surrender? Impossible! Traitor! We'd been taught, and firmly believed, that we Okinawans, Great Japanese all, must never fall into the hands of the enemy. Despite that, a Japanese soldier was walking right into the sea. Another soldier, crouching behind a rock near us, shot him. The sea water was dyed red. Thus I saw Japanese murdering Japanese for the first time."[15]

Civilians, driven by the martial spirit produced throughout Japan in the previous two decades, and by fear of the supposedly barbaric Allied soldiers, were just as fanatic. Again on Okinawa, there is a hor-rific recollection by Kinjo Shigeaki, now a Christian minister but 16 at the time: "My memory tells me the first one we laid hands on was Mother....When we raised our hands against the mother who bore us, we wailed in our grief. I remember that. In the end we must have used stones. To the head. We took care of Mother that way. Then my broth-er and I turned against our younger brother and younger sister. Hell engulfed us there."[16]

This Japanese assumption of dishonour being intimately related to surrender was displayed dramatically as recently as 1971, when the dis-tinguished Japanese novelist, Ooka Shohei, refused to accept a presti-gious literary award because of the shame he felt over having been a prisoner of war.[17] And Nishihara Wakana, a widow of an IJA soldier, has noted that some members of an anti-war soldiers' association became POWs at the end of the war. "Yet even their colleagues say things like, 'How can they speak about war when they ended up prisoners?'"[18]

> It had been a practice for Japanese who were taken prisoner to call them-selves by false names. Because of the shame, we took every precaution to see that our captors did not find out our real names. Lance Corporal Uehara, who had been an Assistant Station-Master for Japan National Railways in civilian life at Utsunomiya, called himself Toshi Uehara after a popular Japanese singer.[19]

In his memoir, an IJA corporal on Angaur Island, at the tip of the Palau Islands, remembered the comrades who fought and fell with him. "I can say that I'm proud to have belonged to that unit....At that time, the most earnest desire of us young men was simply and innocently to 'die for our homeland.' Especially in the Utsunomiya 14th Division, composed mostly of country boys, almost everyone had this simple faith."[20]

Bushido is a cultural phenomenon. There were other cultural differences between Japanese soldiers and their western prisoners that may have played a role here. One difficulty that westerners have in understanding their Japanese captors was the apparent inconsistency in attitude; for example, at least at times the Japanese guards were demonstrably kind to children, yet gratuitously cruel to animals.

We may forget that cruelty to animals is by no means extinct in our own culture. The various prevention-of-cruelty-to-animals groups sprang up relatively recently—the Cruelty to Animals Act in the United Kingdom, which represents the beginnings of general recognition in the English-speaking world that such cruelty should be prevented, dates only from 1876.[21] This was just 60 years before World War Two, only a moment in terms of human history. Moreover, the first societies that sprang up in the nineteenth century did so for the obvious reason that in those countries—England, Scotland, Wales, Ireland, Canada, the United States—a great deal of cruelty was practised against animals (and children). That is, violence of this type was so common in western countries that societies had to be created and legislation passed to attempt to control it. Thus the Japanese may not be so culpable if they have, in this respect, lagged some part of a century behind the western world in creating a general climate of disapproval for such acts.

But our concern here is with cruelty to humans—a practice well-established in the Japanese armed forces, principally by the process of enforced participation until the acts became mundane. Tominaga Shozo, a recruit in the IJA sent to China in 1941, remembered some of the details of his training. The day before it ended, an officer took the men to a detention centre. One room contained a group of Chinese prisoners. Lt. Tanaka announced that these were the raw materials for their trial of courage: "He said that it was to be a test to see if we were qualified to be platoon leaders. He said we wouldn't be qualified if we couldn't chop off a head....When my turn came, the only thought I had was 'Don't do anything unseemly!' I didn't want to disgrace myself."[22] Tominaga bowed to his regimental commander and stepped forward. Blindfolded, one thin prisoner knelt at the edge of the pit:

> I unsheathed my sword, a gift from my brother-in-law, wet it down as the lieutenant had demonstrated, and stood behind the man. The prisoner didn't move. He kept his head lowered. Perhaps he was resigned to his fate. I was tense, thinking I couldn't afford to fail. I took a deep breath and recovered my composure. I steadied myself, holding the sword at a point above my right shoulder, and swung down with one breath. The head flew away and the body tumbled down, spouting

blood. The air reeked from all that blood. I washed blood off the blade then wiped it with the paper provided. Fat stuck to it and wouldn't come off. I noticed, when I sheathed it, that my sword was slightly bent. At that moment, I felt something change inside me. I don't know how to put it, but I gained strength somewhere in my gut.[23]

If Tominaga is truly representative, some elements of the brutality experienced by Allied soldiers and POWs is the result of classical Pavlovian conditioning. All armies train soldiers to fight to survive. Not all—indeed, probably very few—explicitly train men to bayonet children. But My Lai has shown publically what every combatant knows: it happens. Tominaga himself passed the "exam" just described. He went on to train other Japanese soldiers, at a time when the enemy were Chinese, British, American, Indian, Australian, and others: "A new conscript became a full-fledged soldier in three months in the battle area. We planned exercises for these men. As the last stage of their training, we made them bayonet a living human."[24]

Another former IJA soldier has revealed how the banality of murder could grow to become an obsession:

I personally severed more than forty heads. Today, I no longer remember each of them well. It might sound extreme, but I can almost say that if more than two weeks went by without my taking a head, I didn't feel right. Physically, I needed to be refreshed. I would go to the stockade and bring someone out, one who looked as if he wouldn't live long. I'd do it on the riverbank, by the regimental headquarters, or by the side of the road. I'd order the one I planned to kill to dig a hole, then cut him down and cover him over.[25]

That such attitudes were being nurtured in the IJA boded ill for their future POWs.

Japanese Treatment of Their Own Servicemen

Trained in the grim philosophy of death, compelled to sell his life against impossible odds, condemned to blow himself to pieces with his last grenade retained for the purpose...rather than submit to capture, the Japanese soldier was brutalized from the day he entered the service....For all the shame which the Japanese nation was to endure for its treatment of others, yet no greater condemnation could be made than of the manner in which it allowed a system to develop which condemned its own sons to live and die in a mockery of human dignity.[26]

To help to understand the way Japan treated Allied POWs, we must inquire into their treatment of their own men. The Japanese attitude towards their own casualties is relevant because of the insight it may give into how they would regard Allied casualties. The record seems dismaying, for there is much evidence of behaviour ranging from callousness to brutality. For example, a Japanese train returning to Singapore from Burma was crowded with Japanese sick and wounded. They had been

> shut up in steel ten-ton trucks for many hours, without food or water, and with their wounds, all serious, untended. Many of the POWs were moved to pity and offered them water and even a cigarette; the stench was enough to knock you down. Little wonder that the Japanese High Command were callous to us, if that was how they treated their own people.[27]

Nohara Teishin, who was a soldier in China in the 1930s, experienced a cholera epidemic there. The men with cholera were moved to a bamboo grove that was surrounded by a rope. The patients had to promise not to leave. Nobody prepared food for them. "So I'd take my friend's rice and cook it for him. It was said that if you got too close, you'd be infected. But I passed things to him on the end of a bamboo."[28]

Equally unfortunate were Japanese casualties under treatment in forward hospitals when Allied military pressure forced retreat. During withdrawal under pressure, available evidence indicates that casualties who were too weak to walk were killed by the medical staff of the hospitals. The following order issued by the Chief of Staff of the 17th Division prior to its withdrawal from Gavuvu, New Britain, in January 1944, throws further light on this practice. "Arrangements to send the sick and wounded to the rear are being made, but if this causes an obstruction to the efficient execution of the withdrawal, unavoidable instances when the wounded and sick must be disposed of are to be expected."[29]

In the campaign on Bataan, American surgeons performed a careful plastic repair of the shattered arm of a Japanese soldier, captured while wounded. The technique required wiring the fingertips in place, coupled with continuous traction and other methods. When the hospital was captured by the Japanese, an IJA medical officer began to take down the traction; in reply to an American protest, he indicated that the method was too much trouble—the arm would be amputated.[30]

Ashton observed similar indifference, even cruelty, by Japanese against Japanese. Just after the surrender on Bataan a Japanese soldier was brought to No. 1 Hospital, having fallen and suffered a severe head injury. Dr. Ashton treated him and advised that he be taken to the nearby Japanese military hospital. He was picked up by the Japanese and literally thrown under the edge of the American hospital, to be collected later.[31]

In Japan, POWs saw many instances of this institutionalized insensitivity. Once they saw a badly injured Japanese worker in the mine, totally ignored by their Japanese *hancho,* who later explained that when "a Jap falls ill or is injured, he is considered a fool, who has offended the National Spirit and the War Effort."[32]

A soldier wounded late in the Philippines campaign of 1945 remembered the response of a medical orderly to his fear of death by gangrene:

> I had seen with my own eyes countless examples of the terror of a wound becoming gangrenous. Because of the hot sticky climate, the progression of gangrene was extremely rapid....Screwing up my face and twisting my body in agony, I tried to appeal to the medic, "Can't you at least do something to prevent gangrene?" The medic, who had not spoken a word, slowly and deliberately brought something out and placed it on my shoulder so it wouldn't drop. This was neither medicine nor a bandage. Giving off a dim black lustre in the deepening gloom, with a heavy feeling like lead, it was a hand grenade. The honourable doctor did not need to say it in words. I guessed it meant, "Military order: the best path for you is immediate suicide." I would never have imagined that the prescription for a serious injury would be a hand grenade. It was as final as receiving a death sentence.[33]

Deep-rooted differences between Japanese customs and beliefs and those of the western nations produced predictable conflict. Where national custom differed from the provisions of the Geneva Convention, it should not surprise us to find that the Convention was frequently ignored. One of these basic differences concerned corporal punishment, most commonly manifested to POWs as a slap in the face to punctuate and emphasize discipline. The Japanese in the 1930s and 1940s seemed to accept this as expected behaviour—unpleasant but inevitable and appropriate; many Allied POWs found it a gross insult, and a few died for reacting to it.

Justice was dispensed in the IJA in a manner quite different from western armies, where charges must be laid, forms filled, and courts martial conducted, and where the use of violence against another serviceman is forbidden. In the IJA, it was routine for derelictions of duty to be punished instantly, on the spot, by striking the offender. How much violence could be used, and what kind, depended to some degree on the offence, as well as on the enthusiasm of the punisher and on his certainty at being correct himself, since he was in turn at risk from someone higher ranking.

That such punishment was a routine is attested to widely. Here is the account of a Japanese soldier of an episode from his days in training in China:

One of my friends refused to bayonet a prisoner on command. For about a week, every day he was ordered to appear before senior soldiers. Each time he came back mangled. For this reason, even when the target was a child, when ordered to thrust, we obeyed.[34]

Nor need the cause of disciplinary action be so substantial as refusing to obey an order. Another former soldier remembered that once, while on active duty, he let some article of equipment slip off his horse's back: "one of the older soldiers strode up to me and, screaming that I was a no-good, struck me dozens of times with a length of green bamboo. When he had finished with this he began beating me in the face with a canteen."[35] Ooka, in his well-known novel, *Fires on the Plain (Nobi)*, refers to "the military tendency to raise one's temper automatically as one raised one's voice."[36]

At Hong Kong, Lewis Bush was watching some Japanese soldiers just after the surrender in December 1941. He had noticed that the ordinary soldiers were never seen with loot.

A young Japanese guard picked up a children's picture book from a heap of rubbish and was reading aloud in English, "Twinkle, twinkle, little star," when he was pounced upon by a "kempei" corporal, knocked down, kicked and beaten by a dozen of these monsters until he was covered with blood from head to foot and had to be carried away by his comrades. His oppressors laughed and thought they had had a great joke. My friends said: "Well, bad enough to be a prisoner, but thank God we are not Japanese soldiers."[37]

Kumagaya Tokuichi wrote: "People knew that military duty was as hard as a prison sentence."[38]

Many POWs observed such occurrences; their memoirs frequently mention beatings of Japanese guards by their own non-commissioned officers for what the POWs viewed as entirely trivial or non-existent offences. They also made the equation between this behaviour and their own ill-usage by their captors. One example will illustrate the point: a young Australian 2nd Lieutenant, captured at Singapore and imprisoned at Changi Camp, could see IJA infantry in training on an adjacent golf course; the young soldiers were "beaten and slapped by their NCOs if they made the smallest mistake in negotiating the difficult course."[39] After the war, the Minister of War, Tojo Hideki, rationalized this method of chastisement. He stated that face-slapping had been a common form of training among the ill-educated classes of the Japanese. In the IJA the use of slapping was forbidden, but it continued "because of the influence of the customs of the people."[40]

Not all Europeans, nor all Japanese, reacted similarly to being slapped. Frank Harding, Winnipeg Grenadiers, found that his response was contempt. "Their culture is entirely different from ours and I thought to myself, 'Ignorant people.' I suppose they thought it was the ultimate insult, but as far as I was concerned, I just thought, 'Do your worst—one day I'm going to get out of here.'"[41] But slapping was taught to the Japanese—forced upon them—at an early age. One teenager in the 1940s, Sato Hideo, disagreed with Tojo's self-serving assessment; she found the process repugnant:

> The thing I hated most was the habit of slapping among the pupils themselves. Again it was just like the military. All these customs entered our lives in 1944 and 1945. Everything then was done by group. If one member of the group forgot something important, or did-n't do his homework, everyone in the group was responsible. We'd be made to line up in the hall, two lines facing each other. The teacher would order us to deliver a blow to the student standing opposite us. I hated that....If you didn't do it at full force, both of you would be beaten by the teacher.[42]

Of course, much brutality was tied to the pragmatic reality that you *can* make some sick men work if you beat them enough, or if you withhold their food for as long as they are out of the working force. Here are the instructions expressed by War Minister Tojo Hideki on 30 May 1942, when he was inspecting the Zentsuji Division, which had responsibility for large numbers of POWs:

> To this Division is attached a prisoner of war camp. Prisoners of war must be placed under strict discipline as far as it does not contravene the law of humanity. It is necessary to take care not to be obsessed with a mistaken idea of humanitarianism or swayed by personal feelings towards those prisoners of war which may grow in the long time of their imprisonment. The present situation of affairs in this country does not permit anyone to lie idle doing nothing but eating freely. With that in view, in dealing with the prisoners of war, too, I hope you will see that they may be usefully employed.[43]

Some brutality to patients stemmed from the suspicion—sometimes justified—that MOs might assist the well in pretending to be sick. If so, beating up a few might help keep them all honest.

In the Far East during World War Two, the worst kinds of direct brutality were meted out by members of the *Kempeitai*. With these men, roughly the Japanese equivalent of the Gestapo, torture was routine. Post-war trials contain innumerable horrific descriptions by survivors of the cruel brutality that characterized the *Kempeitai* in action. Uno Shintaro, former *Kempeitai* member, has testified recently: "The major means of getting intelligence, though, was to extract information by interrogating prisoners. They don't say anything if you don't ask. Even threatened, they often didn't speak. If you torture them, some will talk. Others won't. Torture was an unavoidable necessity. Murdering and burying them follows naturally. You do it so you won't be found out."[44] This same former soldier for Imperial Japan candidly described the frighteningly banal motivation of a torturer:

> We tried to secure the needed information by using torture. I gathered capable soldiers and noncoms who understood Chinese and trained them. I was sure this was my purpose for living. I believed and acted in this way because I was convinced of what I was doing. We carried out our duty as instructed by our masters. We did it for the sake of our country. From our filial obligations to our ancestors. On the battlefield, we never really considered the Chinese [to be] humans. When you're winning, the losers look really miserable.[45]

Among Allied POWs, the most miserable were often those forced to work for the Japanese, usually too hard. In 1942, Minister of War Tojo Hideki admonished the newly appointed commanders of POW camps to "not let them [POWs] remain idle even for a single day, so as to utilize most effectively their manpower and technical ability for the expansion of our industries and to contribute to the execution of the great Eastern Asia War."[46] Such a statement could be translated into harsh action by overzealous or inhumane persons, who might well consider themselves to be following Tojo's instructions assiduously.

Many situations combined to promote the occurrence of brutality. An indirect cause was the logistical collapse that sometimes resulted from overwhelming military success occurring unexpectedly quickly. The IJA was quite unprepared to cope with the masses of POWs at Singapore and in the Philippines, for example. Another source of brutal behaviour was desperation. To give one instance, the Haruku Island airfield-construction project was doomed without tools, but for the Japanese in command, who were forced to show progress, any seeming advance was better than nothing. So they drove the POWs mercilessly.[47] Another all too common cause for brutality towards the sick could be categorized as incomprehensible stupidity. It seems the most basic kind of common sense to realize that feeding the sick usually helps them get better; thus, pragmatically, they could do more work. But the Japanese refused to feed ill and injured POWs adequately.

Failure to communicate is a category that perhaps should be placed at the head of the list, for the brutality experienced by the average POW, intent on minding his own business and getting home safely, was largely related to this failure. And it occurred at least partly because few Japanese spoke English (including, unfortunately, some of their interpreters) and fewer westerners spoke Japanese. But the failure had predictable and unpleasant consequences. Here is the quite typical experience of one Canadian: "I was in the convalescent ward and I got up in the morning to go out and wash and this Japanese gave me the end of his rifle butt right in the chest. I hadn't done anything that I could figure out, but he gave me another whomp, but I finally found out that all he wanted me to do was salute him."[48]

At least one POW seems to have made a successful attempt to breach the wall of misunderstanding that separated captor and captive:

> I decided to risk it. "In our army we do not strike or beat people as pun-ishment. Ito is always doing so and this blackens my thoughts about him." The little man's eyes opened wide. He wasn't angry—just amazed. He was a front-line soldier without experience of guard duty until he boarded the ship three weeks ago. For the next ten minutes he cross-examined me about this astonishing revelation. How did we pun-ish our soldiers then? How was discipline maintained in our army? How did we force our men to fight? He'd always understood that only our politicians and the officer-class wanted war with Japan and that the sol-diers and ordinary people had to be driven into battle at pistol-point. His obviously genuine notions about the position in Britain seemed even more incredible when he added later that he had gained an economics degree at Tokyo University and was also (as he put it) a "serious student of world history." From this time on, Ito's attitude to prisoners under-went a profound change. He was still as noisy as ever, but never again raised a hand against any of us.[49]

An unquestioned source of Japanese frustration and anger, often contributing to brutal behaviour, was the recognition that they were seen as having "inferior" status in the eyes of the west. This stigma was applied in Canada just as it was throughout the western world. Here is just one pre-war evidence of it.

The Hong Kong POWs experienced the direct result of Canadian inter-war racial prejudices through their effect on one Japanese-Canadian. This was the interpreter, Inouye Kanao, known without affection as "The Kamloops Kid" because Inouye had lived in that city in British Columbia. He seemed to delight in abusing prisoners, espe-cially Canadians. Later, as an interpreter for the *Kempeitai*, he became involved in the torture of suspects. But in Sham Shui Po, in 1942, "[w]e enjoyed, in an odd way, the sight of a fellow Canadian, free and well fed. His boots were beautifully polished and he smelled of clean, strong soap—perfume to me. Slender and sleek, he fascinated me and drew me with the hypnotic power of a handsome, magical boa constrictor."[50]

When Maj. Cecil Boon, regarded by many of the POWs as an arch traitor, was orderly officer in Sham Shui Po he sometimes made the rounds at night with "The Kamloops Kid." The two seemed to delight in interrogating Canadians. "The Kid said he had been ridiculed as a child in B.C. and he swore Canadians would pay for it; he was partic-ularly vindictive."[51]

Inouye had the perhaps unique experience, after the war, of being sentenced to death by two different jurisdictions. He was tried first as an ordinary Japanese war criminal, at Hong Kong, by a British court that had Canadian representation. After sentencing, his conviction was dismissed because the courts had no right to try a Canadian citizen. But he was promptly rearrested and tried by Canada for treason. That conviction was carried out in August 1947.[52]

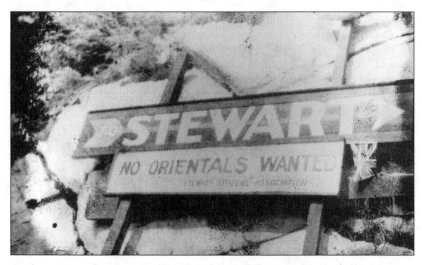

Figure 9.1. Sign at Stewart, BC, July 1929. (Provincial Archives of Manitoba, Canadian Airways Collection #1809.)

Dr. Anthony Coombes, an ex-POW in Hong Kong, was the Port Medical Officer there after the war. His colleague, the Police Medical Officer, was summoned to witness the judicial execution of Inouye Kanao after his conviction for treason. This doctor was a conscientious objector and refused to do this, so Coombes was asked to go in his place. He did so with no compunction and, I sensed at the time of our interview almost 50 years later, some relish.

> Inouye yes. I went to his hanging. I had to. The doctor who was in medical charge of Stanley Jail was a conscientious objector and he refused point blank to attend the hanging. A medical officer had to attend. And Newton, Isaac Newton who was the Director of Medical Services then rang me up. (I was doing Port Health,) rang me up and said, "I've got a job for you Coombes. I'm sure you'll enjoy it." I said, "Oh, what?" He said, "You've got to attend the hanging and do an official post mortem on a Japanese prisoner." And I said, "Oh, who's that?" And he said, "Oh a chap named Inouye." And I said, "OK. I'll do it." So I attended. In a way, well I hadn't personally much to do with him, but he used to swagger about and swat people, and throw them onto the ground. A nasty chap....But he went to his death shouting "Banzai!"[53]

Many ex-POWs have suggested in their memoirs that the Japanese (or all Asians) were by nature brutal and barbaric; that they were different from Europeans and North Americans. Thus the brutality that these POWs observed during captivity they regarded as inevitable; indeed, some of these writers carried the argument to its logical conclusion, often seeming to excuse heinous behaviour as being "natural" and unavoidable on the part of their captors.

Common sense suggests that such a solution is unlikely, for in terms of human behaviour there seems, to the student of history, little to differentiate any nationality or race from any other. But common sense carries slight weight as historical evidence. Nevertheless, the intimation that the Japanese are inherently and inevitably cruel and barbaric—that is, demonstrably more so than other national or racial groups—can readily be shown to be untrue by examining the history of their treatment of prisoners of war before World War Two.

In the Russo-Japanese War of 1904-1905, Japan inflicted a decisive defeat on the Russians, to the shocked surprise not only of the Czar and his countrymen, but also to all the western world and, perhaps, to the Japanese. Thousands of Russian soldiers and sailors were prisoners of the Japanese. How were these men treated? The evidence, as summarized by Veith,[54] reveals a situation quite different from what we might have expected on the basis of events in the 1940s. Medical treatment offered was excellent, with the result that only 2.4 percent of the wounded POWs died.[55] Camps were well-organized and complaints seem to have been minimal. The world was favourably surprised and impressed. "The Japanese themselves were quite aware and proud of the extent to which they followed the laws of the Geneva and Hague Conventions and their own literature on the Russo-Japanese war is full of this fact."[56]

> My grandfather took great interest in the Japanese Red Cross, and he served as its president from 1903 for ten years, after retiring from active participation in the government. During the Russo-Japanese War the Red Cross was very active; Japanese women proved their competence as nurses and volunteers; and several thousand of them ministered to over a million Japanese and Russian wounded soldiers and prisoners. For the assistance given the Russians, the Tsar in 1909 awarded a Red Cross decoration to my grandfather.[57]

In World War One, Japan was an ally of Britain and, ultimately, the USA. In the course of that war, Japan held as POWs a substantial number of Germans captured at Tsingtau in 1914, after a siege lasting some weeks. These men were held captive in Japan till the war ended; how were they treated?

An American observer recorded in 1916 that "the Imperial Japanese Government had shown a desire to safeguard every prisoner's health and welfare,"[58] though certainly there were complaints and problems. These were corrected, and in at least one camp, constructed in Bando in 1917 and amalgamating several previous camps, conditions seem to have been idyllic (if that word can be used to describe any prisoner-of-war camp).[59] But all camps improved, so that late in the war they all had "sports facilities, libraries, instructions in all types of academic and non-academic subjects and theater groups."[60] Perhaps the ultimate statistic is mortality. Of 4,592 German and Austrian POWs captured in 1914,[61] only 82 died before the men were released five years later, and of these 82 a number died of the worldwide influenza pandemic.[62] This is a mortality rate of 1.8 percent, to be compared with figures for World War Two of 4 percent for Allied POWs in Europe and 27 percent for Allied POWs in Asia.

Nogi Harumichi was convicted by the Allies of war crimes committed in Indonesia. In his judgment:

> Today, Japan's government justifies what the military did during those war years. I'm saying this because I'm receiving a pension today. The time I spent in Sugamo prison as a war criminal is included in my service. This is the Japanese state saying, "Thank you very much for your efforts. You acted for the sake of Japan." Although I was given thirty years by America for a crime I committed, it's treated as just a foreign sentence, unimportant. After I left Sugamo, nobody looked at me strangely."[63]

The situation may be different today, but in the 1940s American soldiers (and those of other nations) often had their own taste of institutionalized brutality as a routine part of the training process. William Manchester has described his indoctrination into the US Marine Corps.

> Boot camp is a profound shock to most recruits because the Corps begins its job of building men by destroying the identity they brought with them. Their heads are shaved. They are assigned numbers. The DI is their god. He treats them with utter contempt....in my day it was quite common to see a DI bloody a man's nose, and some boots were gravely injured, though I know of none who actually died." And he goes on to describe a discipline involving men alternately trying to hit a partner on the forehead with the butt of one's rifle. Too contrived a miss brought the DI to demonstrate, following which concussions were not uncommon.[64]

The Japanese People

> I know the Japanese intimately. The Japanese will not crack. They will not crack morally or psychologically or economically, even when eventual defeat stares them in the face. They will pull in their belts another notch, reduce their rations from a bowl to a half bowl of rice, and fight to the bitter end.[65]

In the 1930s, visitors to Japan were sometimes perceptive enough to sense what was going on. One Canadian family, living in Shanghai, holidayed near Nagasaki. Though they had a happy vacation, they also noticed many signs of change. Even in their vacation town, photography was prohibited. In the village stores, all toys were military: tanks, fighter planes, guns, cannons, gas masks, swords. "[T]he dolls were dressed as soldiers or nurses." Periodically, all work stopped while the villagers had mock air raid alerts, did calisthenics, or went through motions "which looked like the loading of an imaginary gun, perhaps anti-aircraft, for they looked frequently skyward."[66]

A Japanese novel portrays the impact on high school. The day began for the students with roll call, the flag-raising ceremony, then reading aloud the Imperial Rescript declaring war. The girls then marched to their classrooms. Every day Hanako, the young heroine of the novel, sewed collars on soldiers' uniforms; her classroom had become a sewing factory. Academic work was a thing of the past. "It was an assembly line method of production: those who sewed sleeves sewed only sleeves, while others sewed only trousers, or pockets, buttons, or buttonholes." The students did this work all day long.

> Even while attending school in Tokyo, Hanako without fail used to fall ill once a week and have to miss school. After transferring to Wakayama Girls' School, she found herself spending each day sewing on khaki collars, work which she detested. Her constitution was such that, if she had to do something she disliked, she would conveniently develop a fever. For this reason, she missed three consecutive days of school. When she returned to school, however, she was reprimanded severely by the teacher in charge. He said that if she had been in the army, her punishment would have been a long imprisonment. Hanako was the only one in her group who sewed on collars; therefore, as a result of her absence, there were over a hundred uniforms without collars. Illness was no excuse for being absent, she was told. Japan was now fighting to the bitter end, and anyone who fell ill was showing weakness of spirit.[67]

A European diplomat's wife observed some of the pre-war Japanese attitudes and beliefs:

> [F]rom the time they can begin to understand anything, axioms of honour, kindness, filial duty, and above all patriotism, are repeated and explained to them with a good faith and solemnity which would send our English schoolboys off into fits of scoffing laughter. The nursery catechism takes somewhat this form in Japan. "What do you love best in the world?" "The Emperor, of course." "Better than father and mother?" "He is the Lord of Heaven, the father of my father and mother." "What will you give the Emperor?" "All my best toys, and my life when he wants it."[68]

Here is an extract from a letter, Niwa Naomi (14) to Setsuko: "We're not schoolgirls now—I'm a farmhand and you're a factory apprentice. I think we ought to be clearer about that in our minds. In this emergency, Japan needs us to produce rather than study. I think we should concentrate on working in earnest."[69]

There is much that can be admired in this attitude. Unhappily, carried to extremes, it contributed to the misery of life in the Far East in the early 1940s—for, among many others, tens of thousands of prisoners of war.

Chapter 10

The Journey Ends—But It

Never Does

*A*t Hong Kong, there was a delay of almost four weeks between the apparent surrender of Japan and the arrival of Allied relieving forces. The ex-POWs had difficulty coping. One noted in his diary as late as 4 September: "All of us are just going on our nerves, drinking too much, too much entertainment all of a sudden."[1]

Finally, the war ended officially on 16 September 1945. On that date, Maj.Gen. Okada Umekichi, Occupation Commander, and Vice-Adm. Fujita Ruitaro, C in C, South China Fleet, signed the capitulation documents and surrendered their swords to Rear-Admiral Sir Cecil Harcourt, RN. This long-awaited ceremony took place at Government House in Hong Kong.[2]

A nurse who spent the last three years of the war in Stanley internment Camp recalled: "We heard later, that we only had about 8 days to live as we were going to be killed in groups of 30, as we were becoming a liability. We were saved by the atom bomb."[3] This assessment of the effect of the atom bomb is common among former Far East POWs. Whether civilian internees distant from the Home Islands would have been killed is uncertain, but it seems unlikely that POWs in Japan would have survived an Allied invasion.

Casualties

As it was, Canadian losses at Hong Kong were heavy. A total of 23 officers and 267 Other Ranks were killed or died of wounds: 5 officers and 16 Other Ranks of Brigade Headquarters, 7 and 123 of the Royal Rifles, and 11 and 128 of the Winnipeg Grenadiers. Inclusive in these num-

---

Notes to Chapter 10 are on pp. 373.

bers are those who were murdered by the Japanese when trying to surrender or after they had surrendered. Twenty-eight Canadian officers and 465 Other Ranks were reported wounded.[4]

Until 1943, all Canadian prisoners of war were kept in camps at Hong Kong. As a result of previous injury or of conditions there, 4 officers and 124 Other Ranks died. In addition, four POWs from the Winnipeg Grenadiers were shot by the Japanese, probably without formal trial, when captured attempting to escape. The diphtheria epidemic in the summer and autumn of 1942 caused 58 deaths. Ironically, regarding the survivors, some Canadian medical officers believed that this epidemic actually may have saved some lives, as the Japanese isolated for months men who were carriers of the disease and who would otherwise have been forced to labour on Kai Tak aerodrome to their physical detriment.[5]

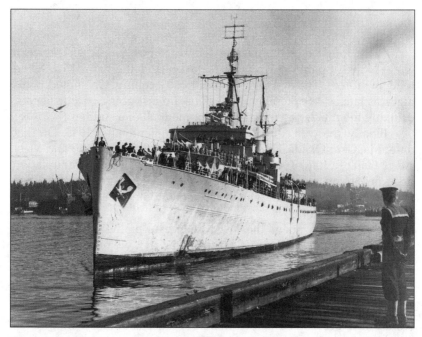

Figure 10.1. HMCS *Prince Robert* entering harbour at Esquimalt, BC, carrying Canadian ex-prisoners of war home to Canada, October 1945. (National Archives of Canada, National Photographic Collection PA. 116788.)

Beginning in January 1943 a single Canadian officer and 1,183 Other Ranks were taken on one or another of four drafts to Japan, where they were forced to labour in various industries, chiefly mining. This left a total of only 369 Canadian POWs in Hong Kong for the last two years of the war, a high proportion of whom were officers. In Japan, conditions were extremely bad because of the exhausting labour, and an additional 136 men died. Thus, of the 1,975 Canadians who sailed from Vancouver in October 1941, 557 were buried or cremated in the Far East.[6] Ironically, when those Canadians who had remained in Hong Kong were ready to be sent home, it was an old friend that did the job. HMCS *Prince Robert*, one of the ships that had brought them to the Far East, was charged with the responsibility of seeing the sickly, emaciated survivors home again.[7] She arrived in Esquimalt on 20 October 1945.[8]

The Medical Cost of Imprisonment

One US medical officer stationed at Guam examined 325 ex-POWs from Japan during September 1945. All were seen 12 to 15 days after release. Of the 325 ex-POWs, there were 129 US ORs, 48 US officers, 135 Canadian ORs, and one Canadian officer (all originally from Hong Kong, so the officer must have been Capt. John Reid, RCAMC), and 12 civilians. A table cites diseases suffered during captivity: the top six conditions were dysentery (184 – 56.4%), beriberi (136 – 42%), malaria (77 – 24%), avitaminosis (49 – 15%), diphtheria (40 – 12%)—Canadians from Sham Shui Po—and pneumonia (37 – 11.4%).[9] Ninety-nine of the men were infested with *Ascaris lumbricoides*, or the common tapeworm; average weight loss was 45 pounds.[10] Moreover, as the author pointed out, the men included in this study represented the more physically fit of the liberated prisoners, and of course it considers neither those internees who died in prison, nor those prisoners who were seriously ill and required immediate medical care before their evacuation to any distant hospital.

One pleasing event took place on the way home, in Hawaii. There, some of the Canadian POWs had the pleasure of finding one of the nursing sisters whom they had last seen three years before in Hong Kong. This was Nursing Sister May Waters, who was on the Canadian hospital ship *Letitia*, which was in Hawaii for repairs.[11]

After the war, medical assessments and tests of all kinds were performed on the former prisoners, a process that, in some jurisdictions, continues to the present day. Given the appalling conditions, it is perhaps worth noting that some men survived captivity in a relatively healthy state. Relative, not necessarily to fortunate men who had not been imprisoned, but rather to the remainder of their POW comrades.

> Perhaps the finding from the present study that was most surprising was the fact that 48 men, almost 10 per cent of our population, survived the malnutrition, hazardous working conditions, frequent beatings, et cetera, throughout the entire period, with no illness or accident that resulted in either hospitalization or lost working days.[12]

In 1950, former POW MO John Crawford examined medical files for the first 400 (alphabetically) of 1,400 HK veterans for the presence of various symptoms, the changes in incidence since the war's end, and the distribution of these symptoms in the various military districts of Canada. There were four complaints in which there was no significant difference in distribution in the six military districts. Two—optic atrophy and edema—are measurable, as is one aspect of a third, GI disturbances. Associated with these three in evenness of distribution was fatiguability, even though there is no test or objective way of measuring this complaint. But it has been observed in experimental starvation; therefore "one must assume that the complaint of fatiguability in the group under study is a 'true bill.'"[13] Crawford cites one case history of a man who had had some paresthesias, died suddenly from another cause, and was found at autopsy to have major neurological changes: "One should therefore guard against the assumption that the complaint of paresthesia is entirely or even mainly psychogenic in origin."[14] By 1949 it had become apparent that rehabilitation of these former prisoners of the Japanese had not proceeded as well as had been hoped or expected.[15]

The mental aspect was more severe than anticipated. One man, decades later, recalled with revulsion, "I still have nightmares about stepping in human waste and seeing big rats."[16] The post-war toll has been high, though that large subject is outside the scope of this book.

Retribution

There were, of course, war crimes trials for those Japanese, Koreans, Formosans, and others who had behaved particularly badly and who could be located. The results of some of these trials have been mentioned earlier. At least one Canadian believed the trials served a useful purpose. A member of the Royal Rifles was brought back to Japan to testify after the war, when the trials began. This was Sgt. Joseph M. "Red" McCarron (E29838):

> Some justice was done—seemed to be done. In a democratic fashion, they were brought to trial and had a fair hearing and no resentment when they presented their side. A real court. It wasn't just a travesty. It was a show, I think, for democracy and some justice was meted out eventually.[17]

However, there has been much debate as to how much justice was meted out. Some sentences seemed remarkably lenient, and the general shortening or cancellation of prison terms smacks more of politics than it does of justice. A legal historian, examining the trials relevant to Canadians after the war, concluded that "there was a superabundance of pragmatism and too little justice."[18]

There were Allied POWs who also had, at least in the eyes of some of their fellows, behaved dishonourably. A substantial number of complaints were described by men during interrogation after the war, and a few trials resulted. Maj. Boon was exonerated. CSM Tugby and the others from Oeyama were tried in Winnipeg in 1946 and were either acquitted or, at most, received reprimands.

Maj. Bowie expressed his feelings on this topic:

> I took part in some discussions on any action to be taken to report on the conduct of individuals while prisoners and I took the view that adverse reports should only be made in cases of the grossest neglect of duty and I made no report of this kind. Our staff and patients, apart from an occasional minor misdemeanour by one or two, conducted themselves splendidly.[19]

And note the feelings of Lt. Harry White, Winnipeg Grenadiers, and some at least of his fellow Canadian ex-POWs. Regarding some Japanese POWs at Manila: "on the whole we have a very tolerant attitude towards them. I don't know why it is after the treatment we got but we somehow feel sort of sorry for the little Bastards.[20]

Pensions

The struggle to convince reluctant governments to award pensions appropriate to service and to conditions experienced has been carried on by POW organizations in many countries.[21] The Canadian ex-POWs from Hong Kong have been leaders in this effort, achieving results that satisfy many of the men though, by the nature of such things, universal contentment will not occur.[22] One veteran has praised the government: "Canada has to be very proud of the way they helped veterans of the Second World War, more so than any other country."[23] In an attempt to wrest more adequate compensation from the Government of Japan, the Canadians have led an approach to the United Nations.[24] This ultimately failed to achieve any monetary results, as did an appeal to Japanese courts.

Postlude

Of the camps themselves, there remains little physical evidence, no matter how permanently they are stamped into the lives and memories of the survivors. In Hong Kong the best preserved former POW site undoubtedly is the Bowen Road British Military Hospital. No longer a hospital, it lives on vigorously as a school, the general physical entity unchanged in more than half a century.

Of North Point Camp not a shard now exists. One might almost say that North Point itself has vanished in the tumultuous drive to expand Hong Kong, which on the north shore of Hong Kong Island has meant the "reclamation" of as much as one-half mile of stone and cement into the harbour towards Kowloon. Immediately after the war,

North Point Camp continued in service. Dr. Selwyn-Clarke described, in 1946, what was then called the North Point Convalescent Home:

> This institution was opened towards the end of April, 1946, in rehabilitated buildings of what had originally been a refugee camp before the Pacific War and, subsequently, in turn a prisoner-of-war camp for British and Imperial troops and, lastly, for Chinese awaiting forcible "repatriation" by the Japanese.[25]

Sham Shui Po similarly evades discovery. Its position on the shore opposite Stonecutter's Island has become displaced inland almost half a mile, as the surface area of Hong Kong is pushed ever further into the surrounding waters. The Hong Kong Urban Council has constructed the large Sham Shui Po Park more or less on the POW camp site. In 1990 the Hong Kong Volunteers, and in 1991 the two Canadian regiments, had memorial plaques erected on a tiny plot adjacent to the children's playground. The Volunteers planted two trees that are flourishing: a camphor tree (*Cinnamomum camphora*) on the left as you look at the Volunteers' memorial, and a Casuarina tree (*Casuarina stricta*) on the right; sadly, the two maples planted by the Canadians were less successful. In December 1995 only one maple still graced the area, and it was stunted, broken, and offering no promise of long and vigorous life.

Of Ma Tau Chung Camp for Indian POWs there is no trace. It was located somewhere between the street of that name to the south and Argyle St. to the north, and it is in this portion of Kowloon that several prisoner-of-war sites were located. In the area bound by Prince Edward Rd. on the north, Lomond St. on the west, and Argyle St. on the south was the Argyle Street Camp which, during 1942-1945 held most of the officers (excluding the Indians) of the captured regiments and headquarters. After the war the camp was in continuous use until recent times, most recently housing Vietnamese refugees. During the war there were 16 or 17 huts; in 1995, only five remained, standing empty, doors ajar, the floor of one littered with children's school books in Vietnamese. The Hong Kong Eye Hospital and its nurses' residence and school almost surround the barbed wire fences and the huts, and given the modern cost of land in Hong Kong, the last remnants surely will disappear soon.

Just a block away, at the corner of Argyle St. and Forfar Rd., northeast corner, behind a six-foot tall heavy stone wall, lies the building that was used as the Imperial Japanese Army Prisoner of War Headquarters. Part of the building apparently was torn down during the construction of The Arcadia, 8 Forfar Road, a luxury high-rise of the type so much seen in Hong Kong in the 1980s and 1990s. The entrance into the property off Argyle St. is graced by quite a magnificent iron peacock six feet in height and spread across both halves of the gate. It is a modest two-storey building and one wonders how long it can withstand the pressure, so characteristic of Hong Kong, to build multi-storey apartment complexes.

Finally in this area, one other structure continues in active use and apparently permanent existence. What was the Central British School, now King George V School, is on Tin Kwong Road just south of Argyle St. and within eyesight of the POWs in the Argyle Street Camp. As Central British School, the building served as a POW hospital from April to September 1945. The Japanese closed down Bowen Road Hospital in March of that year, sending patients and staff to Sham Shui Po. The following month, after an alternative site had been ruled out as unsuitable, the patients were moved into the school.

In Japan, there seem to be no former POW campsites still in existence. The place in Niigata where Camp 5B was located, for example, is completely built up with apartment buildings.

Conclusions

Japanese prisoner-of-war camps throughout the Far East in World War Two can be seen as if they were a series of huge, ill-organized, badly equipped hospital wards containing tens of thousands of individuals. At any given moment most of the POWs were not classified as "patients," though most would have been so labelled at home in normal times.

For too many their undoubted illnesses and injuries, coupled with the impact of climate, starvation, and overwork, ended in death. For almost all, recurring ill health and hunger kept them miserable and unhappy, relieved far too infrequently by entertainments, Red Cross parcels, news from home, and the rare, clandestine joy of putting one over on their captors.

The vast majority of those who survived their ordeal did so with honour. That is, they did not give in, they did not collaborate, they behaved reasonably decently to their fellow sufferers, and they made it home. But too often they arrived home with unwanted and sometimes unrecognized baggage. They brought nicotine addiction and intestinal parasites. They carried the seeds of restless dissatisfactions and dysfunctions that, for many, led to broken marriages, alcohol problems, difficulty in the workplace, and premature death. Many of the long-term survivors, fast leaving us now, still grapple with the consequences of almost four years as guests of the Emperor.

They survived their long night's journey into day—but the day was not the triumphant, glorious nirvana visualized on the long grey days in Sham Shui Po or Niigata or Oeyama. Their experience deserves to be better known among those of us who have benefited from their sacrifices.

Notes

Preface

1 Cited in Telford Taylor, *The Anatomy of the Nuremberg Trials* (New York: Alfred A. Knopf, 1992), 9.
2 For a recent edition, see Henri Dunant, *A Memory of Solferino* (Washington: The American Red Cross, 1959).
3 Throughout this book, Japanese names are cited in the Japanese style: family name first followed by given name, except names within quotations, which have not been altered.
4 Shimomura was later War Minister to the last pre-occupation Japanese government, which lasted 16 August to 24 September 1945. See Richard Fuller, *Shokan: Hirohito's Samurai.* (London: Arms and Armour, 1992), 196.
5 Anonymous, *International Convention Relative to the Treatment of Prisoners of War, Geneva, July 27, 1929* (Ottawa: King's Printer, 1931), 31.
6 International Military Tribunal for the Far East (IMTFE), Defence Exhibits, Document 3044, Secret Memorandum of 6 September 1934, Hashimoto Toranosuke, Vice-Minister of War, to Shigemitsu Mamory, Vice-Minister of Foreign Affairs.
7 IMTFE, Defence Exhibits, Document 3043, Secret Memorandum of 15 November 1934, Vice-Minister of Navy to Vice-Minister of Foreign Affairs.
8 This process is outlined in Charles G. Roland, "Allied POWs, Japanese Captors, and the Geneva Convention," *War and Society* 9 (1991): 83-101.
9 IMTFE, Defence Exhibits, Document 1494.
10 IMTFE, Defence Exhibits, Document 1490.
11 IMTFE, Defence Exhibits, Document 1493, Togo to Swiss Minister, 2 March 1942.

Abbreviations

1 Between World War One and World War Two, the officer corps of the Indian Army, formerly exclusively British, was being altered rapidly to include increasing numbers of Indian officers. These men were of three types, KCOs (who had been through Sandhurst), ICOs (who had studied at Dehra Dun in India, and VCOs. The first two groups were treated as equivalent to British officers. But, according to Elphick and Smith, "[t]he vast majority of Indian officers were VCOs and, no matter how senior, were subordinate to the most junior of British officers. (Peter Elphick and Michael Smith, *Odd Man Out: The Story of Singapore Traitor* (London: Coronet Books, Hodder and Stoughton, 1994), 97.

Chapter 1

1 Gabriel Guitard, notebook kept, in pencil, at Niigata POW Camp 5B, October 1943 to February 1944. Copy in possession of the author.

2 C. Miller Fisher, "Residual Neuropathological Changes in Canadians Held Prisoners of War by the Japanese (Strachan's Disease)," *Canadian Services Medical Journal* 11 (1955): 157-99; see pp. 167-68, where he is identified simply as "A.C.T."; among "C" Force personnel, only Arthur C. Thomas, H6185, Winnipeg Grenadiers, had these initials.

3 C.P. Stacey, *Official History of the Canadian Army in the Second World War,* Vol. I: *Six Years of War* (Ottawa: Edmond Cloutier, 1955), 455; Oliver Lindsay, *The Lasting Honour: The Fall of Hong Kong 1941* (London: Hamish Hamilton, 1978), 15-16.

4 George Beer Endacott, *Hong Kong Eclipse* (Hong Kong: Oxford University Press, 1978), 57-58.

5 Stacey, *Six Years of War,* 457; Lindsay, *The Lasting Honour,* 17-19.

6 Endacott, *Hong Kong Eclipse,* 48.

7 Peter H. Starling, *In Oriente Fidelis: The Army Medical Services in the Battle of Hong Kong, December 1941* (Aldershot: RAMC Historical Museum [1986]), 3.

8 Starling, *In Oriente,* 3.

9 Norman J. Leath, "Report Prepared for C.G. Roland on 1st February 1988," 6.

10 Public Record Office (PRO), London, WO 222/20A, War Diary of Lt. Col. C.O. Shackleton, RAMC, OC, Military Hospital, Bowen Road, Hong Kong, 3.

11 Imperial War Museum (IWM), London, Item 93/18/1, Papers of Mrs. D. Ingram [Sister D. Van Wart], Hong Kong, 2.

12 Donald C. Bowie, "Captive Surgeon in Hong Kong: The Story of the British Military Hospital, Hong Kong, 1942-1945," *Journal of the Hong Kong Branch of the Royal Asiatic Society* 15 (1975): 158.

13 Starling, *In Oriente,* 4.

14 "In morning Bevan, Mrs. Cook and I went per Mr. Bevan's car to Bacteriological Institute to have blood tests. Dr. Beggie took the test—it was dark brown (venous)....They won't take the actual blood till it is wanted." IWM, London, Department of Documents, Item 73/671, Papers of Barbara C. Redwood, entry of 21 November 1941.

15 IWM, Redwood Papers, entry of 30 November 1941.

16 John Luff, *The Hidden Years* (Hong Kong: South China Morning Post, 1967), 8.

17 For biographical details see the entry, "Henry Duncan Graham [Harry] Crerar," Daniel J. Bercuson and J.L. Granatstein, *Dictionary of Canadian Military History* (Toronto: Oxford University Press, 1992), 55-56.

18 Sir Lyman P. Duff, *Report on the Canadian Expeditionary Force to the Crown Colony of Hong Kong* (Ottawa: King's Printer, 1942), 14.

19 Stacey, *Six Years of War,* 441.

20 Stacey, *Six Years of War,* 443.

21 Anonymous, *The Royal Rifles of Canada in Hong Kong, 1941-1945* (Sherbrooke: Hong Kong Veterans' Association of Canada, Quebec-Maritimes Branch, 1980), 7.

22 Stacey, *Six Years of War,* 444; Lindsay, *The Lasting Honour,* 9.

23 Stacey, *Six Years of War,* 444-45.

24 Stacey, *Six Years of War,* 445-47.

25 Galen Roger Perras, "'Our Position in the Far East Would Be Stronger without This Unsatisfactory Commitment': Britain and the Reinforcement of Hong Kong, 1941," *Canadian Journal of History* 30 (1995): 257.

26 C.R. Shelley, "HMCS *Prince Robert*: The Career of an Armed Merchant Cruiser," *Canadian Military History* 4 (1995): 47-60.

27 For biographical details, see Bercuson and Granatstein, *Dictionary of Canadian Military History*, 114.
28 H/Capt. Uriah Laite, MC, United Church; H/Capt. James Barnett, Church of England; and H/Capt. F.J. Deloughery, Roman Catholic.
29 Stacey, *Six Years of War*, 448.
30 Anonymous, *Canadian Prisoners of War and Missing Personnel in the Far East* (Ottawa: King's Printer, 1945), 59.
31 Kay Christie, "Behind Japanese Barbed Wire—A Canadian Nursing Sister in Hong Kong," *Royal Canadian Military Institute Year Book* (Toronto: RCMI, 1979), 11-13.
32 Dr. S. Martin Banfill, interview by C. Roland, Hannah Chair for the History of Medicine, Oral History Archive, McMaster University, Hamilton, Ontario, HCM 27-83, Montreal, PQ, 14 July 1983 (hereafter, all interviews in this archive are referred to simply as CGR, HCM); see p. 8 for his account of this unfortunate instance.
33 Lindsay, *The Lasting Honour*, 13.
34 Colin Standish, cited in Anonymous, *Royal Rifles of Canada*, 15.
35 Stacey, *Six Years of War*, 449.
36 National Archives of Canada (NAC), Ottawa, MG 30 E181, Tom Forsyth, "Hong Kong Diary and Memories of Japan: Gleanings from the Diary of a Winnipeg Grenadier," entries for 1 and 3 December 1941.
37 NAC MG 30 E181, Forsyth Diary, entry for 28 November 1941.
38 IWM, File PP/MCR/243, Diary of A.J. Alsey, 1942.
39 J.N.B. Crawford, "A Medical Officer in Hong Kong," *Manitoba Medical Review* 26 (1946): 63-68.
40 William Allister, *Where Life and Death Hold Hands* (Toronto: Stoddart, 1989), 16.
41 Crawford, "A Medical Officer in Hong Kong," 63.
42 Banfill interview, HCM 27-83, 10.
43 Capt. Daniel Bergsma, cited in Peter Neary, "Venereal Disease and Public Health Administration in Newfoundland in the 1930s and 1940s," *Canadian Bulletin of Medical History/Bulletin canadien d'histoire de la médicine* 15 (1998): 144.
44 Bowie, "Captive Surgeon," 157.
45 Crawford, "A Medical Officer," 63.
46 Allister, *Where Life and Death*, 17.

Chapter 2

1 C.P. Stacey, *Six Years of War*, 458-60; Lindsay, *The Lasting Honour*, 20-22.
2 John Luff, *The Hidden Years*, vii-viii, Appendix B.
3 J.N.B. Crawford, "A Medical Officer in Hong Kong," 63.
4 IWM, London, Item P324, Papers of Mrs. Day Joyce, Hong Kong, 40.
5 Donald C. Bowie, "Captive Surgeon," 159.
6 Thomas F. Ryan, *Jesuits under Fire in the Siege of Hong Kong, 1941* (London: Burns Oates & Washbourne, 1945), 75-76.
7 Australian War Memorial (AWM), Canberra, Personal Records, PR 83, File 32, Report of Service from December 1941 to September 1945, of Captain J.J. Woodward, IMS/IAMC, 1.
8 Rhodes House Library, Oxford, MSS.Ind.Ocn.s.233, Dr. K.H. Uttley, Hong Kong, "My Internment Diary: December 8th, 1941-August 1945," entry for 12 December 1941, 6.
9 Rhodes House Library, Uttley Diary, entry for 12 December 1941, 7.
10 Government Records Service, Public Record Office (PRO), Hong Kong, Ref. No. AB/920, Acc. No. 4462 (B), Copy of Diary Kept by Dr. Isaac Newton, entry for 15 December 1941.

11 Greenhous has shown how precarious the water supply was, yet how ignorant of the problem the London planners were. See Brereton Greenhous, "C" *Force to Hong Kong: A Canadian Catastrophe, 1941-1945* (Toronto: Dundurn Press, 1997), 40-41.

12 Greenhous, *"C": Force*, 40-41.

13 Rhodes House Library, Uttley Diary, entry for 15 December 1941, 10.

14 PRO, Hong Kong, Newton Diary, entry for 22 December 1941.

15 Rhodes House Library, Uttley Diary, entry for 15 December 1941, 11-12.

16 IWM, Joyce Papers, 6.

17 IWM, Joyce Papers, 12.

18 IWM, Joyce Papers, 13.

19 Rhodes House Library, Uttley Diary

20 Rhodes House Library, Uttley Diary

21 IWM, Joyce Papers, entry for 8 December 1941, 2.

22 IWM, Joyce Papers, entry for 8 December 1941, 3.

23 Rhodes House Library, Uttley Diary

24 Rhodes House Library, Uttley Diary

25 IWM, Joyce Papers, entry for 10 December 1941, 5-6.

26 IWM, Joyce Papers, 18-19.

27 Rhodes House Library, Oxford, MSS.Ind.Ocn.s.76, Lance A. Searle, Diary, Wartime and Stanley Gaol, 1941-1943, 57.

28 Rhodes House Library, Uttley Diary, entry for 24 December 1941, 16.

29 PRO, Hong Kong. Hong Kong Record Series No. 225, War Diary of Maj. E.G. Stewart, D & S No. 1/48(2), notes for 22 December 1941.

30 Cited in Alan Birch and Martin Cole, *Captive Christmas: The Battle of Hong Kong, December 1941* (Hong Kong: Heinemann Asia, 1979), 110.

31 Walter T. Steven, *In This Sign* (Toronto: Ryerson Press, n.d.), 63.

32 Marsman records that Japanese artillery destroyed the water mains on Hong Kong Island on 19 December. Jan H. Marsman, *I Escaped from Hong Kong* (New York: Reynal & Hitchcock, 1942), 27-28.

33 Bowie, "Captive Surgeon," 159.

34 Bowie, "Captive Surgeon," 159.

35 Data from lists maintained by Cpl. N.J. Leath as part of his duties as chief clerk at Bowen Road Hospital; copies sent by Leath to C.G. Roland, 1990.

36 IWM, London, Item 93/18/1, Papers of Mrs. D. Ingram [Sister D. Van Wort], 3.

37 Ryan, *Jesuits under Fire*, 143-44.

38 IWM, Department of Documents, London, Item 73/671, Papers of Barbara C. Redwood, entry for 30 November 1941.

39 IWM, London, Item PP/MCR/25, Memoirs of Mrs. M.W. (Barbara) Redwood, Microfilm of TLS, MS entitled "Incident at Jockey Club, Happy Valley, Hong Kong, Dec. '41," 4.

40 Birch and Cole, *Captive Christmas*, 74.

41 Birch and Cole, *Captive Christmas*, 17.

42 Birch and Cole, *Captive Christmas*, 21.

43 Birch and Cole, *Captive Christmas*, 25.

44 Birch and Cole, *Captive Christmas*, 27.

45 Birch and Cole, *Captive Christmas*, 28.

46 Birch and Cole, *Captive Christmas*, 31.

47 Birch and Cole, *Captive Christmas*, 36-37.

48 PRO, London, War Crimes Papers, Judge Advocate General's Office, WO 235, File 1107, Trial of Lt.Gen. Ito Takeo, IJA, testimony of Miss Amy Williams, 62ff.

49 Amy Williams testimony, 64.

50 IWM, Redwood memoirs, 44.

51 Phillip Bruce, *Second to None: The Story of the Hong Kong Volunteers* (Hong Kong: Oxford University Press, 1991), 272.
52 IWM, Redwood Papers, entry for 23 December 1941.
53 IWM, Ingram Papers, 3.
54 IWM, Ingram Papers, 3.
55 IWM, Ingram Papers, 4.
56 Personal communication, (typed letter, signed), Muriel Jean (McCaw) Channing to author, 11 March 1996, 2.
57 IWM, Ingram Papers, 4.
58 IWM, Ingram Papers, 4.
59 IWM, Ingram Papers, 4-5.
60 Rhodes House Library, Uttley Diary, 30.
61 Rhodes House Library, Uttley Diary, 30-31.
62 George Beer Endacott, *Fragrant Harbour: A Short History of Hong Kong* (Hong Kong: Oxford University Press, 1962), 164.
63 Wellcome Institute for the History of Medicine, London, Contemporary Medical Archives Collection (CMAC), Medical Women's Federation Collection, SA/MWF, Box 21, C/195, Work of British Medical Women in POW Camps, TLS Report by Dr. Annie Sydenham, Nethersole Hospital, Hong Kong, 9 April 1950, 1.
64 Wellcome Institute, Sydenham Report, 1.
65 Wellcome Institute, Sydenham Report, 1.
66 Wellcome Institute, Sydenham Report, 1.
67 Endacott, *Fragrant Harbour*, 161.
68 I.D. Zia, *The Unforgettable Epoch (1937-1945)* (Hong Kong: Chi Sheng Publishing, 1971), 41-42.
69 Cited in Haruko Taya Cook and Theodore F. Cook, *Japan at War: An Oral History* (New York: The New Press, 1992), 462.
70 Imperial Military Tribunal for the Far East (IMTFE), Exhibit No. 1982A, Extract from Testimony of Hideki Tojo, 27 March 1946, 5 pp. Translation of section marked by Tojo in book published 8 January 1941, *Senjin Kun* (*Teachings for the Battlefield*), 2-3.
71 PRO, WO 235, File 1015, Trial of Shoji Toshishige; affidavit of L/Cpl. Gordon Edward Williamson, 2 March 1946, 2.
72 Much of the remainder of this chapter is based on an article by the author, "Massacre and Rape in Hong Kong: Two Case Studies Involving Medical Personnel and Patients," *Journal of Contemporary History* 32 (1997): 43-61.
73 Starling, *In Oriente*, 4.
74 Bruce, *Second to None*, 235.
75 Stacey, *Six Years of War*, 488.
76 These men were QMS R. Buchan, MM, Sgt. E. Watt, Cpl. A. Newton, Cpl. Norman J. Leath, Pte. H.L. Mohan, Pte. J.C. Dunne, Pte. A.C. Williams, Pte. G. McFarquhar, Pte. I. Langley, and Pte. R. Reid.
77 These names and numbers derive from PRO WO 222/20A, War Diary of Lt Col. C.O. Shackleton, RAMC, Appendix D: List of Personnel at Salesian Mission House; and from PRO WO 235, File 1107, Testimony of Miss Lois Fearon, 109-14.
78 IMTFE, Defence Counsel Evidence, Vol. 37, No. 1595A, Summary of Examination of Capt. Osler Thomas, 9 March 1946, 1.
79 PRO, WO 235, File 1030, Trial of Maj.Gen. Tanaka Ryosaburo for war crimes in December 1941, Testimony of Miss Lois Fearon, 203.
80 PRO, WO 235, File 1030, Testimony of S. Martin Banfill, 19.
81 Personal communication, letter from Dr. Banfill to author, 24 January 1995.
82 PRO, WO 235, File 1030, Examination of Mary Suffiad, 1.

83 NAC, Ottawa. RG 24, C 2 (f), Vol. 8018, file TOK-1-2-5, part 1, Letter by E.H. Tinson, 4 April 1946, re: Events at Shau Kie Wan on 19 December 1941, 2.

84 Personal communication, S. Martin Banfill to author, 1983.

85 IMTFE, Vol. 37, No. 1594, Affidavit of Capt. S. Martin Banfill, 1-2.

86 Much of the detail given here is from an affidavit sworn by Cpl. Norman John Leath, Wilton, UK, 23 January 1946.

87 IMTFE, Vol. 37, No. 1594, Banfill Affidavit, 3.

88 PRO, WO 235, File 1030, Prosecution Exhibit 5, Affidavit of Capt. Osler Thomas, 1.

89 PRO, WO 235, File 1107, Trial of Ito Takeo, Testimony of Miss Lois Fearon, 112.

90 PRO, WO 235, File 1030, Prosecution Exhibit Q, Affidavit of Cpl. N. Leath, 2.

91 Personal communication, Norman Leath to author, 18 January 1995.

92 Leath, "Report Prepared for C.G. Roland," 25-26.

93 Leath, "Report Prepared for C.G. Roland," 27.

94 Leath, "Report Prepared for C.G. Roland," 18.

95 PRO, WO 235, File 1030, Affidavit of Capt. Osler Thomas, 1.

96 Edwin Ride, *BAAG: Hong Kong Resistance, 1942-1945* (Hong Kong: Oxford University Press, 1981), 3.

97 PRO WO 235, File 1030, 63.

98 IMTFE, Vol. 37, No. 1594, Affidavit of S. Martin Banfill, 3.

99 Communication did exist between the Far East POW world and Canada. Not only did Mrs. Banfill hear of her husband's "death," but in turn he knew of her sad end. On 22 March 1943, Sgt. Ray Squires noted in his diary that Capt. Banfill had received the tragic news; "he is a very fine man and carries it well." Raymond Squires, "War Diary, Hong Kong and Kowloon, 1941-1945," 28.

100 Charles G. Roland, "Allied POWs, Japanese Captors, and the Geneva Convention," *War & Society* 9 (1991): 83-101.

101 Telford Taylor, *The Anatomy of the Nuremberg Trials* (New York: Alfred A. Knopf, 1992), 10.

102 PRO, WO 235, File 1107, Testimony of Tanaka Ryusaburo, 154.

103 PRO, WO 235, File 1107, Affidavit of S. Martin Banfill, 3.

104 PRO, WO 222/20A, Shackleton War Diary, 4.

105 PRO, WO 235, File 1107, Testimony of S.D. Begg, 69.

106 Anonymous, *A Record of the Actions of the Hongkong Volunteer Defence Corps in the Battle for Hong Kong, December, 1941* (Hong Kong [1954]), 53.

107 PRO, WO 235, File 1107, Testimony of Mrs. E.A. Fidoe, 53-61, and Mr. S.D. Begg, 66-72.

108 Anonymous, *A Record of the Actions*, 54.

109 Luff, *Hidden Years*, 143.

110 PRO, WO 222/20A, Shackleton War Diary, 18 December 1941, 13.

111 IMTFE, Exhibit 1591A, Statement of Sister Miss A.F. Gordon of Events That Occurred at St. Stephen's College Hospital During the Period 23–26 December 1941, 2.

112 Freddie Guest, *Escape from the Bloodied Sun* (London: Hutchinson's Universal Book Club, 1957), 41.

113 PRO, WO 235, File 1107, Testimony of S.D. Begg, 72.

114 Randolph Steele, "With the Royal Rifles of Canada in Hong Kong and Japan," MS memoir in possession of the author, 6.

115 Lewis Bush, *Clutch of Circumstance* (Tokyo: Okuyama, 1956), 23.

116 PRO, WO 222/20A, Appendix F, Statement of Sgt. H. Peasegood, RAMC, on Events at St. Stephen's College, 1.

117 PRO, WO 222/20A, Appendix F, Statement of Sgt J.H. Anderson, 2.

118 National Archives and Records Administration (NARA), Washington, RG 153, File 35-552, Trial of Lt. Nichizawa Masao, Affidavit of Capt. J.A.G. Reid, 1.

119 Steele, "With the Royal Rifles," 5.

120 Steele, "With the Royal Rifles," 5.

121 Wenzell Brown, *Hong Kong Aftermath* (New York: Smith & Durrell, 1943), 97-98.

122 Brown, *Hong Kong Aftermath*, 112-13.

123 Personal communication, meeting of Arthur Gomes and the author, 4 December 1995, Hong Kong.

124 Shu-Fan Li, *Hong Kong Surgeon* (New York: E.P. Dutton, 1964), 102ff.

125 Zia, *Unforgettable Epoch*, 45.

126 Zia, *Unforgettable Epoch*, 52-29.

127 Susan Brownmiller, *Against Our Will: Men, Women, and Rape* (New York: Simon and Schuster, 1975), 37.

128 In English, three principal sources document these experiences. The literature in Japanese is much more extensive. See the following: Soka Gakkai Youth Division, *Peace Is Our Duty: Accounts of What War Can Do to Man*, trans. Richard L. Gage (Tokyo: Japan Times, 1982); Soka Gakkai Youth Division, *Cries for Peace: Experiences of Japanese Victims of World War II* (Tokyo: Japan Times, 1978); and Haruko Taya Cook and Theodore F. Cook, *Japan at War: An Oral History* (New York: New Press, 1992).

129 Soka Gakkai, *Peace Is Our Duty*, 129.

130 Ruth Seifert, "War and Rape: A Preliminary Analysis," in Alexandra Stiglmayer, ed., *Mass Rape: The War against Women in Bosnia-Herzegovina*, trans. Marion Faber (Lincoln: University of Nebraska Press, 1993), 58 and 64.

131 A useful history of these events is: Iris Chang, *The Rape of Nanking: The Forgotten Holocaust of World War II* (New York: Penguin Books, 1998), 290.

132 Bruce, *Second to None*, 272.

133 PRO, WO 235, File 1015, Trial of Shoji Toshishige, Affidavit of L/Cpl. Charles Bradbury, 9 March 1946, 1.

134 Les Canivet, Interview, CGR, HCM 60-85, Grand Valley, ON, 11-12.

135 Bowie, "Captive Surgeon," 160.

136 William Allister, *Where Life and Death Hold Hands* (Toronto: Stoddart, 1989), 44. Italics in original.

137 James Bertram, *Beneath the Shadows: A New Zealander in the Far East, 1939-46* (New York: John Day, 1947), 98.

138 Zia, *Unforgettable Epoch*, 62-63.

139 University of Alberta Archives, Edmonton, Accession No. 77-1, Dr. Benjamin Wheeler Papers, Box 1, File 5, Memoir, "Some Experiences as a Prisoner-of-War of the Japanese," 1-2.

Chapter Three

1 David Bosanquet, *Escape through China: Survival after the Fall of Hong Kong* (London: Robert Hale, 1983), 125.

2 David A. Golden, Interview, CGR, HCM, 1-84, Ottawa, ON, 12 January 1984, 8.

3 These dates and times are taken from Martyn's diary, kept throughout his captivity: Canadian War Museum, Ottawa, (CWM) F.D.F. Martyn Papers, Acc. 1981-276/10, cat. no. 60-6-52.

4 PRO, WO 235, File 1015, Trial of Shoji Toshishige; Affidavit of Cpl. Sydney Hiscox, WG, 11 March 1946, 2.

5 PRO, WO 235, File 1015, Affidavit of Cpl. Samuel Kravinchuk, WG, 19 January 1946.

6 Itinerary based on interview with Arthur Gomes, Hong Kong, December 1995.

7 Alice Y. Lan and Betty M. Hu, *We Flee from Hong Kong* (Grand Rapids, MI: Zondervan Publishing House, 1944), 42-43.

8 NAC, Ottawa, MG 30 E181, Forsyth Diary, entry for 18 April 1942.

9 NAC, Forsyth Diary, entry for 20 January 1942.

10 John N.B. Crawford, Interview, CGR, HCM 6-83, Ottawa, ON, 26 April 1983, 7.

11 PRO, WO 224, File 188, Hong Kong, Interrogation Report SKP/5/44, Lt. R.B. Goodwin, 20 October 1944, 16.

12 Shu-Fan Li, *Hong Kong Surgeon*, 103-104.

13 John Luff, *The Hidden Years*, 172.

14 Richard Fuller, *Shokan: Hirohito's Samurai* (London: Arms and Armour, 1992): for Isogai, see 117; Sakai, 185; Tanaka, 210.

15 NAC, RG 24, Vol. 12,839, File 392-46, Affidavit of Maj. S.R. Kerr, 15 February 1946, 1.

16 IWM, File PP/MCR/243, Alsey Diary.

17 CWM, 58 A1 24.4, White Diary, entry for 12 September 1942, 14.

18 Lewis Bush, *Clutch of Circumstance*, 92-93.

19 NAC, Papers of Frank William Ebdon, MG 30, E 328, Ebdon Diary, entry for 8 January 1943.

20 Les Fisher, *I Will Remember: Recollections and Reflections on Hong Kong 1941 to 1945—Internment and Freedom* (Totton, Hampshire: A.L. Fisher, 1996), 119.

21 Donald C. Bowie, "Captive Surgeon."

22 Bowie, "Captive Surgeon," 164.

23 Bowie, "Captive Surgeon," 246.

24 Bowie, "Captive Surgeon," 270.

25 Liam Nolan, *Small Man of Nanataki: The True Story of a Japanese Who Risked His Life to Provide Comfort for His Enemies* (New York: E.P. Dutton, 1966), 82.

26 IWM, Alsey Diary.

27 IWM, Alsey Diary.

28 Luff, *Hidden Years*, 160.

29 Luff, *Hidden Years*, 167.

30 Wellcome Institute for the History of Medicine, London, Contemporary Medical Archives Centre (CMAC), RAMC Collection, RAMC 729/10.

31 Norman J. Leath, "Report Prepared for C.G. Roland on 1 February 1988," 37.

32 Royal Army Medical College Library, Millbank. Muniment Room, Item 1291, Bowie Papers. One item in the papers is a copy of the newsletter, 8 pp.

33 Solomon Bard, Interview, CGR, HCM 7-87, Hong Kong, 7 September 1987, 21.

34 John Crawford, Interview, CGR, HCM 6-83, Ottawa, ON, 26 April 1983, 13.

35 Bowie, "Captive Surgeon," 234.

36 PRO, WO 235, File 1012, Exh. L, Deposition of Capt. Arthur Strahan, 28 June 1946, 7.

37 CWM, White Diary, entry for 15 July 1945, 40.

38 Bowie, "Captive Surgeon," 209.

39 PRO, WO 222/20A, Shackleton War Diary, 4.

40 Kathleen G. Christie, Interview, CGR, HCM 28-82, Toronto, ON, 8 December 1982, 32-33.

41 Bowie, "Captive Surgeon," 203-204.

42 IWM, Item 86/67/1, Papers of Albert Kettleborough. The poem, by Lt. R.S. Rothwell, 1/Middlesex, is part of an unbound collection of poetry written in many hands.

43 Leath, "Report Prepared for C.G. Roland," 39.

44 CWM, White Diary, entry for 12 April 1945, 37.

45 IWM, Ingram Papers, 5.

46 IWM, Ingram Papers, 6.

47 Personal communication, Muriel Jean (McCaw) Channing to Roland, 3.

48 Wellcome Institute, CMAC, GC/131/18, Papers of Surg/Cmdr. J.A. Page, 1.
49 IWM, Ingram Papers, 7.
50 Personal communication, Channing to Roland, 3.
51 Personal communication, Channing to Roland, 4.
52 PRO, WO 235, File 1012, Trial of Tokunaga, testimony of J.N.B. Crawford, 5.
53 Bosanquet, *Escape through China*, 41.
54 IMTFE, Defense Counsel Evidence, Vol. 37, no. 1600A, deposition of W.A. Hall, 4.
55 Bosanquet, *Escape through China*, 42.
56 CWM, White Diary, entry for 27 January 1942, 6.
57 Steele, "With the Royal Rifles," MS memoir in possession of the author, 6.
58 George Orwell, *Down and Out in Paris and London* (Harmondsworth, Middlesex: Penguin, 1970), 91.
59 CWM, White Diary, entry for 6 February 1942, 7.
60 Heather MacDougall, *Activists and Advocates: Toronto's Health Department, 1883-1983* (Toronto: Dundurn Press, 1990), 102.
61 William Burrill, *Hemingway: The Toronto Years* (Toronto: Doubleday Canada, 1994), 47.
62 Anthony H. Coombes, Interview, CGR, HCM 4-94, Sussex, England, 4 May 1994, 36-37.
63 Kenneth G. Cambon, Interview, CGR, HCM 23-83, Vancouver, BC, 10 June 1983, 7.
64 Bosanquet, *Escape through China*, 41.
65 A.J.N. Warrack, "Conditions Experienced as a Prisoner of War from a Medical Point of View," *Journal of the Royal Army Medical Corps* 87 (1946): 209-10.
66 PRO, WO 235, File 1012, Testimony of J.N.B. Crawford, 6.
67 NAC, MG 30 E181, Forsyth Diary, entry for 16 February 1942.
68 Warrack, "Conditions Experienced," 210.
69 Luff, *Hidden Years*, 160.
70 CWM, White Diary, entry for 18 April 1942, 10.
71 CWM, White Diary, entry for 2 February 1942, 7.
72 CWM, White Diary, entry for 4 February 1942, 7.
73 Ralph Goodwin, *Hongkong Escape* (London: Arthur Barker, 1953), 23.
74 Bush, *Clutch of Circumstance*, 43.
75 J.E.C. Robinson, "Work and Problems of a Medical Officer Prisoner of War in the Far East," *Journal of the Royal Army Medical Corps* 91 (1948): 55.
76 Kenneth Cambon, *Guest of Hirohito* (Vancouver: PW Press 1990), 36.
77 William Allister, *Where Life and Death Hold Hands* (Toronto: Stoddart, 1989), 52.
78 Henry Lyons, Interview, in Gustave Gingras and Carol Chapman, *The Sequelae of Inhuman Conditions and Slave Labour Experienced by Members of the Canadian Components of the Hong Kong Forces, 1941-45, While Prisoners of the Japanese Government* (Toronto: War Amps of Canada, 1987), 7.
79 James Bertram, *Beneath the Shadows: A New Zealander in the Far East* (New York: John Day, 1947), 111.
80 Sham Shui Po is spelled several ways, the most common of the variations being Shamshuipo, Shumshuipo, Shum-Shui-Pu, Sham Sui Po, Shamshuio Po, Shamshimpo, and Shamshyupo. However, it is spelled "Sham Shui Po" in most sources, in government maps and documents, and in contemporary Hong Kong itself, and that spelling will be used here. Within quotations all original spellings have been retained.
81 Bertram, *Beneath the Shadows*, 109.
82 IWM, PP/MCR/121, Billings Diary, 21.
83 IWM, Billings Diary, entry for 2 February 1945.

84 Australian War Memorial (AWM), Canberra, AWM 54, File 779/1/21, Diary of Major H.G.G. Robertson, RAMC, Shamshuipo Camp.

85 CWM, White Diary, entry for 30 December 1941, 1.

86 CWM, White Diary, 2.

87 Public Record Office (PRO), London, WO 235, File 1012, Exhibit, 1 April 1942: "The Administrative Regulations for the Prisoners of War in the Hong Kong Prisoners of War Camp," issued over the name of Col. Tokunaga, OC.

88 Bosanquet, *Escape through China*, 47.

89 IWM, Alsey Diary.

90 PRO, WO 224, File 188, Hong Kong.

91 IWM, Newton Diary, entry for 24 January 42.

92 IWM, Alsey Diary.

93 IWM, Item 86/89/1, Papers of A. Dandie, "The Story of 'J' Force," 71.

94 IWM, Alsey Diary.

95 IWM, Billings Diary, 28.

96 IWM, Alsey Diary.

97 Nolan, *Small Man of Nanataki*, 73.

98 Julien Goodman, *M.D.P.O.W.* (New York: Exposition Press, 1972), 163.

99 Luff, *Hidden Years*, 187.

100 IWM, Billings Diary, 22-23.

101 Bush, *Clutch of Circumstance*, 77.

102 Luff, *Hidden Years*, 187.

103 Luff, *Hidden Years*, 190.

104 Bowen Road Hospital on the Island was the hospital location for non-Indian troops, whereas the Indian troops had a hospital in Whitfield Barracks, Kowloon, with 120 beds, in buildings that now form part of the Hong Kong Museum of History.

105 CWM, White Diary, entry for 7 November 1942, 16.

106 IWM, MS Diary of Major W.T. Carden re: His Service as an NCO with Royal Army Pay Corps at Hong Kong.

107 PRO, London, WO 235, File 892, Trial of Niimori Genchiro, testimony of Med.Capt. Saito Shunichi, 235.

108 AWM, Canberra, Personal Records, PR 83, File 32, Report of Service from December 1941 to September 1945 of Capt. J.J. Woodward, 13-14.

109 AWM, Woodward Report, 24.

110 Coombes Interview, HCM 45-94, 10.

111 Luff, *Hidden Years*, 191.

112 Jonathan F. Vance, *Objects of Concern: Canadian Prisoners of War through the Twentieth Century* (Vancouver: UBC Press, 1994), 184.

113 Vance, *Objects of Concern*, 185.

114 CWM, White Diary, entry for 22 November 1942, 16.

115 PRO, WO 224, File 188, Hong Kong, 1.

116 The efforts of the Canadian government to persuade Japan to permit shipments of Red Cross supplies have been scrutinized by Vance, in *Objects of Concern*, 195-205.

117 CWM, White Diary, entry for 4 September 1944, 30.

118 CWM, White Diary, entry for 27 February 1945.

119 CWM, White Diary, entry for 27 May 1943, 21.

120 Anonymous, *The Register of the George Cross* (Cheltenham: This England Books, 1985), 61.

121 CWM, White Diary, entry for 20 August 1943, 23.

122 Sir Selwyn Selwyn-Clarke, *Footprints: The Memoirs of Sir Selwyn Selwyn-Clarke*, 78.

123 Interview with Arthur Gomes, Hong Kong, December 1995.

124 Ken Cuthbertson, *Nobody Said Not to Go: The Life, Loves, and Adventures of Emily Hahn* (Boston: Faber and Faber, 1998), 259.

125 Cuthbertson, *Nobody Said Not to Go*, 295.

126 CWM, White Diary, entry for 16 February 1943, 19.

127 CWM, White Diary, entry for 7 April 1943, 20.

128 John N.B. Crawford and John A.G. Reid, "Nutritional Disease Affecting Canadian Troops Held Prisoner of War by the Japanese," *Canadian Journal of Research* 25 (1947): 78.

129 IWM, Billings Diary, 51-52.

130 IWM, Billings Diary, entry for 18 April 1942.

131 IWM, Billings Diary, entry for 14 September 1942.

132 IWM, Billings Diary, entry for 7 August 1942.

133 IWM, Alsey Diary, entry for 7 February 1942.

134 Coombes Interview, HCM 45-94, 29.

135 Coombes Interview, HCM 45-94, 27-28.

136 IWM, Billings Diary, 63.

137 CWM, White Diary, entry for 17 August 1944, 29.

138 IWM, Billings Diary, 66.

139 William Allister, *A Handful of Rice* (London: Secker & Warburg, 1961).

140 Allan S. Walker, *Medical Services of the R.A.N. and R.A.A.F. with a Section on Women in the Army Medical Services* (Canberra: Australian War Memorial, 1961), 91.

141 Joan Beaumont, *Gull Force: Survival and Leadership in Captivity, 1941-1945* (North Sydney: Allen & Unwin, 1988), Table 8.5.

142 The Canadian figures are calculated from data in Carl Vincent, *No Reason Why: The Canadian Hong Kong Tragedy, an Examination* (Stittsville: Canada's Wings, 1981), Appendix A, 252-53.

143 IWM, MS Diary of Maj. W.T. Carden.

144 IWM, Alsey Diary, entry for 16 April 1942.

145 PRO, WO 224, File 188, Hong Kong, 25.

146 IWM, Item 85/36/1, Diary of Lt.Col. R.J.L. Penfold, entry for 23 July 1944.

147 Goodwin, *Hongkong Escape*, 10.

148 IWM, Carden Diary.

149 IWM, Alsey Diary.

150 PRO, Hong Kong, Newton Diary, entry for 24 December 1941.

151 Early in 1942 Captain Ashton-Rose was named Major (Acting). Exactly when that occurred is unknown.

152 Government Records Service, PRO, Hong Kong, Ref. No. AB/920, Acc. No. 4462(B), Copy of Diary kept by Dr. Isaac Newton, entry for 25 December 1941.

153 Newton Diary, entry for 26 December 1941.

154 Newton Diary, entry for 28 December 1941.

155 Newton Diary, entry for 31 December 1941.

156 Newton Diary, entry for 3 January 1942.

157 Newton Diary, entry for 16 January 1942.

158 Newton Diary, entry for 20 January 1942.

159 PRO, WO 235, File 1012, Trial of Col. Tokunaga Isao, Capt. Saito Shunkishi, Lt. Tanaka Hitochi, Interpreter Tsutada Itsuo, and Sgt. Harada Jotaro.

160 NAC, RG 24, Vol. 12,839, File 392-46, Affidavit of Maj. S.R. Kerr, 15 February 1946, 1-2.

161 Luff, *Hidden Years*, 162.

162 AWM, Woodward Report, 9.

163 AWM, Woodward Report, 10.

164 Warrack, "Conditions Experienced," 213.

165 Warrack, "Conditions Experienced," 214.

166 AWM, Woodward Report, 14.
167 Warrack, "Conditions Experienced," 213.
168 AWM, Woodward Report, 12.
169 AWM, Woodward Report, 13.
170 Warrack, "Conditions Experienced," 214.
171 Warrack, "Conditions Experienced," 217.
172 PRO, London, WO 222, File 22, Z.233, POW Camps in Hong Kong and Japan, by Capt. A.J.N. Warrack, 12-13.
173 Warrack, "Conditions Experienced," 211.
174 Warrack, "Conditions Experienced," 212.
175 Warrack, "Conditions Experienced," 213.
176 PRO, WO 224, File 188, Hong Kong, 13.
177 Warrack, "Conditions Experienced," 215.
178 Warrack, "Conditions Experienced," 216.
179 IWM, Penfold Diary, entry for 4 October 1942.
180 Penfold Diary, entry for 24 January 1943.
181 Warrack, "Conditions Experienced," 215.
182 IWM, Penfold Diary, entries for 7 May and 14 May 1944.
183 Penfold Diary, entry for 27 August 1944. Underlining in original.
184 CWM, White Diary, entry for 26 April 1945, 38.
185 White Diary, entry for 28 April 1945, 38.
186 White Diary, entry for 7 May 1945, 38.
187 Endacott, *Hong Kong Eclipse*, 11.
188 IWM, Penfold Diary, entry for 25 January 1942.
189 Endacott, *Hong Kong Eclipse*, 175.
190 Endacott, *Hong Kong Eclipse*, 177.
191 Bertram, *Beneath the Shadows*, 113.
192 IWM, Billings Diary, 56.
193 Endacott, *Hong Kong Eclipse*, 176.
194 Endacott, *Hong Kong Eclipse*, 176.
195 AWM, Woodward Report, 7.
196 AWM, Woodward Report, 9.
197 AWM, Woodward Report, 14.
198 NAC, RG 24, Vol. 11251, Miscellaneous Reports on POW Camps in Germany, Italy, and the Far East.
199 Banfill Interview, CGR, HCM 27-83, 23.
200 Endacott, *Hong Kong Eclipse*, 176.
201 Anonymous, *The Register of the George Cross*, 13.
202 Mahmood Khan Durrani, *The Sixth Column: The Heroic Personal Story of Lt.-Col. Mahmood Khan Durrani, G.C.* (London: Cassell, 1955), 219.
203 NAC, Forsyth Diary, entry for 5 March 1943.
204 Endacott, *Hong Kong Eclipse*, 194.
205 Endacott, *Hong Kong Eclipse*, 177.
206 Selwyn Selwyn-Clarke, *Hong Kong Government: Annual Report of the Medical Department for 1946* (Hong Kong: Local Printing Press, 1947), 24.

Chapter Four

1 AWM, Canberra, Personal Records, PR 83, File 32, Report of Service from December 1941 to September 1945, of Captain J.J. Woodward Report, 5.
2 IWM, Alsey Diary, File PP/MCR/243, 1942.
3 NAC, Ottawa, MG30, E181, Tom Forsyth, "Hong Kong Diary and Memories of Japan: Gleanings from the Diary of a Winnipeg Grenadier," entry for 29 May 1942.
4 Forsyth Diary, entries for 1-3 June, 1942.

5 G.P. Shearer, "Stanley, Hong Kong: The First Three Years," *Royal Engineers Journal* 58 (1944): 170.

6 Albert Coates and Newman Rosenthal, *The Albert Coates Story: The Will That Found the Way* (Melbourne: Hyland House, 1977), 89.

7 Diary of Sgt. Lancelot Ross, quoted in Anonymous, *The Royal Rifles of Canada in Hong Kong, 1941-1945* (Sherbrooke: Hong Kong Veterans' Association of Canada, Quebec-Maritimes Branch, 1980), 297.

8 CWM, Ottawa, Item 58 A1 24.4, Diary of Lt. Harry L. White, Winnipeg Grenadiers, 30 December 1941-20 October 1945, 15.

9 IWM, Alsey Diary, entry for 24 January 1942: "Paraded with 200 men at 8:30, numbered off endless times and went on lorries to Kai Tak aerodrome....Started digging and filling holes in on K 'drome."

10 IWM, Alsey Diary.

11 NAC, Forsyth Diary, entry for 25 June 1942.

12 Randolph Steele, "With the Royal Rifles of Canada in Hong Kong and Japan," MS memoir in possession of the author, 9.

13 A.H. Delbridge, Interview, in Gustave Gingras and Carol Chapman, *The Sequelae of Inhuman Conditions*, 7.

14 CWM, White Diary, entry of 12 November 1943, 25.

15 J.E.C. Robinson, "Work and Problems of a Medical Officer Prisoner of War in the Far East," *Journal of the Royal Army Medical Corps* 91 (1948): 51.

16 John N.B. Crawford and John A.G. Reid, "Nutritional Disease Affecting Canadian Troops Held Prisoner of War by the Japanese," Canadian Journal of Research 25 (1947): 59.

17 NAC, Forsyth Diary, entry for 6 January 1942.

18 IWM, Alsey Diary.

19 Luigi Ribiero, [Reminiscences of a POW at Hong Kong] MS, 10.

20 IWM, Alsey Diary.

21 IWM, Alsey Diary.

22 IWM, Alsey Diary.

23 IWM, Alsey Diary.

24 IWM, Alsey Diary.

25 IWM, Alsey Diary.

26 CWM, White Diary, entry for 9 September 1942, 14.

27 NAC, Forsyth Diary, entry for 7 August 1942.

28 IWM, Alsey Diary.

29 NAC, Forsyth Diary, entry for 25 July 1942.

30 IWM, Item 85/42/1, Papers of CSM Ronald Alfred Edwards, HKUDC, 31.

31 IWM, Edwards Papers, 33.

32 Sir Albert Rodrigues, Interview, CGR, HCM 8-87, Hong Kong, 8 September 1987, 20-21.

33 NAC, Papers of Frank William Ebdon, MG 30, E 28. Diary kept by CSM Ebdon 26 December 1942 to 26 December 1943 at Sham Shui Po, Hong Kong, and Omine Camp, Japan, entry for 2 January 1943.

34 William Allister, *Where Life and Death Hold Hands* (Toronto: Stoddart, 1989), 74.

35 CWM, White Diary, entry for 29 January 1944, 26.

36 NAC, Forsyth Diary, entry for 2 April 1943.

37 Ribiero, [*Reminiscences*], 19.

38 Miranda, born in Portugal but raised in Brazil, had left Rio de Janeiro for Broadway and then Hollywood in the 1930s. "Bahia" was one of her classic numbers; a trademark was the "basket-of-fruit" headdress, as well as her vivacity and remarkably expressive eyes.

39 CWM, White Diary, entry for 21 May 1943, 21.

40 Personal communication, Arthur Gomes to author, 1991.

41 IWM, Edwards Papers, 124.

42 Edwards Papers, 124.

43 Coombes, Interview, CGR, HCM 4-94, 30.

44 Ribiero, [*Reminiscences*], 23.

45 IWM, Edwards Papers.

46 From "Berrigan," in Gary Geddes, *Hong Kong Poems* (Oberon Press, 1987), 49.

47 Russell Braddon, *The Naked Island* (London: Werner Laurie, 1952), 161.

48 Public Record Office (PRO), Hong Kong, Government Records Service, Ref. No. AB/920, Acc. No. 4462 (B), Copy of Diary kept by Dr. Isaac Newton, Hong Kong, 7 Dec 41 until 1 June 42, entry for 3 January 1942.

49 IWM, Alsey Diary.

50 CWM, White Diary, entry for 10 December 1943, 25.

51 Bard Interview, CGR, HCM 1-90, Burlington, ON, 7 May 1990, 28-29.

52 IWM, Alsey Diary.

53 NAC, MG 30, E 437, Papers of Charles E. Price, "Notes on Contract Bridge," compiled by W.F. Nugent.

54 Roussel Interview, HCM 38-85, 21-23.

55 CWM, White Diary, entry for 6 January 1942, 3.

56 IWM, Alsey Diary, entry for 11 January 1942.

57 University of Alberta Archives, Edmonton, Accession No. 77-1, Dr. Benjamin Wheeler Papers, Box 1, File 5, Memoir, "Some Experiences as a Prisoner-of-War of the Japanese," 2-3.

58 Roy H. Whitecross, *Slaves of the Son of Heaven* (Sydney: Dymock's Book Arcade, 1953), 117.

59 Preston John Hubbard, *Apocalypse Undone: My Survival of Japanese Imprisonment during World War II* (Nashville: Vanderbilt University Press, 1990), 72.

60 Hank Nelson, "'A Bowl of Rice for Seven Camels': The Dynamics of Prisoner-of-War Camps," *Journal of the Australian War Memorial* 14 (1989): 33-42.

61 The following paragraphs owe much to R.A. Radford, "The Economic Organisation of a POW Camp," *Economica* 12 (1945): 189-201.

62 Radford, "The Economic Organisation," 194.

63 IWM, Alsey Diary, entry for 31 January 1942.

64 Arthur Raymond Squires, "War Diary, Hong Kong and Kowloon, 1941-1945," MS unnumbered pp., entry for 6 March 1942.

65 NAC, Forsyth Diary, entry for 23 July 1942.

66 A. Kenneth Pifher, Interview, CGR, HCM 1-89, Grimsby, ON, 10 February 1989, 27.

67 AWM, Woodward Report, 29.

68 Roy Robinson, Interview, CGR, HCM 10-83, Winnipeg, MB, 27 May 1983, 9.

69 IWM, Alsey Diary, 1942.

70 Liam Nolan, *Small Man of Nanataki*, 123.

71 Wenzell Brown, *Hong Kong Aftermath* (New York: Smith & Durrell, 1943), 147.

72 James Allan Ford, *Season of Escape* (London: Hodder & Stoughton, 1963), 123-24.

73 Harold Atkinson, Interview, CGR, HCM 7-83, Winnipeg, MB, 27 May 1983, 31-32.

74 Don Wall, ed., *Singapore and Beyond: The Story of the Men of the 2/20 Battalion, Told by the Survivors* (East Hills, Australia: 2/20 Battalion Association, 1985), 242.

75 IWM, Item 87/34/1, Papers of Geoffrey C. Hamilton, "Prisoner of War in Hong Kong and Japan, 1941-1945," 6.

76 James Allan Ford, *Season of Escape*, 90.

77 Arthur Raymond Squires, "War Diary," entry for 6 March 1942.

78 Frank Foster, *Comrades in Bondage* (London: Skeffington and Son, 1946), 71.

79 James Bertram, *Beneath the Shadows: A New Zealander in the Far East, 1939-45* (New York: John Day, 1947), 117.

80 Kate Caffrey, *Out in the Midday Sun: Singapore 1941-45* (London: New English Library, 1977), 254.

81 IWM, Alsey Diary, 1942.

82 NAC, RG 24, C 1, HQS 9050-12-15, Reel C-5335, Cigarettes for POWs, 1943; Letter from N.B. Greenleaf, 22 July 1943.

83 CWM, Acc. No. 1983-38/1, Diary of Donald Geraghty, entries for 23 and 27 February 1945, 40.

84 Anonymous, *Report of the International Committee of the Red Cross on Its Activities during the Second World War (September 1, 1939 - June 30, 1947)*, Vol. 1, General Activities (Geneva: International Red Cross, 1948), 463.

85 Archie Lee McMaster, "*Lo Joe*" (MS, United States Military Academy Library, Special Collections, [1942-45]), 184.

86 Philippa Poole, *Of Love and War: The Letters and Diaries of Captain Adrian Curlewis and His Family, 1939-1945* (London: Century, 1983), 166.

87 Adrian Martin, *Brothers from Bataan: POWs, 1942-1945* (Manhattan, KA: Sunflower University Press, 1992), 94.

88 North Americans might call this a Rube Goldberg apparatus.

89 IWM, Billings Diary, 22.

90 Braddon, *Naked Island*, 161-62.

91 H. Robert Charles, *Last Man Out* (Austin, Texas: Eakin Press, 1988), 40.

92 IWM, Billings Diary, entry for 13 October 1944, 71.

93 Billings Diary, 23.

94 John Stewart, *To the River Kwai: Two Journeys—1943, 1979* (London: Bloomsbury, 1988), 46.

95 IWM, Alsey Diary.

96 Gavan Daws, *Prisoners of the Japanese: POWs of World War II in the Pacific* (New York: William Morrow, 1994), 116.

97 Walter Irvine Summons, *Twice Their Prisoner* (Melbourne: Oxford University Press, 1946), 134.

98 Kenneth Cambon, *Guest of Hirohito*, 38.

99 John W. Foote, VC, Interviewed at Norwood, Ontario, 11 June 1981, CGR, HCM 8-81,18-19.

100 Kenneth Harrison, *The Brave Japanese* (Adelaide: Rigby, 1966), 136-37.

101 George Wright-Nooth with Mark Adkin, *Prisoner of the Turnip Heads: Horror, Hunger and Humour in Hong Kong, 1941-1945* (London: Leo Cooper, 1994), 191.

102 IMTFE, Exhibit No. 3137, Deposition of C.R. Jackson re: Conditions in Hamowa POW Camp, 5.

103 PRO, WO 222, File 190, 5.

104 NAC, Federal Records Centre, Locator No. G287-16, Trial of CSM Tugby, Testimony of R.E. Bronson, 126.

105 NAC, RG 24, C 2 (f), Vol. 8018, File TOK-1-2-11, Various Reports by LtCol. Oscar Orr re: War Crimes Trials in the Far East, 1947.

106 PRO, WO 224, File 194, Far East: Java Camps. 304/1/Inf. CSDIC (India), Red Fort, Delhi: Information Section Report No. 85, 16 October 1944, 3.

107 North Texas State University, Denton, TX, Oral History Collection, No. 69, Robert Gregg, 74.

108 R. Jackson Scott, *90 Days of Rice* (Pioneer, CA: California Traveler, 1975), 192-93.

109 PRO, WO 222, File 190, 5.

110 PRO, WO 222, File 190, 5.

111 J. Wellington Wimpy, known simply as Wimpy, was a significant member of the cast of characters in the comic strip, "Popeye the Sailor," written and

drawn by Max and David Fleischer, based on the character created by Elzie
Segar. He became famous for the phrase cited here.

112 Roy H. Whitecross, *Slaves of the Son of Heaven*, 193.

113 David C.C. Hinder, ["Experiences and Conditions in Three Small POW
Parties"], MS Prepared for Australian Government Enquiry, 1973, 10.

114 Donald C. Bowie, "Captive Surgeon, 206.

115 Bowie, "Captive Surgeon," 206.

116 Atkinson Interview, CGR, HCM 7-83, 36-37.

117 Atkinson Interview, CGR, HCM 7-83, 38.

118 H.M. Dekking, "Tropical Nutritional Amblyopia ('Camp Eyes')," *Ophthalmologica*
113 (1947): 87.

119 M.E. Pohlman and E.F. Ritter, Jr., "Observations on Vitamin Deficiencies in an
Eye, Ear, Nose, and Throat Clinic of a Japanese Prison Hospital," *American
Journal of Ophthalmology* 35 (1952): 229.

120 Pohlman and Ritter, "Observations on Vitamin Deficiencies," 230.

121 David C.C. Hinder, "Prisoners of War: Long-Term Effects," *Medical Journal of
Australia* 1 (1981): 565.

122 Cited in *USA Today*, 6 October 1995, 4D.

123 IWM, Item 81/32/1, J.F. Chandler, Diary, 1943-45, re: POW life in Java and the
Spice Islands, 159.

124 Robinson, "Work and Problems," 53.

125 Robert W. Miller, "War Crimes Trials at Yokohama," *Brooklyn Law Review* 15
(1949): 196.

126 NAC, Forsyth Diary, entries for 7-28 March 1944.

127 William Stewart, Interview, CGR, HCM 62-85, Burlington, ON, 6 July 1985, 40-41.

128 Allan S. Walker, *Medical Services of the R.A.N. and R.A.A.F., with a Section on
Women in the Army Medical Services* (Canberra: Australian War Memorial,
1961), 86.

129 IWM, Papers of Geoffrey C. Hamilton, 25-26.

130 Edmund Goldsmid, ed., *A Counter-Blaste to Tobacco. (Written by King James I)*
(Edinburgh: Privately Printed, 1884; originally published in London, 1604), 32.

131 Bush, *Clutch of Circumstance*, 86.

132 J.D. Adamson and D.C. Brereton, "Ultimate disabilities in Hong Kong repatriates," *Treatment Services Bulletin* ser.4, 3 (1948): 8.

133 CWM, White Diary, entry for 26 August 1945, 44.

134 Calvin G. Jackson, *Diary of Col. Calvin G. Jackson, MD, Kept during World War II,
1941-1945* (Ada, OH: Ohio Northern University, 1992), 142.

135 Kenneth Harrison, *The Brave Japanese* (Adelaide: Rigby, 1966), 136.

136 Bush, *Clutch of Circumstance*, 188.

137 IWM, Billings Diary, 73.

138 IWM, Papers of A. Dandie, 68.

139 Allister, *Where Life and Death*, 185-86.

140 Allister, *Where Life and Death*, 198-99.

141 Allister, *Where Life and Death*, 128-29.

142 Allister, *Where Life and Death*, 200-201.

143 IWM, Alsey Diary.

144 In an unofficial census 10 years before the war, the estimated Indian population of Hong Kong was 4,745. See Sir Francis Low, ed., *The Indian Year Book
1944-45: A Statistical and Historical Annual of the Indian Empire, with an
Explanation of the Principal Topics of the Day* (Bombay: Bennett, Coleman & Co.
Ltd., [1945]), 912.

145 Bard Interview, CGR, HCM 7-87, 8-9.

146 See Edwin Ride, *BAAG: Hong Kong Resistance, 1942-1945* (Hong Kong: Oxford
University Press, 1981).

147 IWM, Alsey Diary.
148 IWM, Carden Diary.
149 IWM, Alsey Diary.
150 David Bosanquet, *Escape through China: Survival after the Fall of Hong Kong* (London: Robert Hale, 1983).
151 IWM, Alsey Diary.
152 Bertram, *Beneath the Shadows*, 122.
153 IWM, Alsey Diary.
154 John Luff, *Hidden Years*, 194.
155 CWM, White Diary, entry for 24 May 1942, 11.
156 PRO, WO 222, File 22, Z.233. Capt. A.J.N. Warrack, 11.
157 IWM, Alsey Diary.
158 IWM, Carden Diary.
159 IWM, Alsey Diary.
160 NARA, RG 153, File 35-145, Trial of Yumita Kyogzo, Kondo Shoogo, and Ishige Michiharu, Affidavit of Harold Englehart, 16 January 1946, 2.
161 IMTFE, Defense Counsel Evidence, Vol. 37, No. 1600A, Deposition of W.A. Hall, 3-4.
162 Richard Fuller, *Shokan: Hirohito's Samurai*, 85.
163 Angus A. MacMillan, Interview, in Gingras and Chapman, *The Sequelae of Inhuman Conditions*, 8.
164 Roland, "Allied POWs, Japanese Captors, and the Geneva Convention," *War and Society* 9 (1991).
165 CWM, White Diary, entry for 29 August 1942, 13.
166 AWM, Woodward Report, 17.
167 AWM, Woodward Report, 18.
168 Albert Coates and Neuman Rosenthal, *The Albert Coates Story: The Will That Found the Way* (Melbourne: Hyland House, 1977), 135.
169 Jack Edwards, *Banzai, You Bastards!* (London: Souvenir Press, 1990), 79.
170 These books include: David Bosanquet, *Escape through China*; R.B. Goodwin, *Hongkong Escape*; R.B. Goodwin, *Passport to Eternity*; Freddie Guest, *Escape From the Bloodied Sun*; Anthony Hewitt, *Bridge with Three Men: Across China to the Western Heaven in 1942*; Benjamin A. Proulx, *Underground From Hongkong*; and Jan Henrik Marsman, *I Escaped from Hong Kong*. In addition, Lindsay Ride's escape in January 1942 is described in Edwin Ride, *BAAG: Hong Kong Resistance, 1942-1945*.
171 *Shu-Fan Li*, Hong Kong Surgeon (New York: E.P. Dutton, 1964), 159.

Chapter Five

1 From a poem, "A Prisoner's Prayer," by an unknown author, Sham Shui Po, cited in Randolph Steele, "With the Royal Rifles of Canada in Hong Kong and Japan," MS memoir in possession of the author, 9.
2 NAC, Ottawa, MG30, E181 Tom Forsyth, Hong Kong Diary and Memories of Japan, entry for 13 March 1942.
3 George Orwell, *Down and Out in Paris and London*, 51
4 CWM, Ottawa, Acc. 1981-276/10, cat. no. 60-6-52, F.D.F. Martyn Papers, entry for 17 January 1943.
5 Eating utensils were scarce also. One man "saw one of the Rifles eating his rice out of a large ornamental hub cap off an automobile." NAC, Forsyth Diary, entry for 19 January 1942.
6 IWM, London, File PP/MCR/243, Diary of A.J. Alsey, 1942.
7 CWM, Item 58 A1 24.4, Diary of Lt. Harry L. White, Winnipeg Grenadiers, 30 December 1941-20 October 1945, entry for 14 July 1942, 12.

8 NARA, Washington, RG 153, File 36-489, Trial of Lt. Yanaru Tetsutoshi; Testimony of WO1 Harold B. Shephard, RRC, 10.
9 IWM, Alsey Diary.
10 IWM, Alsey Diary.
11 PRO, London, WO 224, File 188. Interrogation Report of Lt. R.B. Goodwin, 20 October 1944, 5.
12 Sir Selwyn Selwyn-Clarke, *Footprints: The Memoirs of Sir Selwyn Selwyn-Clarke*, 74.
13 Selwyn-Clarke, *Footprints*, 75.
14 AWM, Canberra, Personal Records, PR 83, File 32, Report of Service from December 1941 to September 1945 of Capt. J.J. Woodward, 11.
15 AWM, Woodward Report, 31.
16 John N.B. Crawford and John A.G. Reid, "Nutritional Disease Affecting Canadian Troops Held Prisoner of War by the Japanese," *Canadian Journal of Research* 25 (1947): 56.
17 Crawford and Reid, "Nutritional Disease Affecting Canadian Troops," 53.
18 CWM, Item 58 A1 24.5, Diary of Delbert Louis William, 16 October 1941-5 October 1942, entry for 10 March 1942.
19 IWM, Alsey Diary.
20 James Bertram, *Beneath the Shadows: A New Zealander in the Far East, 1939-46*, 119.
21 IWM, Alsey Diary.
22 IWM, Alsey Diary.
23 AWM, Woodward Report, 26.
24 Kenneth Harrison, *The Brave Japanese*, 245.
25 AWM, Woodward Report, 16.
26 NAC, Forsyth Diary, entry for 5 March 1942.
27 CWM, Martyn Papers, entries for 17 March 1942.
28 AWM, Canberra, AWM 54, File 481/1/24, Items of Medical Interest from Captured Japanese Documents and Interrogations of Prisoners of War; Locations of Disease in Japanese-Occupied Territory, 25.
29 Allan S. Walker, *Middle East and Far East*, 548.
30 Crawford and Reid, "Nutritional Disease," 59.
31 NAC, Forsyth Diary, entry for 20 December 1942.
32 PRO, WO 224, File 188, Interrogation Report of Lt. R.B. Goodwin, 8.
33 Crawford and Reid, "Nutritional Disease," 57.
34 Dr. Anthony Henry Coombes Interview, CGR, 4 May 1994, Sussex, England, HCM 5-94, 33.
35 IWM, Department of Documents, London, Item 85/42/1, Papers of CSM Ronald Alfred Edwards, HKVDC.
36 Arthur Raymond Squires, "War Diary, Hong Kong and Kowloon, 1941-1945," MS, 41.
37 Colin Standish, cited in: Anonymous, *The Royal Rifles of Canada in Hong Kong, 1941-1945*, 382.
38 Albert Coates and Neuman Rosenthal, *The Albert Coates Story* (Melbourne: Hyland House, 1977), 110.
39 Charles G. Roland and Harry Shannon, "Patterns of Disease Among World War 2 Prisoners of the Japanese: Hunger, Weight Loss, and Deficiency Diseases," *Journal of the History of Medicine and Allied Sciences* 46 (1991): 65-85.
40 Government Records Service, PRO, Hong Kong Manuscript Series No 81, . Papers of Dr. A.H.R. Coombes, Shamshuipo Camp Isolation Hospital, Menu, Christmas Day 1942.
41 Roussel Interview, CGR, HCM 38-85, 21-23.
42 John Luff, *The Hidden Years*, 187.

43 NAC, Forsyth Diary, undated entry, 88-89.

44 Ross Diary, in Anonymous, *Royal Rifles of Canada*, 378.

45 Calvin G. Jackson, *Diary of Col. Calvin G. Jackson, MD, Kept during World War II, 1941-1945* (Ada, OH: Ohio Northern University, 1992), 133, 135, 137, and 172.

46 Naval Historical Center, Operational Archives, Washington. R.D. Millar, *Narrative of Personal Experiences in the Far East*, MS Prepared for Historical Records Section, Royal New Zealand Air Force, Wellington, NZ, 13 April 1946, 35; emphasis in the original.

47 Agnes Newton Keith, *Three Came Home* (New York: Time Inc., 1965), 215.

48 Orwell, *Down and Out*, 36.

49 Squires, "War Diary," entry for 15 December 1943, 34.

50 This concept is discussed in Anne Hardy, "Beriberi, Vitamin B[1] and World Food Policy, 1925-1970," *Medical History* 39 (1995): 61-77.

51 IWM, Alsey Diary.

52 C. Miller Fisher, "Residual Neuropathological Changes in Canadians Held Prisoners of War by the Japanese (Strachan's Disease)" *Canadian Services Medical Journal* 11 (1955): 157-99, at 191.

53 John R. Bumgarner, *Parade of the Dead: A US Army Physician's Memoir of Imprisonment by the Japanese, 1942-1945* (Jefferson, NC: McFarland, 1995), 71.

54 Norman J. Leath, "Report Prepared for C.G. Roland, MD, History of Medicine, McMaster University, Hamilton, Ontario, 1 February 1988," 31.

55 C.H.A., "The ABC of Vitamins," in: Wellcome Institute, Contemporary Archives Medical Collection, Dr. Cicely Williams Collection, PP/CDW, Box 8, Folder 9.

56 Anne Hardy, "Beriberi, Vitamin B[1] and World Food Policy, 1925-1970," *Medical History* 39 (1995): 61-77 at 64.

57 W.R. Aykroyd, "Beriberi and Other Food-deficiency Diseases in Newfoundland and Labrador," *Journal of Hygiene* 30 (1930): 366-67.

58 Jean Cantlie Stewart, *The Quality of Mercy: The Lives of Sir James and Lady Cantlie* (London: George Allen & Unwin, 1983), 53.

59 Much of the historical context outlined here is derived from a book written by one of the pioneer students of beriberi: Robert R. Williams, *Toward the Conquest of Beriberi* (Cambridge: Harvard University Press, 1961).

60 Williams, *Toward the Conquest*, 44.

61 Cited in Williams, *Toward the Conquest*, 48.

62 Haru Matsukata Reischauer, *Samurai and Silk: A Japanese and American Heritage* (Cambridge: Belknap Press of Harvard University Press, 1986), 104.

63 Tanizaki Jun'ichiro, *The Makioka Sisters* (New York: Vintage Books, 1995), 5.

64 Tanizaki, *The Makioka Sisters*, 118.

65 From Fig. 8, "Malnutrition and nutrition activities in Japan," *Report of Joint FAO/WHO Nutrition Committee for the South and East Asia Fourth Meeting*, cited in Williams, *Toward the Conquest*, 222.

66 Bertram, *Beneath the Shadows*, 110.

67 W.M. Silliphant, "Under the Japs in Bilibid," MS, Otis Historical Archives of the Armed Forces Medical Museum, 1946.

68 See, for example, the observations of these medical officers: S.E.L. Stening, "Experiences as a Prisoner of War in Japan," *Medical Journal of Australia* 1 (1946): 773-75; A.P. Curtin, "Imprisonment under the Japanese," *British Medical Journal* 2 (1946): 585-86.

69 Williams, *Toward the Conquest*, 63.

70 D. Denny-Brown, "Neurological Conditions Resulting from Prolonged and Severe Dietary Restrictions (Case Reports in Prisoners-of-War and General Review)," *Medicine* 26 (1947): 45.

71 T.M. Pemberton, "Observations on Diseases among British Prisoners of War in Japanese Hands in the Far East (1942-45)," *New Zealand Medical Journal* 48 (1949): 145-50.

72 J.S. Haimsohn, "Avitaminoses as Seen in Japanese Prisoners of War, with Review of Two Cases," *Memphis Medical Journal* 22 (1947): 196-200.

73 IWM, Item PP/MCR/121, Diary of Adrian Richardson Billings, RN, 1941-1945, 29.

74 Williams, *Toward the Conquest*, 23.

75 NARA, RG 153, File 35-136; Deposition of Maj. A.A. Weinstein, 10 June 1947, 3.

76 Weinstein Deposition, 2.

77 Weinstein Deposition, 3.

78 Weinstein Deposition, 4.

79 Russell Braddon, *The Naked Island* (London:Werner Laurie, 1952) 109.

80 J.A. Page, "Painful-feet Syndrome among Prisoners of War in the Far East," *British Medical Journal* 2 (1946): 261.

81 Ralph Hibbs, "Beriberi in Japanese Prison Camp," *Annals of Internal Medicine* 25 (1946): 274.

82 Lewis Bush, *Clutch of Circumstance*, 88.

83 Crawford and Reid, "Nutritional Disease Affecting Canadian Troops," 67.

84 NAC, Forsyth Diary, entry for 25 August 1942.

85 CWM, Acc. No. 1983-381, Diary of Donald Geraghty, 16.

86 NAC, MG 30 E 28, Diary kept by CSM Ebdon, 26 December 1942 to 26 December 1943, at Sham Shui Po, Hong Kong, and Omine Camp, Japan, entry for 1 January 1943.

87 NAC, Ebdon Diary, entry for 4 January 1943.

88 William Allister, *Where Life and Death Hold Hands*, 66.

89 Allister, *Where Life and Death*, 104.

90 Coombes Interview, CGR, HCM 5-94, 36-37.

91 Walter Grey, Interview, in Gustave Gingras and Carol Chapman, *The Sequelae of Inhuman Conditions*, 7.

92 Walter G. Jenkins, Interview, CGR, 9 June 1983, Victoria, BC, HCM 22-83, 29.

93 CWM, White Diary, entry for 23 December 1942, 17.

94 White Diary, entry for 19 February 1943, 19.

95 White Diary, entry of 27 February 1943, 20.

96 Donald C. Bowie, "Captive Surgeon," 174-75.

97 Leath, "Report Prepared for C.G. Roland," 35.

98 Crawford and Reid, "Nutritional Disease Affecting Canadian Troops," 68.

99 IWM, Item P324, Papers of Mrs. Joyce Day, Hong Kong, 5.

100 Dean A. Smith and Michael F.A. Woodruff, *Deficiency Diseases in Japanese Prison Camps* (London: His Majesty's Stationery Office, 1951), 169.

101 Dean A. Smith, "Nutritional Neuropathies in the Civilian Internment Camp, Hong Kong, January, 1942—August, 1945," *Brain* 69 (1946): 211-12.

102 Smith, "Nutritional Neuropathies," 215.

103 Smith, "Nutritional Neuropathies," 215-16.

104 Smith, "Nutritional Neuropathies," 219.

105 Ralph E. Hibbs, "Beriberi in Japanese Prison Camp," 271.

106 Hibbs, "Beriberi in Japanese Prison Camp," 279-81.

107 Hibbs, "Beriberi in Japanese Prison Camp," 282.

108 J.A. Page, "Painful-feet Syndrome among Prisoners of War in the Far East," 261.

109 Frank Evans, *Roll Call at Oeyama: P.O.W. Remembers* (Llandysul, Dyfed: J.D. Lewis & Sons, 1985), 82.

110 S.E.L. Stening, "Experiences as a Prisoner of War in Japan," 774.

111 IMTFE, Exhibit No. 3111, Investigation Squad of Army Medical College, Suggestions Regarding Improvement of Health Conditions of Prisoners of War Camp; Undated [on internal evidence, 1st half of 1943], 4.

112 J. Grierson, "On the Burning in the Feet of Natives," *Transactions of the Medical & Physical Society of Calcutta* 2 (1826): 275-80.

113 Murray Glusman, "The Syndrome of 'Burning Feet' (Nutritional Melalgia) as a Manifestation of Nutritional Deficiency," 212.

114 J.G. Malcolmson, *Observations on Some Forms of Rheumatism* (Madras: Vepery Mission Press, 1835).

115 Gustavo C. Roman, "Epidemic Neuropathies of Jamaica," *Transactions and Studies of the College of Physicians of Philadelphia* ser. 5, 7 (1985): 264.

116 L.R. Sharples, "The Condition of 'Burning Feet' or 'Foot Burning' in Labourers on Sugar Plantations in the Corentyne District of British Guiana," *Journal of Tropical Medicine and Hygiene* 32 (1929): 359.

117 Sharples, "The Condition of 'Burning Feet,'" 359.

118 J.D. Adamson, P.K. Tisdale, D.C. Brereton, and L.W.B. Card, "Residual Disabilities in Hong Kong Repatriates," *CMAJ* 56 (1947): 484.

119 J.D. Adamson and D.C. Brereton, "Ultimate Disabilities in Hong Kong Repatriates," *Treatment Services Bulletin* ser. 4, 3 (1948): 5-10 at 7.

120 John N. Crawford, "A Preliminary Report on a Follow-up Study of Repatriates from Japanese Prisoner of War Camps," *Treatment Services Bulletin* 5 (1950): 166.

121 J.D. Adamson and C.M. Judge, "Residual Disabilities in Hong Kong Prisoners of War," *Canadian Services Medical Journal* 12 (1956): 850.

122 Adamson and Brereton, "Ultimate Disabilities," 23.

123 Glusman, "The Syndrome of 'Burning Feet'," 222.

124 Glusman, "The Syndrome of 'Burning Feet'," 216.

125 Sidney Vernon, "Nutritional Melalgia, a Deficiency Vascular Disease," 799.

126 See "Beriberi Heart Disease Regulation," *The Quan* 49 (February 1995): 1. The article, actually an official US government letter of 22 December 1994, specifies: "No pathophysiologic basis has been established to explain the relationship between the edema and ischemic heart disease." *The Quan* is the newsletter of the American Defenders of Bataan & Corregidor, Inc.

127 David R.W. Haddock, "Neurologic Illness in the Tropics," in Strickland, *Hunter's Tropical Medicine* (Toronto: W.B. Saunders, 1984), 65-66.

128 Stening, "Experiences as a Prisoner."

129 A comprehensive historical consideration of pellagra can be found in a volume that contains many of the seminal papers on the subject reproduced along with editorial analysis: see Kenneth J. Carpenter, ed., *Pellagra* (Stroudsburg, PA: Hutchinson Ross, 1981).

130 Smith and Woodruff, *Deficiency Diseases*, 103-104.

131 Smith and Woodruff, *Deficiency Diseases*, 103-104.

132 Crawford and Reid, "Nutritional Disease," 80.

133 Coombes Interview, CGR, HCM 4-94, 35.

134 Squires, "War Diary," 30.

135 Walter Grey, Interview, in Gingras and Chapman, *The Sequelae of Inhuman Conditions*, 6.

136 Thomas Joseph Dewar, Interview, in Gingras and Chapman, *The Sequelae of Inhuman Conditions*, 5.

137 Frank Arnold Harding, Interview, in Gingras and Chapman, *The Sequelae of Inhuman Conditions*, 5.

138 P.G. Bell and J.C. O'Neill, "Optic Atrophy in Hong Kong Prisoners of War," *CMAJ* 56 (1947): 481.

139 Bell and O'Neill, "Optic Atrophy," 476.
140 John Durran, "Ocular Signs in the Prisoner of War from the Far East," *British Medical Journal* 1 (1946): 626.
141 Bell and O'Neill, "Optic Atrophy," 479.

Chapter Six

1 Kenneth Harrison, *The Brave Japanese* 226-27.
2 Robert Boyd, Interview, CGR HCM 13-83, Winnipeg, Manitoba, 28 May 1983.
3 NAC, Ottawa, MG30 E181 Tom Forsyth, "Hong Kong and Memories of Japan," Diary entry for 12 June 1942.
4 For a discussion of this problem, see A.A. Liebow, P.D. MacLean, J.H. Bumstead, and L.G. Welt, "Tropical Ulcers and Cutaneous Diphtheria," *Archives of Internal Medicine* 78 (1946): 255-95.
5 Dr. S. Martin Banfill, Interview, CGR HCM 27-83, Montreal, Quebec, 14 July 1983, 31.
6 Calvin G. Jackson, *Diary of Col. Calvin G. Jackson* (Ada, OH: Ohio Northern University, 1992), 58 and 60.
7 T.M. Pemberton, "Observations on Diseases among British Prisoners of War in Japanese Hands in the Far East (1942-45)," *New Zealand Medical Journal* 48 (1949): 148.
8 At this same time, spring 1942, doctors in the Warsaw ghetto also observed decreased immunity to infectious diseases. The Jews of the ghetto were trying to survive on rations even less adequate than in the Far East POW camps. Often, at autopsy, pathologists would find evidence of massive infectious disease that had not been detected on the hospital wards because starvation had so badly damaged or destroyed the normal immune responses of the patients. See C.G. Roland, *Courage Under Siege: Disease, Starvation, and Death in the Warsaw Ghetto* (New York: Oxford University Press, 1992), 154-64.
9 NAC, RG 24, C2(f), Vol. 8018, File TOK-1-4, Diary of Maj. H.G.G. Robertson, 1941-1943.
10 IWM, London, File PP/MCR/243, Diary of A.J. Alsey, 1942.
11 CWM, Ottawa, Item 58 A1 24.4, Diary of Lt. Harry L. White, Winnipeg Grenadiers, 30 December 1941-20 October 1945, entry for 16 August 1942, 13.
12 Data from lists maintained by Cpl. N.J. Leath as part of his duties as chief clerk at Bowen Road Hospital; copies sent by Leath to the author in 1990. The data are confirmed in Donald C. Bowie, "Captive Surgeon," 172.
13 Bowie, "Captive Surgeon," 173.
14 Lists maintained by Leath.
15 IWM, Item 93/18/1, Papers of Mrs. D. Ingram [Sister D. Van Wart], Hong Kong, 6.
16 Liam Nolan, *Small Man of Nanataki*, 61.
17 IWM, Ingram Papers, 6.
18 Dr. Anthony Henry Coombes Interview, CGR, HCM 4-94, 4 May 1994, Sussex, England, 21.
19 Dr. James Anderson, Interview, CGR, HCM 43-85, Victoria, BC, 20 April 1985, 28.
20 Bowie, "Captive Surgeon," 173.
21 Bowie, "Captive Surgeon," 173.
22 John N.B. Crawford and John A.G. Reid, "Nutritional Disease Affecting Canadian Troops Held Prisoner of War by the Japanese," 61.
23 Crawford Interview, CGR, HCM 6-83; Banfill Interview , CGR, HCM 27-83.
24 James Bertram, *Beneath the Shadows: A New Zealander in the Far East, 1939-46*, 111.
25 Frank Harding, Interview, in Gustave Gingras and Carol Chapman, *The Sequelae of Inhuman Conditions*, 7.

26 Government Records Service, PRO, Hong Kong, Coombes Papers, Certificate signed by Maj. Ashton-Rose, IMS, SMO, re Failure to Supply Diphtheria Antitoxin, 26 Feb 43.

27 Government Records Service, PRO, Hong Kong, Coombes Papers, Expenditure of Diphtheria Antitoxin, September and October 1942.

28 Government Records Service, PRO, Hong Kong, Coombes Papers, Graph of Diphtheria Cases and Deaths, July to September 1942.

29 IWM, Alsey Diary.

30 Government Records Service, PRO, Hong Kong, Coombes Papers, Handwritten List "Unofficial Antitoxin."

31 Government Records Service, PRO, Hong Kong, Coombes Papers, Graph Summarizing Diphtheria Epidemic, POW Camp "S" Hong Kong (June-Dec) 1942, italics added.

32 Bowie, "Captive Surgeon," 174.

33 Sir Selwyn Selwyn-Clarke, *Footprints: The Memoirs of Sir Selwyn Selwyn-Clark*, 80.

34 US Strategic Bombing Survey, *The Japanese Wartime Standard of Living and Utilization of Manpower* ([Washington, DC]: Manpower, Food and Civilian Supplies Division, 1947), 45.

35 Coombes, Interview, CGR, HCM 4-94, 46.

36 Coombes, Interview, CGR, HCM 4-94, 18-19.

37 Bowie, "Captive Surgeon," 174.

38 Government Records Service, PRO, Hong Kong, Coombes Papers, Graph Summarizing Diphtheria Epidemic, POW Camp "S" Hong Kong (June-Dec) 1942.

39 NAC, Forsyth Diary, entry for 14 August 1942.

40 Dr. Solomon Matthew Bard, Interview, CGR, HCM 7-87, Burlington, ON, 7 May 1990, 11-12.

41 CWM, Item 58 A1 24.5, Diary of Delbert Louis William Welsh, 16 October 1941-5 October 1942, entry for 5 October 1942.

42 Bard Interview, HCM 7-87, 11-12.

43 CWM, White Diary, entry for 17 September 1942, 14.

44 NAC, Forsyth Diary, entry for 14 October 1942.

45 Ross Diary, in Anonymous, *The Royal Rifles of Canada in Hong Kong, 1941-45*, 293.

46 Bard Interview, HCM 7-87, 11-12.

47 NAC, Forsyth Diary, undated entry, 94.

48 Banfill Interview, HCM 27-83, 1983.

49 No criticism should be inferred from this observation, which is an indication of the severity of the Depression these young men had just survived, requiring many to leave school and attempt to earn a living. The observation was made by many who were there, including one of the Canadian medical officers. See remarks of Dr. Gordon Gray in Daniel G. Dancocks, *In Enemy Hands: Canadian Prisoners of War, 1939-45* (Edmonton: Hurtig, 1983), 238. Also see Bertram, *Beneath the Shadows*, p. 106, "It had been a shock to find a score or more illiterate Canadians, all from the province of Quebec." Some Grenadiers were illiterate also, as noted in the file of one man interrogated after the war in connection with a war crimes investigation of a Japanese guard. See NAC, Ottawa, RG 24, C2(f), Vol. 8018, File TOK-1-2-5, part 2, Despatches, R.O.G. Morton to Secretary, DND (Army), 22 November 1946.

50 Terry Lockhart, *A Colonial Boy* (Devonport, Tasmania: Terry Lockhart, 1989), 85-86.

51 Ross Diary, in Anonymous, *Royal Rifles of Canada*, 292.

52 Ross Diary, in Anonymous, *Royal Rifles of Canada*, 293.

53 Kenneth Cambon, *Guest of Hirohito*, 42.
54 Jonathan F. Vance, *Objects of Concern*, 187.
55 Arriving at this decision occasioned much heartache amongst the medical officers responsible. Dr. Banfill stated: "We had a meeting in which we condemned all these people to death, the four of us." Banfill Interview, HCM 27-83, 30.
56 CWM, Ottawa, Acc. No. 1983-38/1, Diary of Donald Geraghty, Hong Kong POW, 13.
57 Colin Standish, Interview, CGR, HCM 3-90, Cookshire, PQ, 8 May 1990, 1.
58 Arthur Raymond Squires, "War Diary, Hong Kong and Kowloon, 1941-1945," MS unnumbered pp., 25.
59 S. Martin Banfill, "Shamshuipo," in Anonymous, *Royal Rifles of Canada*, 310.
60 These figures are derived from the nominal rolls maintained for each draft by the office of the SMO of "C" Force, Maj. J.N.B. Crawford: NAC, Ottawa, MG30, E213, John Crawford Papers.
61 IWM, Alsey Diary.
62 E. Lionel Hurd, War Diary, entry for 6-10 October 1942, cited in Anonymous, *Royal Rifles of Canada*, 189.
63 IWM, Department of Documents, London, Item PP/MCR/121, Diary of Adrian Richardson Billings, RN, 1941-1945, 104 pp., 31-32.
64 Australian War Memorial (AWM), Canberra, Personal Records, PR 83, File 32, Report of Service from December 1941 to September 1945 of Captain J.J. Woodward, 13.
65 K.W. Todd, "European into Coolie: Ps.O.W. Adapt Themselves to the Tropical Villagers' Diseases," *Journal of the Royal Army Medical Corps* 86 (1946): 184.
66 Banfill Interview, HCM 27-83, 32.
67 Atkinson Interview, HCM 7-83, 4.
68 Atkinson Interview, HCM 7-83, 8.
69 J.M.S. Dixon, "Diphtheria in North America," *Journal of Hygiene* 93 (1934): 419-21
70 See, among other studies: D.T. Fraser and K.C. Halpern, "Diphtheria Studies, Toronto," *American Journal of Public Health* 30 (1940): 44-46; W. Goldie and E.C.G. Maddock, "A Milk-borne Outbreak of Diphtheria," *Lancet* 1 (1943): 285-86; A. Groulx, "The Diphtheria Situation in Montreal and the Immunization Campaign," *L'Union Médicale du Canada* 72 (1943): 923-24; Arthur Gryfe, "The Taming of Diphtheria: Ontario's Role," *Annals RCPSC* 20 (1987): 115-19; and P.S. Campbell, "The Occurrence of Diphtheria in Halifax from October 1, 1940 to January 31, 1941," *Canadian Public Health Journal* 32 (1941): 404-409.
71 The Schick Test was a skin test designed to show whether or not the tested individual had ever had an attack of diphtheria.
72 NAC, Ottawa, Department of National Defence, RG 24, Vol. 15290, War Diary, Winnipeg Grenadiers, entries for 19, 21, and 22 January and 1 February 1940.
73 Winnipeg Grenadiers War Diary, entry for January 1941.
74 Lewis Bush, *Clutch of Circumstance*, 78.
75 IWM, Alsey Diary.
76 IWM, Department of Documents, London, Item 85/36/1, Diary of Lt. Col. R.J.L. Penfold, entries of 1, 8, 15, and 22 November 1942.
77 IWM, Penfold Diary, 5 January 1942 to 12 August 1945, entry for 19 November 1944.
78 PRO, London, WO 235, File 1012, Trial of Tokunaga et al., 191.
79 PRO, London, WO 235, File 1012, Trial of Tokunaga et al., 193-95.
80 Rhodes House Library, Oxford, MSS. Ind. Ocn. S.233, Dr. K.H. Uttley, MD, Hong Kong. "My Internment Diary: December 8th 1941-August 1945," 22.

81 For example, Deighton points out that the Imperial Japanese Army built its own submarine fleet, and both services constructed separate merchant fleets. Len Deighton, *Blood, Tears and Folly: In the Darkest Hour of the Second World War* (London: Cape, 1993), 546. Van der Vat confirms this remarkable occurrence, stating that the IJA built 20 large submarines intended as cargo-carriers; Dan van der Vat, *Stealth at Sea: The History of the Submarine* (Boston, New York: Houghton Mifflin, 1994), 150.

82 PRO, London, WO 235, File 1012, Trial of Tokunaga et al.

83 PRO, WO 235, File 1012. Both letters, each two pages in length, are attached to the review of the case by DJAG, 9 May 1947.

84 S.E.L. Stening, "Experiences as a Prisoner of War in Japan," 774.

85 Julien M. Goodman, *M.D.P.O.W.* (New York: Exposition Press, 1972), 71.

86 Emetine is an alkaloid made from the roots of the ipecacuanha plant; it has been supplanted by more effective amoebicidal drugs since World War Two.

87 Goodman, *M.D.P.O.W.*, 71.

88 Albert Coates and Newman Rosenthal, *The Albert Coates Story: The Will That Found the Way*, 115.

89 PRO, London, War Office, Medical Historian's Papers, WO 222, File 22, Z.233, "POW Camps in Hong Kong and Japan," Capt. A.J.N. Warrack, RAMC, 63 pp, 23 January 1946, 4-5.

90 AWM,Canberra, AWM 54 File 779/1/21, Report from Diary of Major H.C.G. Robertson, RAMC, Shamshuipo Camp, entries for 6 January and 16 February 1942.

91 Palmer Interview, in Gingras and Chapman, *Sequelae of Inhuman Conditions*, 4.

92 Pemberton, "Observations on Diseases," 147.

93 Squires Interview, CGR, HCM 21-83.

94 Crawford and Reid, "Nutritional Disease," 60.

95 Bush, *Clutch of Circumstance*, 88.

96 IWM, Alsey Diary.

97 IWM, Alsey Diary.

98 Bowie, "Captive Surgeon," 173.

99 C.W. Maisey, "Some Observations On, and Methods of Dealing With, Medical Problems when a Prisoner of War of the Japanese, 1942-1945," *Journal of the Royal Army Medical Corps* 92 (1949): 260.

100 William Allister, *Where Life and Death Hold Hands*, 48.

101 IWM, Billings Diary, 48.

102 Coates and Rosenthal, *Albert Coates Story*, 134.

103 Bush, *Clutch of Circumstance*, 130-31.

104 University of Alberta Archives, Edmonton, Accession No. 77-1, Dr. Benjamin Wheeler Papers, Box 1, File 5, Memoir "Some Experiences as a Prisoner-of-War of the Japanese," n.d., 7.

105 Jackson, *Diary of Col. Calvin G. Jackson*, 70.

106 Jackson, *Diary of Col. Calvin G. Jackson*, 77.

107 Stan Arneil, *One Man's War*, 106.

108 Jean Cantile Stewart, *The Quality of Mercy: The Lives of Sir James and Lady Cantile*, 41.

109 Anonymous, "Quinine." http://www.bev.net/education/schools/ahsscience/apbiol/quinine.html.

110 John Herbert Hardy, Interview, HCM 9-83, 11.

111 David Bosanquet, *Escape through China: Survival after the Fall of Hong Kong*, 126.

112 G.P. Shearer, "Stanley, Hong Kong: The First Three Years," *Royal Engineering Journal* 58 (1944): 167-68.

113 Anonymous, *A Record of Actions of the Hongkong Volunteer Defence Corps in the Battle for Hong Kong, December 1941* (Hong Kong: Ye Olde Printerie, [1954]), 5.

114 Augustus Muir, *The First of Foot: The History of the Royal Scots (The Royal Regiment)* (Edinburgh: Royal Scots History Committee, 1961), 93.
115 Muir, *First of Foot*, 103
116 Bowie, "Captive Surgeon," 158.
117 Joyce Hibbert, "Biscuit, Book, and Candle in Hong Kong," in *Fragments of War: Stories from Survivors of World War II* (Toronto: Dundurn Press, 1985), 115-19.
118 C. G. Roland, "'Sunk under the Taxation of Nature': Malaria in Upper Canada," in C.G. Roland, *Health, Disease and Medicine: Essays in Canadian History* (Toronto: Hannah Institute for the History of Medicine, 1984), 154-70; Roland, "Medical Aspects of War in the West, 1812-1813," in K.G. Pryke and L.L. Kulisek, eds., *The Western District* (Windsor, Ontario: Essex County Historical Society, 1983), 49-60.
119 Mary Ellen Condon-Rall, "Allied Cooperation in Malaria Prevention and Control: The World War II Southwest Pacific Experience," *Journal of the History of Medicine and Allied Sciences* 46 (1991): 496.
120 Crawford and Reid, "Nutritional Disease," 61.
121 Angus A, MacMillan, in Gingras and Chapman, *Sequelae of Inhuman Conditions*, 8.
122 MacMillan, in Gingras and Chapman, *Sequelae of Inhuman Conditions*, 8.
123 NAC, Forsyth Diary, 31.
124 CWM, White Diary, entry for 27 February 1943, 20.
125 Squires, "War Diary," 37.
126 Walter G. Jenkins, Interview, CGR, HCM 22-83, Victoria, BC, 9 June 1983, 19.
127 Todd, "European into Coolie," 182-83.
128 IWM, Department of Documents, London, MS Diary of Major W.T. Carden re his services as an NCO with Royal Army Pay Corps at Hong Kong, entry for 48th week of captivity [1st week of December 1942].
129 John Stroud, Interview, CGR, HCM 19-85, Toronto, ON, 26 February 1985, 12-13.
130 AWM, Woodward Report, 23.
131 George Beer Endacott, *Hong Kong Eclipse*, 145.
132 Shu-Fan Li, *Hong Kong Surgeon*, 103-104.
133 Colin Standish Interview, CGR, HCHM/OHA, HCM 9-89, Cookshire, QC, 30 May 1989, 20-21.
134 A.J.N. Warrack, "Conditions Experienced as a Prisoner of War from a Medical Point of View," 219.
135 NAC, Ottawa, Department of National Defence, Directorate of History, Ottawa. File 593(D17), Debriefing of Capt. John A.G. Reid, 31 October 1945, 73.
136 National Archives and Records Administration (NARA), Washington, RG 153, File 35-215, Trial of Ino Masaji and Onodera Chosuke; Exhibit 64, Deposition of Byron Duwayne Wood, 5 July 1946.
137 John E. Moss, "A Medical Survey of Allied Repatriates after Liberation from Japanese Prisons," *US Naval Medical Bulletin* 47 (1947): 599.
138 Larry M. Dean, Frank N. Willis, and Robert Obourn, "Health Records of American Prisoners of the Japanese during World War II," *Military Medicine* 145 (1980): 840.
139 G. Bras (trans. F.W. Klutzow), "Ziekten en hun behandeling in kampen langs de rivier de Kwai," *Nederlands Tijdschrift voor Geneeskunde* 129 (1985): 1530
140 C. G. Roland, "Stripping Away the Veneer: POW Survival in the Far East as an Index of Cultural Atavism," *Journal of Military History* 53 (1989): 79-94.
141 Todd, "European into Coolie," 179.
142 Matome Ugaki, *Fading Victory: The Diary of Admiral Matome Ugaki, 1941-1945,* trans. Chihaya Masataka (Pittsburgh: University of Pittsburgh Press, 1991), 301.
143 IWM, Billings Diary, 99.

144 Winston Ross Cunningham, Interview, CGR, HCM 18-83, London, ON, 28 June 1983, 24-26.
145 These paragraphs rely heavily on the article by John Murray and Anne Murray, "Suppression of Infection by Famine and Its Activation by Refeeding—A Paradox?" *Perspectives in Biology and Medicine* 20 (1977): 471-83.
146 Murray and Murray, "Suppression of Infection," 472-73.
147 Murray and Murray, "Suppression of Infection," 477.
148 Harold Rifkin, "Dengue Fever (Breakbone Fever)," in Max Pinner and Benjamin F. Miller, eds., *When Doctors Are Patients* (New York: Norton, 1962), 119-23.
149 AWM, AWM 54, File 481/1/24, Items of Medical Interest from Captured Japanese Documents and Interrogations of Prisoners of War, 19.
150 Joseph Ateah, Interview, CGR, HCM 16-83, Winnipeg, MB, 28 May 1983, 7.
151 William Ashton Interview, in Gingras and Chapman, *Sequelae of Inhuman Conditions*, 5.
152 Ella Louise May, "Parasitologic Study of 400 Soldiers Interned by the Japanese," *American Journal of Tropical Medicine* 27 (1947).
153 Hugh J. Morgan, Irving S. Wright, and Arie van Ravenswaay, "Health of Repatriated Prisoners of War from the Far East," *JAMA* 130 (1946): 997.
154 Geoffrey V. Gill and Dion R. Bell, "Persisting Tropical Diseases amongst Former Prisoners of War of the Japanese," *Practitioner* 224 (1980): 803.
155 Anthony Henry Coombes, Interview, CGR, HCM 4 May 1994, 5-94, 37-38.
156 Winnipeg Grenadiers War Diary, entries for 26 August 1940 and January 1941.
157 Silliphant, "Under the Japs in Bilibid," 61.
158 George Hicks, *The Comfort Women: Sex Slaves of the Japanese Imperial Forces*, 66.
159 Hicks, *The Comfort Women*, 67.
160 AWM, Woodward Report, 16.
161 IWM, Alsey Diary, entries for 9, 11, 12, 14, and 19 August 1942.
162 Squires, "War Diary," 32.
163 IWM, Billings Diary, 37-38.
164 CWM, White Diary, entry for 9 November 1944, 31.
165 IWM, Penfold Diary, entry for 31 December 1944.
166 Arthur Squires Interview, CGR, HCM 21-83, Victoria, BC, 9 June 1983, 19.
167 Moss, "A Medical Survey," 603.
168 Morgan, Wright, and van Ravenswaay, "Health of Repatriated Prisoners," 999.
169 H.H.W. Brooke, "Chest X-ray Survey of Repatriated Prisoners of War from Japanese Camps," *Canadian Medical Association Journal* 54 (1946): 142.
170 University of Alberta Archives, Wheeler Papers, Box 3, file 15, "Classification of Diseases, No. 4 Branch Camp," 31 August 1945.
171 AWM 54, Written Records, 1939-45 War, 481/8/10, Final Summary of the Medical Staff, August 10, 1943 - August 28, 1945, Fukuoka Camp 17.
172 NARA, RG 153, File 35-1168, Deposition of Sgt. Joseph Pase, 28 August 1946, 2.
173 William James Overton, Interview, in Gingras and Chapman, *Sequelae of Inhuman Conditions*, 5.
174 Leonard J. Birchall, Interview, CGR, HCM 5-86, Kingston, ON, 22 February 1986, 33.
175 PRO, London, WO 224, File 192, Far East: Tokyo Group.
176 NARA, RG 153, File 33-15, Report on Visit of the Delegates of the Swiss Legation to Shinagawa POW Hospital (Higashi), 19 February 1945, 3.
177 NARA, Washington, Office of the Judge Advocate General (Army), RG 338, Records of the US Eighth Army, Sugamo Prison Records, 1945-1952, 8132nd Army Unit, Sugamo Sup. Det., Box 231, File: Tokuda Hisakichi.

178 C. G. Roland, "Human Vivisection: The Intoxication of Limitless Power in Wartime," in Bob Moore and Kent Fedorowich, eds., *Prisoners of War and their Captors in World War II* (Manchester: Manchester University Press, 1996), 152-56.

179 PRO, WO 222, Warrack Report, 44.

180 AWM 54, Items of Medical Interest, 17.

181 United States Strategic Bombing Survey, *Japanese Wartime Standard of Living*, 101.

182 Immunization against typhoid fever and paratyphoid A and B.

183 IWM, Alsey Diary, 1942.

184 Colin Standish, in Anonymous, *Royal Rifles of Canada*, 305.

185 Luigi Ribiero, [*Reminiscences of a POW at Hong Kong*], MS, 1987, 20.

186 Squires, "War Diary," 31.

187 Squires, "War Diary," 33.

188 IWM, Alsey Diary.

189 Dr. Winston Ross Cunningham, Interview, CGR, HCM 18-83, London, ON, 28 June 1983, 19.

190 Coombes Interview, CGR, HCM 4-94, 38.

191 Coombes Interview, 7.

192 Walter Grey, Interview, in Gingras and Chapman, *Sequelae of Inhuman Conditions*, 8.

193 John Simcoe, Interview, in Gingras and Chapman, *Sequelae of Inhuman Conditions*, 7.

194 Frank Harding, Interview, in Gingras and Chapman, *Sequelae of Inhuman Conditions*, 7.

195 Primo Levi, "October 1944," *Survival in Auschwitz*, cited in Mordecai Richler, ed., *Writers on World War II: An Anthology*, (Toronto: Penguin Books, 1993), 577.

196 MacMillan Interview, in Gingras and Chapman, *Sequelae of Inhuman Conditions*, 7.

197 Thomas Joseph Dewar, Interview, in Gingras and Chapman, *Sequelae of Inhuman Conditions*, 7.

198 IWM, Billings Diary, 65.

199 IWM, Billings Diary, 36.

200 IWM, Billings Diary, 65.

201 IWM, Billings Diary, 87.

202 Dewar Interview, in Gingras and Chapman, *Sequelae of Inhuman Conditions*, 7.

203 Grey Interview, in Gingras and Chapman, *Sequelae of Inhuman Conditions*, 8.

204 Raymond Richard Sellers, Interview, in Gingras and Chapman, *Sequelae of Inhuman Conditions*, 7.

205 Steele, "With the Royal Rifles of Canada," 6.

206 Ribiero, [*Reminiscences*], 21.

207 Endacott, *Hong Kong Eclipse*, 241.

208 Agnes Newton Keith, *Three Came Home*, 57-58.

209 Sir Selwyn Selwyn-Clarke, *Hong Kong Government: Annual Report of the Medical Department for 1946* (Hong Kong: Local Printing Press Ltd., 1947), 19.

210 Walt Whitman, *Leaves of Grass*, Harold W. Blodgett and Sculley Bradley, eds., section 33, line 845, 67.

211 Bertram, *Beneath the Shadows*, 114.

212 IWM, Alsey Diary.

213 Arneil, *One Man's War*, 164.

214 AWM, Woodward Report, 5.

215 IWM, Item 88/33/1, Papers of Don Peacock: MS "Banjo Mickey Mouse: An Erk's Diary of 1276 Incredible Days as Guest of the Emperor," 123-24.

216 Coombes Interview, CGR, HCM 5-94, 42.

217 IWM, Alsey Diary, entry for 29 August 1942.
218 IWM, Alsey Diary, entry for 21 July 1942.
219 Cambon, *Guest of Hirohito*, 44.
220 Coombes Interview, CGR, HCM 5-94, 39.
221 Allister, *Where Life and Death*, 137.
222 Rudolf Zindel was born in Sargans, St. Gallen, Switzerland, 5 February 1900; his date of death was not available from the ICRC. Personal Communication, Fabrizio Bensi, Archives Division, Comitè International de la Croix-Rouge, to C.G. Roland, 21 August 1996.
223 Anonymous, *Report of the International Committee of the Red Cross*, Vol. 1, 479.
224 Selwyn-Clarke, *Footprints*, 71.
225 Bowie, "Captive Surgeon," 164.
226 Bowie, "Captive Surgeon," 182.
227 Bowie, "Captive Surgeon," 183-84.
228 Rhodes House Library, Oxford, Uttley Diary, 59.
229 IWM, Item 84/42/1, Diary of Maj. Cecil Templer, 8.
230 Anonymous, *Report of the International Committee on Its Activities during the Second World War* (September 1, 1939-June 30, 1947), Vol. 1 General Activities (Geneva: International Red Cross, 1948), 461.
231 Anonymous, *Report of the International Committee*, Vol. 1, 463.
232 Anonymous, *Report of the International Committee*, Vol. 1, 463.
233 Anonymous, *Report of the International Committee*, Vol. 1, 482.
234 PRO, War Office, WO 224, File 188, Hong Kong; Supplementary Report.
235 CWM, White Diary, entry for 28 May 1943, 22.
236 CWM, White Diary, entry for 18 August 1945, 43.
237 Allan S. Walker, *Medical Services of the R.A.N. and R.A.A.F.*, 520.
238 Anonymous, *Report of the International Committee*, Vol. 1, 69.
239 Wellcome Institute for the History of Medicine, CMAC, GC/131/18, Acc. no. 413, Papers of Surgeon/Commander J.A. Page, RN, 3.
240 Anonymous, *Report of the International Committee*, Vol. 1, 437.
241 Anonymous, *Report of the International Committee*, Vol. 1, 446.
242 Anonymous, *Report of the International Committee*, Vol. 1, 451.
243 Anonymous, *Report of the International Committee*, Vol. 1, 465-66.
244 Roger Dingman, *Ghost of War: The Sinking of the* Awa Maru *and Japanese-American Relations, 1945-1995* (Annapolis: Naval Institute Press, 1997), 23.
245 Dingman, *Ghost of War*, 33.
246 Dingman, *Ghost of War*, 33.
247 For details see, for example, Sheldon Harris, *Factories of Death: Japanese Biological Warfare 1932-45 and the American Cover-up* (New York: Routledge, 1994).
248 C.P. Brady, "Happy Valley Race Track," in Anonymous, *Royal Rifles of Canada*, 306-307.
249 Bertram, *Beneath the Shadows*, 112-13.
250 Bush, *Clutch of Circumstance*, 96.
251 Henry Wadsworth Longfellow, "A Psalm of Life," 1839.
252 IWM, Carden Diary, entry for Sixth Week of 1942 (i.e., period including 13 February, the date on which the man being buried had died); pages unnumbered.
253 IWM, Alsey Diary.
254 IWM, Alsey Diary.
255 Bertram, *Beneath the Shadows*, 111.
256 CWM, White Diary, entry for 12 November 1943, 25.
257 Harold Englehart, Interview, CGR, HCM 37-85, Montreal, QC, 10 April 1985, 14-15.
258 CWM, White Diary, entry for 7 August 1943, 24.

Chapter Seven

1 IMTFE, Exhibits No. 1967, 1969, and 1971A: 1967, Memorandum from Yeiichi Tatsumi to Tojo Hideki Re: POW Labour, 2 October 1942; 1969, Memorandum from Kondo Kaitaro to Nakamura Kotaro, same subject, 7 October 1942; 1971A, Excerpt from *Foreign Affairs Monthly Report*, September 1942, re: POW Labour. Quotation is from 1971A, 1.
2 US Strategic Bombing Survey, *The Japanese Wartime Standard of Living and Utilization of Manpower* ([Washington, DC]: Manpower, Food and Civilian Supplies Division, 1947), 63-64.
3 US Strategic Bombing Survey, *Japanese Wartime Standard of Living*, 103.
4 S.P. MacKenzie, "The Treatment of Prisoners of War in World War II," *Journal of Modern History* 66 (1994): 500.
5 IMTFE, Exhibit No. 1971A, 2.
6 US Strategic Bombing Survey, *Japanese Wartime Standard of Living*, 78.
7 US Strategic Bombing Survey, *Japanese Wartime Standard of Living*, 130.
8 US Strategic Bombing Survey, *Japanese Wartime Standard of Living*, 78.
9 US Strategic Bombing Survey, *Japanese Wartime Standard of Living*, 132.
10 James Bertram, *Beneath the Shadows*, 123.
11 IWM, London, File PP/MCR/243, Diary of A.J. Alsey, 1942.
12 IWM, Alsey Diary.
13 IWM, Alsey Diary.
14 IWM, Alsey Diary.
15 IWM, Redwood Papers, entry of 8 October 1942.
16 IWM, Redwood Papers, entry of 12 October 1942.
17 Dr. Anthony Henry Coombes, Interview, CGR, HCM 5-94, 4 May 1994, Sussex, England, 55.
18 AWM, Canberra, AWM 54, File 779/1/21, Report from Diary of Maj. H.G.G. Robertson, 19 January 1943.
19 Bertram, *Beneath the Shadows*, 123.
20 NAC, Ottawa, MG 30, E 328, Ebdon Papers, entry for 11 January 1943.
21 NAC, Ebdon Papers, entry for 13 January 1943.
22 NAC, Ebdon Papers, entry for 16 January 1943.
23 NAC, Ebdon Papers, entry for 17 January 1943.
24 NAC, Ebdon Papers, entry for 19 January 1943; underlining in original.
25 Lewis Bush, *Clutch of Circumstance*, 108-109.
26 Bush, *Clutch of Circumstance*, 136-37.
27 Bush, *Clutch of Circumstance*, 138.
28 IWM, London, Item PP/MCR/121, Diary of Adrian Richard Billings, RN, 1941-1945, 43.
29 IWM, Billings Diary, 46.
30 Bertram, *Beneath the Shadows*, 124.
31 Bertram, *Beneath the Shadows*, 125.
32 PRO, London, War Office, Medical Historian's Papers, WO 222, File 22, Z.233: POW Camps in Hong Kong and Japan, by Capt. A.J.N. Warrack, RAMC, 23 January 1946, 26.
33 Warrack Report, 26.
34 A.J.N. Warrack, "Conditions Experienced as a Prisoner of War from a Medical Point of View," 218-19.
35 Jonathan Cott, *Wandering Ghost*, 375-76.
36 J.M. Gibbs, "Prisoner of War Camps in Japan and Japanese Controlled Areas as Taken from Reports of Interned American Prisoners. Osaka No. 3 Oeyema, Japan," *Laison & Research, American Prisoner of War Information Bureau* (31 July 1946), 1-3.

37 Bertram, *Beneath the Shadows*, 153-54.
38 US Strategic Bombing Survey, *Japanese Wartime Standard of Living*, 2.
39 William M. Silliphant, "Under the Japs in Bilibid," MS, Otis Historical Archives of the Armed Forces Medical Museum, 1946.
40 M.L. Gottlieb, "Impressions of POW Medical Officer in Japanese concentration camps," 669.
41 J.E. Nardini, "Survival Factors in American Prisoners of War of the Japanese," *American Journal of Psychiatry* 109 (1952): 241.
42 Louis Allen, *The End of the War in Asia* (London: Hart-Davis, MacGibbon, 1976), 43-44.
43 Frank Evans, *Roll Call at Oeyama*, 86.
44 Evans, *Roll Call at Oeyama*, 90.
45 Evans, *Roll Call at Oeyama*, 99.
46 US Strategic Bombing Survey, *Japanese Wartime Standard of Living*, 1.
47 US Strategic Bombing Survey, *Japanese Wartime Standard of Living*, 1.
48 US Strategic Bombing Survey, *Japanese Wartime Standard of Living*, 3.
49 US Strategic Bombing Survey, *Japanese Wartime Standard of Living*, 9.
50 US Strategic Bombing Survey, *Japanese Wartime Standard of Living*, 23.
51 US Strategic Bombing Survey, *Japanese Wartime Standard of Living*, 16.
52 US Strategic Bombing Survey, *Japanese Wartime Standard of Living*, 18.
53 J.E.C. Robinson, "Work and Problems of a Medical Officer Prisoner of War in the Far East," 52.
54 Robinson, "Work and Problems," 53.
55 Calvin G. Jackson, *Diary of Col. Calvin G. Jackson, MD, Kept during World War II, 1941-1945*, 194, entry for 23 September 1944.
56 Jackson, *Diary of Col. Calvin G. Jackson*, 25.
57 Jackson, *Diary of Col. Calvin G. Jackson*, 28.
58 A.P. Curtin, "Imprisonment under the Japanese," 585.
59 Gottlieb, "Impressions," 668.
60 Bertram, *Beneath the Shadows*, 150-51.
61 Larry M. Dean, Frank N. Willis, and Robert Obourn, "Health Records of American Prisoners of the Japanese during World War II," 838-41
62 AWM, Canberra, AWM 54, Written Records, 1939-45 War, 481/18/10 "Final Summary of the Medical Staff, August 10 1943-August 28, 1945, Fukuoka Camp 17," 11.
63 Dr. Gerrit Bras, Interview, CGR, HCM 24-86, Wageningen, Netherlands, 2 September 1986, 19.
64 Ernest O. Norquist, *Our Paradise: A GI's War Diary* (Hancock, WI: Pearl-Win Publishing, 1989), 339.
65 R. Jackson Scott, *90 Days of Rice* (Pioneer, CA: California Traveler, 1975), 164-70, 181.
66 North Texas State University, Interview with John Breckenridge Garrison, 57.
67 Charles Huxtable, *From the Somme to Singapore: A Medical Officer in Two World Wars* (Kenthurst, Australia: Kangaroo Press, 1987), 155.
68 Robert S. LaForte, and Ronald E. Marcello, *Building the Death Railway: The Ordeal of American POWs in Burma, 1942-1945* (Wilmington, DE: Scholarly Resources, 1993), 162-63.
69 Kenneth Harrison, *The Brave Japanese*, 229.
70 IWM, Item 86/89/1, Papers of A. Dandie, "The Story of 'J' Force," 187-88.
71 Wellcome Institute for the History of Medicine, London, Current Medical Archives Collection, File GC/131/18, Acc. No. 413, Papers of Surgeon/Commander J.A. Page, RN.
72 US Strategic Bombing Survey, *Japanese Wartime Standard of Living*, 35.
73 Dr. Saul Jarcho, Interview, CGR, HCM 10-86, Rochester, NY, 2 May 1986, 23.

74 US Strategic Bombing Survey, *Japanese Wartime Standard of Living*, 45.
75 US Strategic Bombing Survey, *Japanese Wartime Standard of Living*, 46.
76 US Strategic Bombing Survey, *Japanese Wartime Standard of Living*, 36.
77 US Strategic Bombing Survey, *Japanese Wartime Standard of Living*, 99.
78 US Strategic Bombing Survey, *Japanese Wartime Standard of Living*, 100.
79 US Strategic Bombing Survey, *Japanese Wartime Standard of Living*, 101.
80 US Strategic Bombing Survey, *Japanese Wartime Standard of Living*, 102.
81 CWM, Acc. 1981-276/10, Martyn Papers.
82 CWM, Martyn Papers.
83 Harry Atkinson, Interview, in Gingras and Chapman, *Sequelae of Inhuman Conditions*, 8.
84 Albert Delbridge, Interview in Gingras and Chapman, *Sequelae of Inhuman Conditions*, 2.
85 Delbridge, Interview in Gingras and Chapman, *Sequelae of Inhuman Conditions*, 6.
86 Sato Hideo, in Haruko Taya Cook and Theodore F. Cook, *Japan at War*, 236.

Chapter Eight

1 The number is not capable of precision because camps existed for varying periods of time and often, confusingly, names were changed and rechanged to designate the same camp.
2 Frank Evans, *Roll Call at Oeyama*, 146.
3 John M. Gibbs, "Prisoner of War Camps in Japan and Japanese Controlled Area as Taken from Reports of Interned American Prisoners, Osaka No. 3 Oeyama, Japan," *Liaison & Research American Prisoner of War Information Bureau* (31 July 1946), 3.
4 NARA, Records of the Office of the Judge Advocate General (Army), War Crimes Section, RG 153, File 35-483, Case No. 143, Trial of Lt. Hazama Kosaku; Testimony of LtCol. William B. Reardon, 282.
5 CWM, Ottawa, Acc. 1981-276/10, Cat. No. 60-6-52 F.D.F. Martyn Papers; Martyn was in the third draft from Hong Kong, a portion of which went to Oeyama.
6 AWM, Canberra, AWM 54, File 779/1/19, Papers of L.A.R. Evans Concerning His Time as a POW in Singapore and Japan; 9 Parts; see Folder 2—Evans was OC Rations at Oeyama and worked as a cook.
7 NARA, RG 153, File 35-483, Deposition of Surg.Lt.Cmdr. S.E.L. Stening, 2.
8 NARA, RG 153, File 35-483, Deposition of Maj. H.M.S.G. Beadnell, 2 January 1946, 6.
9 NARA, RG 153, File 35-483, Trial of Lt. Hazama Kosaku.
10 CWM, Martyn Papers.
11 NARA, RG 153, File 35-483, Deposition of Stening, 5.
12 NARA, RG 153, File 35-483, Deposition of Stening, 12.
13 Allan S. Walker, *Medical Services of the R.A.N and R.A.A.F.*, 86.
14 IWM, Department of Documents, London, Item 85/42/1, Papers of CSM Ronald Alfred Edwards HKVDC, Scrapbook "Entertainment a la Shumshuipo," seriatim.
15 NAC, Federal Records Centre, Ottawa, Locator No. G287-15, Trial of Cpl. (acting Sgt.) John Hugh Harvey; NAC, Federal Records Centre, Locator No. G287-16, Trial of CSM Marcus Charles Tugby, Winnipeg Grenadiers.
16 Evans, *Roll Call at Oeyama*, 85.
17 NAC, Tugby Trial, Testimony of Pte. Joseph Podosky, 14.
18 NAC, Tugby Trial, Testimony of Sgt. Kenneth Edward Porter, 55.
19 NAC, Tugby Trial, Testimony of John Andrew Krog, 176.
20 NAC, Tugby Trial, Testimony of Sydney Edward Varcoe, 135.

21 Arthur Thomas Ballingall, Interview, in Gustave Gingras and Carol Chapman, *The Sequelae of Inhuman Conditions,* 5.

22 NAC, Tugby Trial, Testimony of J. Murray, 146.

23 NAC, Tugby Trial, Testimony of J. Murray, 142.

24 NAC, Tugby Trial, Testimony of Maj. H.M.S.G. Beadnell, 234.

25 IWM, Item 87/34/1, Papers of Geoffrey C. Hamilton, "Prisoner of War in Hong Kong and Japan, 1941-1945," 25-26.

26 NAC, Tugby Trial, Testimony of Pte. Brownie Lewicki, 52.

27 NAC, Tugby Trial, Testimony of Major Beadnell, 230.

28 Stening, "Experiences as a Prisoner," 774.

29 Stening, "Experiences as a Prisoner," 775.

30 There are additional caveats. The material available is a series of data sheets typed by Dr. Bleich immediately after he returned to the United States in 1945; since there are no sheets for men who died in the camp, we have no data for these men at all, thus skewing all the results. Also, for years after the war Dr. Bleich made his data sheets freely available to any former POW who requested them (usually to support a case when seeking a medical pension). Thus an unknown number of data sheets is missing from the original whole; there is no way to know whether these missing sheets were representative or whether their absence meaningfully skews the Oeyama data.

31 Flora Ricciuti, "Disease Statistics in Japanese Prisoners of War during World War Two," MS. The sources of data were medical casebooks maintained at Oeyama by Capt. LaMoyne Bleich, US Medical Corps, and at Niigata by Maj. William Stewart, RAMC.

32 W.H. Everts, "Nutritional Disorders in Allied Repatriates and Japanese Prisoners of War," *Journal of Nervous and Mental Diseases* 106 (1947): 393-400.

33 Evans, *Roll Call at Oeyama,* 86.

34 Flora Ricciuti, "Disease Statistics in Japanese Prisoners of War during World War Two." Manuscript presented on completion of a summer Hannah Studentship under the guidance of Dr. Charles G. Roland, September 1987.

35 Ricciuti, "Disease Statistics in Japanese Prisoners."

36 NARA, RG 153, File 35-997, Trial of Med.2/Lt. Fujii Hiroshi; Testimony of Accused, 612.

37 Evans, *Roll Call at Oeyama,* 84.

38 Evans, *Roll Call at Oeyama,* 85.

39 NARA, RG 153, File 35-483, Deposition of Pte. Robert John Dukelow, 4.

40 NARA, RG 153, File 35-483, Testimony of Accused, 709.

41 NARA, RG 153, File 35-483, Deposition of Maj. H.M.S.G. Beadnell, 4.

42 NARA, RG 153, File 35-483, Deposition of Pte. R. Dalzell, 3-4.

43 NARA, RG 153, File 35-1097, Trial of Kojima Itchisaku; the application is Prosecution Exhibit 2, 25 May 1943.

44 Harry E. Steen, "Recollections of Experiences as a POW in the Far East" (Dictated September 1992); HCM 11-92, 41.

45 C. G. Roland and H. S. Shannon, "Patterns of Disease among World War II Prisoners of the Japanese: Hunger, Weight Loss, and Deficiency Diseases in Two Camps," *Journal of the History of Medicine & Allied Sciences* 46 (1991): 72.

46 NARA, RG 153, File 33-76; Deposition of Cpl. Elton Summers, 7 October 1945, 1.

47 NARA, RG 153, File 33-76, Testimony of Accused, 576.

48 Atkinson Interview, in Gingras and Chapman, *Sequelae of Inhuman Conditions,* 5.

49 NARA, RG 153, File 35-1097, Trial of Kojima Itchisaku, Maj. Stewart's Testimony, 145.

50 Personal communication, W. Stewart to C. Roland, 1 May 1995.

51 NARA, RG 153, File 35-997, Trial of Med. 2/Lt. Fujii Hiroshi, Testimony of Accused, 575.

52 The initial after a camp number indicated the administrative category of the camp. A "D" indicated a Dispatch camp, "B" a branch camp. Administratively, these two classes of camps were handled quite differently. In a branch camp all medical matters were conducted by branch camp military personnel, that is to say, by IJA military medical staff. In a dispatch camp the company for which the men were working assumed the responsibility for treating the prisoners of war according to the pertinent medical regulations. See NARA, RG 153, File 35-997, Trial of Med.2/Lt. Fujii Hiroshi, Testimony of Dr. Tokuda Hisakichi, 384.

53 NARA, RG 153, File 35-1097, Trial of Kojima Itchisaku, Testimony of W.M. Stewart, 181.

54 NARA, RG 153, File 35-997, Trial of Fujii Hiroshi, Testimony of W.M. Stewart, 28.

55 NARA, RG 153, File 35-205, Trial of Fujita Tatsuro and others; Deposition by Fellows, 12 September 1945.

56 NARA, RG 153, File 35-205, Fellows Deposition, 13-14.

57 Though many POWs came to have a functional knowledge of basic Japanese, most of the Japanese phrases and sentences that appear in memoirs, depositions, affidavits in court testimony are based on phonetic interpretations rendered arbitrary by the lack of expertise in the language, not only by POWs but also by typists. This sentence is not stylish Japanese, though its meaning was clear to the prisoners.

58 Randolph Steele, "With the Royal Rifles," 11.

59 NARA, RG 153, File 35-997, Trial of Fujii Hiroshi, Testimony of Accused, 569.

60 NARA, RG 153, File 35-205, Trial of Fujita Tatsuro and Others, Fellows Deposition, 6.

61 NARA, RG 153, File 35-997, Trial of Fujii Hiroshi, Review of Staff Advocate General, 29 April 1949, 5-6.

62 NARA, RG 153, File 35-997, Testimony of Dr. Fujimake Shigeo, 424.

63 NARA, RG 153, File 35-997, Testimony of Dr. Fujimake Shigeo, 425.

64 NAC, MG30 E181 Tom Forsyth, "Hong Kong Diary and Memories of Japan: Gleanings from the Diary of a Winnipeg Grenadier," entry for 28 March 1944.

65 Steele, "With the Royal Rifles," 11-12.

66 NARA, RG 153, File 35-205, Trial of Fujita Tatsuro, Fellows Deposition, 8.

67 NARA, RG 153, File 35-205, Trial of Fujita Tatsuro, Fellows Deposition, 8.

68 NAC, Forsyth Diary, entry for 26 May 1944.

69 NAC, Forsyth Diary, entry for 26 May 1944.

70 NAC, Forsyth Diary, entry for 26 May 1944.

71 NARA, RG 153, File 35-1097, Trial of Kojima Itchisaku, Testimony of Maynard Lee, 228.

72 NARA, RG 153, File 35-1097, Trial of Kojima Itchisaku, Testimony of Maynard Lee, 229.

73 NARA, RG 153, File 35-1097, Trial of Kojima Itchisaku, Testimony of Maynard Lee, 254.

74 NAC, Forsyth Diary, entry for 27 March 1944.

75 NARA, RG 153, File 35-1097, Trial of Kojima Itchisaku, Testimony of Maynard Lee, 231.

76 Kenneth Hourigan, quoted by Studs Terkel in *The Good War*, cited in Mordecai Richler, ed., *Writers on World War II: An Anthology* (Toronto: Penguin Books, 1993), 282.

77 NARA, RG 153, File 35-1097, Trial of Kojima Itchisaku, Testimony of Maynard Lee, 232.

78 US Strategic Bombing Survey, *The Japanese Wartime Standard of Living and Utilization of Manpower* ([Washington, DC]: Manpower, Food and Civilian Supplies Division, 1947), 15.

79 Atkinson Interview, in Gingras and Chapman, *Sequelae of Inhuman Conditions*, 2.
80 Atkinson Interview, 2.
81 Atkinson Interview, 2.
82 Atkinson Interview, 3.
83 Steele, "With the Royal Rifles," 15-16.
84 NAC, Forsyth Diary, undated entry, 83-85.
85 NARA, RG 153, File 33-54, File of Affidavits Relating to Niigata POW Camp No. 15D, Shintetsu. Deposition of LtCol. John Francis Breslin, 1.
86 NARA, RG 153, File 33-54. Breslin Deposition, 1.
87 NARA, RG 153, File 33-54. Breslin Deposition, 2.
88 NARA, RG 153, File 33-54. Breslin Deposition, 2.
89 NARA, RG 153, File 33-54. Breslin Deposition, 3.
90 NARA, RG 153, File 33-54. Breslin Deposition, 16-17.
91 NAC, Forsyth Diary, undated entry, 87.
92 Steele, "With the Royal Rifles," 12.
93 William Allister, *Where Life and Death Hold Hands*, 106.
94 Allister, *Where Life and Death*, 112.
95 Allister, *Where Life and Death*, 14.
96 NARA, RG 153, File 35-205, Fellows Deposition, 4.
97 NARA, RG 153, File 35-997, Trial of Med. 2/Lt. Fujii Hiroshi, Testimony of Accused, 570-71.
98 Atkinson Interview, in Gingras and Chapman, *Sequelae of Inhuman Conditions*, 4.
99 NAC, Forsyth Diary, 94.
100 Ross Diary, in Anonymous, *The Royal Rifles of Canada in Hong Kong, 1941- 1945*, 369.
101 Ross Diary, in Anonymous, *Royal Rifles*, 375.
102 NAC, Forsyth Diary, entry for 3 April 1944.
103 NAC, Forsyth Diary, 93.
104 NAC, Forsyth Diary, 92.
105 Atkinson Interview, in Gingras and Chapman, *Sequelae of Inhuman Conditions*, 7.
106 NARA, RG 153, File 35-1097, Trial of Kojima Itchisaku, Testimony of W.M. Stewart, 152.
107 Gabriel Guitard, "Notebook kept in pencil at Niigata POW Camp 5B, October 1943 to February 1944."
108 NARA, RG 153, File 35-997, Trial of Med. 2/Lt. Fujii Hiroshi, Testimony of Fujii Hiroshi, 631.
109 NARA, RG 153, File 35-205, Trial of Fujita Tatsuro and others, Fellows Deposition, 7.
110 Atkinson Interview, in Gingras and Chapman, *Sequelae of Inhuman Conditions*, 7.
111 NARA, RG 153, File 35-205, Trial of Fujita Tatsuro and others, Fellows Deposition, 15.
112 NARA, RG 153, File 35-205, Trial of Fujita Tatsuro and others, Fellows Deposition, 16.
113 Flora Ricciuti, "Disease Statistics in Japanese Prisoners."
114 William M. Silliphant, "Under the Japs in Bilibid," also S.E.L. Stening, "Experiences as a Prisoner of War in Japan," 773-75.
115 Brig. (ret'd) William Stewart, Personal Communication.
116 Larry M. Dean, Frank N. Willis, and Robert Obourn, "Health Records of American Prisoners of the Japanese during World War II," 840.
117 Steele, "With the Royal Rifles," 11.

118 NAC, Forsyth Diary, 94-95.
119 NAC, Forsyth Diary, 102.
120 NAC, Forsyth Diary, 102.
121 NAC, Forsyth Diary, 101-102.
122 NAC, Forsyth Diary, entry for 1 January 1944.
123 Steele, "With the Royal Rifles," 11.
124 Calvin G. Jackson, *Diary of Col. Calvin G. Jackson MD*, 200.
125 Anonymous, *Royal Rifles of Canada*, 366.
126 Anonymous, *Royal Rifles of Canada*, 366.
127 Anonymous, *Royal Rifles of Canada*, 366.
128 NARA, RG 153, File 35-997, Trial of Fujii Hiroshi, Deposition of 2/Lt. Richard P. Fulmer, 7.
129 NAC, Ottawa, Department of National Defence, Directorate of History, File 593(D17), Debriefing of Capt. John A. Reid, 31 October 1945, 81.
130 DND, File 593(D17), Debriefing of Capt. Reid, 31.
131 DND, File 593(D17), Debriefing of Capt. Reid, 34-35.
132 DND, File 593(D17), Debriefing of Capt. Reid, 81.
133 DND, File 593(D17), Debriefing of Capt. Reid, 108.
134 DND, File 593(D17), Debriefing of Capt. Reid, 18.
135 Roy Robinson Interview by Charles G. Roland (CGR), HCHm/OHA, HCM 10-83, Winnipeg, MB, 27 May 1983, 11.
136 DND, File 593(D17), Debriefing of Capt. Reid, 32ff.
137 Allister, *Where Life and Death*, 124.
138 DND, File 593(D17), Debriefing of Capt. Reid, 61.
139 NARA, RG 153, File 35-868, Trial of Kondo Kanechi, accused of war crimes against several Canadian POWs at Tokyo Area 3D POW Camp, Yokohama, in 1943.
140 NARA, RG 153, File 35-868, Statement by the Accused, Kondo, 17 December 1946, 2.
141 Derived from testimony and various other documents throughout this case transcript: NARA, RG 153, File 35-868, Trial of Kondo Kanechi.
142 Angus McRitchie, Interview, CGR, HCM 25-85, Winnipeg, MB, 9 March 1985, 25-26.
143 Pat Poirier, Interview, CGR, HCM 6-90, Montreal, QC, n.d., 18-19.
144 Poirier Interview, CGR, HCM 6-90, 18-19.
145 DND, File 593(D17), Reid Debriefing, 74-75.
146 DND, File 593(D17), Reid Debriefing, 80.
147 IMTFE, Exhibit No. 3111, Investigation Squad of Army Medical College, Suggestions Regarding Improvement of Health Conditions of Prisoners of War Camp, 1.
148 Allister, *Where Life and Death*, 103.
149 Poirier Interview, CGR, HCM 6-90, 12-13.
150 Lionel Speller Interview, CGR, HCM 2-90, Victoria, BC, 27 May 1990.
151 DND, File 593(D17), Reid Debriefing, 69.
152 DND, File 593(D17), Reid Debriefing, 67.
153 DND, File 593(D17), Reid Debriefing, 88.
154 DND, File 593(D17), Reid Debriefing, 95.
155 DND, File 593(D17), Reid Debriefing, 97.
156 Harold Wilfred Englehart Interview, CGR, HCM 37-85, Montreal QC, 10 April 1985, 23-24.
157 DND, File 593(D17), Reid Debriefing, 107.
158 DND, File 593(D17), Reid Debriefing, 116.
159 DND, File 593(D17), Reid Debriefing, 125.
160 DND, File 593(D17), Reid Debriefing, 128.
161 IMTFE, Exhibit No. 3111, Investigation Squad of Army Medical College, 1.

162 IMTFE, Exhibit No. 3111, Investigation Squad of Army Medical College, 2.
163 DND, File 593(D17), Reid Debriefing, 34-35.
164 DND, File 593(D17), Reid Debriefing, 39.
165 DND, File 593(D17), Reid Debriefing, 43.
166 McRitchie Interview, CGR, HCM 25-85, 31.
167 Kenneth M. Gaudin, Interview, in Gingras and Chapman, *Sequelae of Inhuman Conditions*, 5.
168 DND, File 593(D17), Reid Debriefing, 44-45.
169 DND, File 593(D17), Reid Debriefing, 88-89.
170 DND, File 593(D17), Reid Debriefing, 89.
171 DND, File 593(D17), Reid Debriefing, 46.
172 DND, File 593(D17), Reid Debriefing, 47.
173 DND, File 593(D17), Reid Debriefing, 59.
174 DND, File 593(D17), Reid Debriefing, 81.
175 DND, File 593(D17), Reid Debriefing, 100.
176 DND, File 593(D17), Reid Debriefing, 76.
177 DND, File 593(D17), Reid Debriefing, 70.
178 DND, File 593(D17), Reid Debriefing, 79.
179 McRitchie Interview, HCM 25-85, 20.
180 DND, File 593(D17), Reid Debriefing, 108.
181 DND, File 593(D17), Reid Debriefing, 75.
182 DND, File 593(D17), Reid Debriefing, 112.
183 McRitchie Interview, CGR, HCM 25-85, 24.
184 DND, File 593(D17), Reid Debriefing, 120.
185 DND, File 593(D17), Reid Debriefing, 121.
186 DND, File 593(D17), Reid Debriefing, 127.
187 Robinson Interview, CGR, HCM 10-83, 22-23.
188 DND, File 593(D17), Reid Debriefing, 36.
189 DND, File 593(D17), Reid Debriefing, 40.
190 DND, File 593(D17), Reid Debriefing, 53.
191 DND, File 593(D17), Reid Debriefing, 62.
192 DND, File 593(D17), Reid Debriefing, 82.
193 DND, File 593(D17), Reid Debriefing, 112.
194 Anonymous, *Royal Rifles of Canada*, 382.
195 Allister, *Where Life and Death*, 98.
196 DND, File 593(D17), Reid Debriefing, 42.
197 DND, File 593(D17), Reid Debriefing, 114.
198 DND, File 593(D17), Reid Debriefing, 19.
199 Allister, *Where Life and Death*, 168.
200 DND, File 593(D17), Reid Debriefing, 71.
201 DND, File 593(D17), Reid Debriefing, 73.
202 DND, File 593(D17), Reid Debriefing, 47.
203 DND, File 593(D17), Reid Debriefing, 109.
204 DND, File 593(D17), Reid Debriefing, 48-49.
205 Speller Interview, CGR, HCM 2-90, 28-32.
206 NAC, RG 24, C 2 (f), Vol. 8019, file TOK-2-2, "Fukuoka Camp No. 5—Omine."
207 NARA, RG 153, File 36-489, Trial of Lt. Yanaru Tetsutoshi, 7.
208 NARA, RG 153, File 36-489, Testimony of WO1 Harold B. Shephard, RRC, 18.
209 NARA, RG 153, File 36-489, Shephard Testimony, 11.
210 NARA, RG 153, File 36-489, Shephard Testimony, 23.
211 NARA, RG 153, File 36-489, Deposition of John Francis Burns, RRC, 1.
212 NARA, RG 153, File 36-489, Deposition of Lt.Col. H.G.G. Robertson, RAMC, 1.
213 NARA, RG 153, File 36-489, Fukuoka POW Camp No. 5 Branch, Camp Diary, entry for 24 January 1943.

214 NARA, RG 153, File 36-489, Camp Diary, entry for 9 May 1943.

215 NAC, RG 24, C 2 (f), Vol. 8019, file TOK-2-2, "Fukuoka Camp No. 5—Omine."

216 NARA, RG 153, File 36-489, Shephard Testimony, 12.

217 NAC, Diary kept by CSM Ebdon, 26 December 1942 to 26 December 1943, at Sham Shui Po, Hong Kong, and Omine Camp, Japan, entry for 28 January 1943.

218 NAC, Ebdon Diary, entry for 14 February 1943.

219 NARA, RG 153, File 36-489, Camp Diary, entry for 2 February 1943.

220 Ross Diary, in Anonymous, *Royal Rifles,* entry for 3 February 1943.

221 NAC, Ebdon Papers, Regulations for Omine Prisoners' Camp.

222 NARA, RG 153, File 36-489, Diary of Sgt. Ross, entry for 6 April 1943.

223 NAC, Ebdon Diary, entry for 17 April 1943.

224 NARA, RG 153, File 36-489, Shephard Testimony, 28.

225 NARA, RG 153, File 36-489, Deposition of Malcolm Nicholson, 1.

226 George Palmer, Interview in Gingras and Chapman, *Sequelae of Inhuman Conditions,* 2.

227 NARA, RG 153, File 36-489, Deposition of Lt.Col. H.G.G. Robertson, 4.

228 NARA, RG 153, File 36-489, Shephard Testimony, 19.

229 NAC, Ebdon Diary, entry for 31 January 1943.

230 NAC, Ebdon Papers, Regulations for Omine Prisoners' Camp.

231 NARA, RG 153, File 36-489, Deposition of Lt.Col. Robertson, 2.

232 NAC, Ebdon Diary, entry for 26 February 1943.

233 Palmer Interview, in Gingras and Chapman, *Sequelae of Inhuman Conditions,* 3.

234 Tom Blaylock Interview, North Texas State University, Oral History Collection, No. 65, Dallas, TX, 22 March 1971, 67.

235 Blaylock Interview, North Texas State University, 76.

236 NARA, RG 153, File 36-489, Deposition of Clifford Robinson, 2.

237 Palmer Interview, in Gingras and Chapman, *Sequelae of Inhuman Conditions,* 2.

238 NARA, RG 153, File 36-489, Shephard Testimony, 12.

239 NARA, RG 153, File 36-489, Shephard Testimony, 19.

240 North Texas State University, Blaylock Interview, 65.

241 NARA, RG 153, File 35-621, Trial of Tanaka Hiroshi and others, charged with offences against POWs at Narumi POW Camp in 1944 and 1945.

242 Colin Standish, Interview, CGR, HCM 3-90, Cookshire, QC, 8 June 1990, 4-5.

243 Standish Interview, CGR, HCM 3-90, 6.

244 NARA, RG 153, File 35-621, Trial of Tanaka Hiroshi.

245 NARA, RG 153, File 35-61, Trial of Okada Miyoroku, Commandant of Narumi POW Camp, 2B; Review of Staff Judge Advocate, 22 May 1946, 1.

246 Preston John Hubbard, *Apocalypse Undone: My Survival of Japanese Imprisonment during World War II,* 213.

247 IWM, Item 85/42/1, Edwards Papers; Personal Diary, seriatim.

248 IWM, Item 85/42/1, Edwards Papers, Diary.

249 Standish Interview, CGR, HCM 9-89, 31-32.

250 NARA, RG 153, File 35-621, Affidavit of George Allan Watts, 1.

251 Hubbard, *Apocalypse Undone,* 172,

252 NARA, RG 153, File 35-621, Review of Staff Judge Advocate, 31.

253 NARA, RG 153, File 35-621, Review of Staff Judge Advocate, 63.

254 Standish Interview, CGR, HCM 3-90, 12-13.

255 PRO, London, War Crimes Papers, Judge Advocate General's Office, WO 235, file 892, Trial of Niimori Genichiro; Exhibit T, Undated Letter, W. Norman Riley to Maj. J.A. MacDonald.

256 Terry Lockhart, *A Colonial Boy,* 99.

257 Lockhart, *A Colonial Boy,* 99.

258 IWM, Item 85/42/1, Edwards Papers, Diary.

259 NARA, RG 153, File 35-621, Affidavit of Dr. W.N. Riley, 2.

260 NARA, RG 153, File 35-621, Affidavit of Dr. W.N. Riley, 3.

261 Standish Interview, CGR, HCM 3-90, 7-8.

262 Lockhart, *A Colonial Boy*, 106.

263 NARA, RG 153, File 35-621, Affidavit of Dr. Riley, 4.

264 NARA, RG 153, File 35-621, Affidavit of Dr. Riley, 2.

265 NARA, RG 153, File 35-103, Deposition of Capt. Elack Schultz, 2.

266 Elack Schultz was born 25 June 1911 in Wichita, Kansas; he graduated from the University of Lausanne, Switzerland in 1937. He died on 31 May 1979. (All data from the American Medical Association files.)

267 Robert W. Levering, *Horror Trek: A True Story of Bataan, the Death March and Three and One-half Years in Japanese Prison Camps*, 154.

268 Standish Interview, CGR, HCM 9-89, 31-32.

269 NARA, RG 153, File 35-621, Affidavit of Dr. Riley, 4.

270 NARA, RG 153, File 35-621, Affidavit of Dr. Riley, 3.

271 NARA, RG 153, File 35-621, Affidavit of Dr. Riley, 3.

272 NARA, RG 153, File 35-621, Affidavit of Dr. Riley, 4.

273 Hubbard, *Apocalypse Undone*, 176.

274 Hubbard, *Apocalypse Undone*, 192-93.

275 NARA, RG 153, File 35-621, Review of Staff Judge Advocate, 31.

276 Hubbard, *Apocalypse Undone*, 207.

277 Lockhart, *A Colonial Boy*, 109.

278 IWM, Item 85/42/1, Edwards Papers, Diary, seriatim.

279 NARA, RG 153, File 35-621, Affidavit of Dr. Riley, 1.

280 NARA, RG 153, File 35-621, Affidavit of Dr. Riley, 2.

281 NARA, RG 153, File 35-621, Affidavit of Dr. Riley, 6.

282 IWM, Item 85/42/1, Edwards Papers, Diary, seriatim.

283 Hubbard, *Apocalypse Undone*, 186.

284 Standish Interview, CGR, HCM 9-89, 32-33.

285 Standish Interview, CGR, HCM 9-89, 32-33.

286 NARA, RG 153, File 35-621, Affidavit of Dr. Riley, 6.

287 IWM, Item 85/42/1, Edwards Papers, Diary, seriatim.

288 NARA, RG 153, File 35-1697, Trial of Ninomiya Yutaka, Wakamatsu Manzo, and Ozawa Masaharu; Prosecution Opening Statement, 9.

289 NARA, RG 153, File 35-1697, Affidavit of Sgt. Wm. Edward Shayler, WG, 1.

290 NARA, RG 153, File 35-1697, Affidavit of Pte. John Cecil Davies, 1.

291 NARA, RG 153, File 35-1697, Prosecution Opening Statement, 10.

292 NARA, RG 153, File 35-1697, Testimony of Accused, Ninomiya Yutaka, 344.

293 NARA, RG 153, File 35-1697, Review of Staff Judge Advocate, 11.

294 J.W. Chatwell, Interview in Gingras and Chapman, *Sequelae of Inhuman Conditions*, 7.

295 J.W. Chatwell, Interview in Gingras and Chapman, *Sequelae of Inhuman Conditions*, 7.

296 NARA, RG 153, File 35-1697, Affidavit of Carlos Arnulphy, Prosecution Exhibit 3, 1.

297 NARA, RG 153, File 35-1697, Affidavit of Caltano Mario Azedo, Prosecution Exhibit 4, 2.

298 Englehart Interview, CGR, HCM 37-85, 37-38.

299 Reginald Law, Interview, CGR, HCM 7-89, Campbelltown, NB, 28 May 1989, 13.

300 NARA, RG 153, File 35-1697, Affidavit of George Alfred Temple, 1.

301 NARA, RG 153, File 35-1697, Review of Staff Judge Advocate, 13.

302 W.J. Overton, Interview in Gingras and Chapman, *Sequelae of Inhuman Conditions*, 2.

303 NARA, RG 153, File 35-1697, Affidavit of Dr. Patrick M. Cmeyla, 2.

304 NARA, RG 153, File 35-1697, Testimony of Dr. Hironaka Kazuo, 120.

305 Englehart Interview, CGR, HCM 37-85, 26-27.

306 Peterson Interview, in Gingras and Chapman, *Sequelae of Inhuman Conditions*, 3.

307 NARA, RG 153, File 35-1697, Affidavit of Wm. Edward Shayler, 2.

308 Overton Interview, in Gingras and Chapman, *Sequelae of Inhuman Conditions*, 4.

309 NARA, RG 153, File 35-1697, Affidavit of R.C. Wilson, 4.

310 NARA, RG 153, File 35-1697, Testimony of Dr. Hironaka Kazuo, 133.

311 Alfred A. Weinstein, *Barbed-Wire Surgeon*, 234.

312 Leonard Birchall, MS Biographical Notes, in possession of the author, undated but ca. 1970, 36-37.

313 Weinstein, *Barbed-Wire Surgeon*, 222.

314 Ernest O. Norquist, *Our Paradise: A GI's War Diary*, 276.

315 AWM, Canberra, Personal Records, PR 83, File 32, Report of Service from December 1941 to September 1945, of Capt. J.J. Woodward, IMS/IAMC, 28.

316 Weinstein, *Barbed-Wire Surgeon*, 219.

317 NARA, RG 153, File 35-997, Testimony of Lt. Lewis Bush, 532.

318 AWM, PR 83, File 32, Woodward Report, 27.

319 NARA, RG 153, File 35-997, Review of Staff Judge Advocate, 14.

320 Lewis Bush, *Clutch of Circumstance*, 108-109.

321 NARA, RG 153, File 33-76, Deposition of Nelson N. Kaufmann, 3.

322 NARA, RG 153, File 33-76, Deposition of Arthur L. Maher, 13.

323 AWM, PR 83, File 32, Woodward Report, 29-30.

324 AWM, PR 83, File 32, Woodward Report, 31-32.

325 AWM, PR 83, File 32, Woodward Report, 31-32.

326 Sellers Interview, in Gingras and Chapman, *Sequelae of Inhuman Conditions*, 7.

327 James Bertram, *Beneath the Shadows*, 167.

328 Bertram, *Beneath the Shadows*, 146.

329 Bush, *Clutch of Circumstance*, 214.

330 Birchall, MS Biographical Notes, 37-38.

331 Norquist, *Our Paradise*, 296.

332 Weinstein, *Barbed-Wire Surgeon*, 246.

333 NARA, RG 153, File 33-76, Deposition of Nelson N. Kaufmann, 3.

334 Weinstein, *Barbed-Wire Surgeon*, 234.

335 McRitchie Interview, CGR, HCM 25-85, 29.

336 Weinstein, *Barbed-Wire Surgeon*, 239.

337 Bertram, *Beneath the Shadows*, 163.

338 Bertram, *Beneath the Shadows*, 184.

339 Weinstein, *Barbed-Wire Surgeon*, 236.

340 Birchall, MS Biographical Notes, 39.

341 Weinstein, *Barbed-Wire Surgeon*, 245.

342 NARA, RG 153, File 35-997, Pros. Exhibit No. 17, Affidavit of Dr. Lloyd Goad, 1.

343 Weinstein, *Barbed-Wire Surgeon*, 228.

344 NARA, RG 153, File 35-997, Testimony of Dr. Kondo Kinichi, 874-75.

345 Bertram, *Beneath the Shadows*, 153-54.

346 NARA, RG 153, File 35-997, Testimony of Accused, Med.2/Lt. Dr. Fujii Hiroshi, 682.

347 Weinstein, *Barbed-Wire Surgeon*, 225.

348 Bush, *Clutch of Circumstance*, 169-170.

349 Bush, *Clutch of Circumstance*, 169-170.

350 Norquist, *Our Paradise*, 302.

351 McRitchie Interview, CGR, HCM 25-85, 31.

352 Norquist, *Our Paradise*, 284.

353 North Texas State University, Blaylock Interview, 82.

354 NARA, RG 153, File 35-997, Testimony of James Bertram, 3.

355 Bush, *Clutch of Circumstance*, 184. Bush was married to a Japanese woman and had taught school in Japan for several years in the 1930s.
356 Weinstein, *Barbed-Wire Surgeon*, 224.
357 North Texas State University, Blaylock Interview, 76.
358 Weinstein, *Barbed-Wire Surgeon*, 240.
359 Norquist, *Our Paradise*, 293.
360 Richard H. O'Kane, *Clear the Bridge!: The War Patrols of the USS Tang*, 465-66.
361 NAC, RG 24, C 2 (f), Vol. 8020, Affidavit of Albert Alexander Cox, 3.
362 NAC, RG 24, C 2 (f), Vol. 8020, Affidavit of J.W.E. Lawrence, 19.
363 NAC, RG 24, C 2 (f), Vol. 8020, Affidavit of A.A. Cox, 2.
364 NAC, RG 24, C 2 (f), Vol. 8020, Affidavit of A.A. Cox, 2.
365 DND, File 593(D17), Reid Debriefing, 47.
366 NAC, RG 24, C 2 (f), Vol. 8020, Affidavit of Alfred Mansfield, 10-11.
367 NAC, RG 24, C 2 (f), Vol. 8020, Affidavit of Thomas Marr, 19.
368 NAC, RG 24, C 2 (f), Vol. 8020, Affidavit of David Turk, 14.
369 NAC, RG 24, C 2 (f), Vol. 8020, Affidavit of Alexander Gunderson, 7.
370 NAC, RG 24, C 2 (f), Vol. 8020, Affidavit of D. Turk, 15.
371 NAC, RG 24, C 2 (f), Vol. 8020, Affidavit of T.F. Marr, 18.
372 NAC, RG 24, C 2 (f), Vol. 8020, Affidavit of D. Turk, 15.
373 NAC, RG 24, C 2 (f), Vol. 8020, Affidavit of W.A. Moss, 23.
374 NAC, RG 24, C 2 (f), Vol. 8020, Affidavit of A.A. Cox, 4.
375 NAC, RG 24, C 2 (f), Vol. 8020, Affidavit of T.F. Marr, 17.
376 NAC, RG 24, C 2 (f), Vol. 8020, Affidavit of A.A. Cox, 3.
377 PRO, London, War Office, War of 1939-1945: Reports of International Red Cross and Protecting Powers, WO 224, File 192, Far East: Tokyo Group, 3.
378 PRO, London, War Office, Medical Historian's Papers, WO 222, File 22, Z.233: POW Camps in Hong Kong and Japan, by Capt. A.J.N. Warrack RAMC, 23 January 1946, 29.
379 DND, File 593(D17), Reid Debriefing, 82.
380 NARA, RG 153, File 35-997, Testimony of Med.2/Lt. Fujii Hiroshi, 557.
381 NARA, RG 153, File 35-997, Testimony of Med.2/Lt. Fujii Hiroshi, 81.
382 Wellcome Institute for the History of Medicine, London, Current Medical Archives Collection, GC/131/18, Acc. No. 413, Papers of Surg.Cdr. J.A. Page RN, 3.
383 NARA, RG 153, File 35-997, Deposition of Maj. A.A. Weinstein, 10.
384 A.J.N. Warrack, "Conditions Experienced as a Prisoner of War from a Medical Point of View," *Journal of the Royal Army Medical Corps* 87 (1946): 219-20.
385 M.I. Gottlieb, "Impressions of a POW Medical Officer in Japanese Concentration Camps," *US Navy Medical Bulletin* 46 (1946): 68.
386 Gottlieb, "Impressions of a POW Medical Officer," 673.
387 Gottlieb, "Impressions of a POW Medical Officer," 668.
388 Personal Communication, Dr. Lloyd Goad to Author, 3 July 1986.
389 PRO, WO 222, File 22, Z.233, Warrack Report, 31.
390 PRO, WO 222, File 22, Z.233, Warrack Report, 31.
391 PRO, WO 222, File 22, Z.233, Warrack Report, 39.
392 PRO, WO 222, File 22, Z.233, Warrack Report, 40.
393 PRO, WO 222, File 22, Z.233, Warrack Report, 42.
394 PRO, WO 224, File 192, Telegram 26/4/44 re Visit to Shinagawa Hospital 14 April 1944, by ICRC Delegate and Prince Shimadzu, VP Japan Red Cross, and 4-p. Report by Pestalozzi, 2.
395 Gottlieb, "Impressions of a POW Medical Officer," 664.
396 Warrack, "Conditions Experienced," 226.
397 Warrack, "Conditions Experienced," 226.

398 AWM, PR 83, File 32, Woodward Report, 26.

399 AWM, PR 83, File 32, Woodward Report, 30.

400 Warrack, "Conditions Experienced," 221.

401 Warrack, "Conditions Experienced," 221.

402 PRO, WO 222, PR83, File 32, Warrack Report, 44.

403 PRO, WO 222, PR83, File 32, Warrack Report, 44.

404 Gottlieb, "Impressions of a POW Medical Officer," 664.

405 NARA, RG 153, File 35-9, Depositions with Respect to Alleged Brutalities at Shinagawa POW Hospital, Zentsujii POW Camp, and Kawasaki Camp 1B, Deposition of Lt.Cmdr. James Robert Davis, 4.

406 NARA, RG 153, File 35-9, Deposition of Lt.Cmdr. Davis, 5.

407 NARA, RG 153, File 35-9, Deposition of Lt.Cmdr. Davis, 4.

408 NARA, RG 153, File 35-9, Deposition of Lt.Cmdr. Davis, 2.

409 NARA, RG 153, File 35-9, Deposition of Maj. Julian Theodore Saldivar, MD, 1.

410 NARA, RG 153, File 35-399, Trial of Furushima Chotaro; Testimony of Lt. Norman Eugene Churchill, Office of the Adjutant-General, 17.

411 Bush, *Clutch of Circumstance*, 118-19.

412 AWM 54, File 779/1/19, Papers of L.A.R. Evans Concerning His Time as a POW in Singapore and Japan; 9 Parts, Folder 2.

413 Stanley W. Smith, *Prisoner of the Emperor: An American POW in World War II* Duane A. Smith, ed., (Niwot, CO: University Press of Colorado, 1991), 98.

414 Ross Diary, in Anonymous, *Royal Rifles of Canada*, 370-71.

415 Steele, "With the Royal Rifles," 15.

416 Individual patient records, Niigata Camp 5B, 1943-1945, recorded and preserved by Maj. William M. Stewart. Steele is Record No. 105 in the series.

417 NARA, RG 153, File 35-145, Trial of Yumita Kyogzo and others, Testimony of Kondo Shoogo, 148.

418 NARA, RG 153, File 35-145, Trial of Yumita Kyogzo and others, Testimony of Kondo Shoogo, 164.

419 NARA, RG 153, File 35-145, Trial of Yumita Kyogzo and others, Testimony of Kondo Shoogo, 162.

420 NARA, RG 153, File 35-145, Trial of Yumita Kyogzo and others, Testimony of Capt. Newman, 14-15.

421 NARA, RG 153, File 35-145, Trial of Yumita Kyogzo and others, Testimony of Capt. Newman, 18.

422 NARA, RG 153, File 35-145, Trial of Yumita Kyogzo and others, Testimony of Maj. Milton Kramer, 64.

423 NARA, RG 153, File 35-145, Trial of Yumita Kyogzo and others, Testimony of Major Kramer, 68.

424 Bertram, *Beneath the Shadows*, 264.

425 Bertram, *Beneath the Shadows*, 264.

Chapter Nine

1 IMTFE, Exhibit No. 1982A, Extract from Testimony of Hideki Tojo, 27 March 1946; Translation of section marked by Tojo in a book published 8 January 1941, entitled *Senjin Kun* (Teachings for the Battlefield), 5-6.

2 Agnes Newton Keith, *Three Came Home*, 52.

3 James Bertram, *Beneath the Shadows*, 105.

4 Haruko Taya Cook and Theodore F. Cook, *Japan at War: An Oral History*, 114.

5 "Bushido, the code of honor and conduct of the Japanese nobility. Of ancient origin, it grew out of the old feudal bond, which required unwavering loyalty on the part of the vassal....in its fullest expression the code emphasized, besides loyalty to one's superior and personal honor, the virtues of austerity,

self-sacrifice, and indifference to pain; for the warrior, commerce and the profit motive were to be scorned. The code was first formulated in the Kamakura period (1185-1333), put into writing in the 16th cent., and termed *bushido* in the 17th cent. It became the standard of conduct for the DAIMYO and SAMURAI under the Tokugawa shoguns and was taught in state schools as a pre-requisite for government service. After the Meiji restoration (1868), it was the basis for emperor worship." William Bridgwater and Seymour Kurtz, eds., *The Columbia Encyclopedia*, 3rd edition, 303.

6 Arthur Swinson, *Four Samurai: A Quartet of Japanese Army Commanders in the Second World War* (London: Hutchinson, 1968), 24

7 Swinson, *Four Samurai*, 19.

8 Anonymous, *Report of the International Committee of the Red Cross on Its Activities during the Second World War*, Vol. 1 General Activities (Geneva: International Red Cross, 1948), 438-39.

9 Swinson, *Four Samurai*, 21.

10 In a novel about a Japanese officer captured by the Russians in 1945, the author describes the collective suicide of a group of tank crewmen, who wire their tanks together and detonate a massive explosion. The protagonist attempts to persuade them not to kill themselves, but it is significant that his appeal depends on the fact that the Emperor ordered them all to surrender, thus obviating the need for feeling disgrace—not that they should ignore the code itself. Yamasaki Toyoko, *The Barren Zone*, trans. James T. Araki (Tokyo: Kodansha International), 29-30 and 34.

11 IMTFE, Exhibits, Document 1981A, Interrogation of Tojo Hideki, 26 March 1946.

12 Joseph C. Grew, *Report from Tokyo: A Message to the American People* (New York: Simon and Schuster, 1942), 29-30.

13 Swinson, *Four Samurai*, 20.

14 Harriet Sergeant, *Shanghai* (London: John Murray, 1998), 196, quoting General Gao Gu.

15 Miyagi Kikuko, a student nurse in the Himeyuri Student Corps, Okinawa, 1945; cited in Cook and Cook, *Japan at War*, 361.

16 Kinjo Shigeaki, 16-year-old Okinawan youth, cited in *Japan at War*, 365.

17 Agatha Dillard Hahn, *Commentary on Ooka Shohei's Prisoner of War Memoirs (Furyoki)*, 33.

18 Nishihara Wakana, in Cook and Cook, *Japan at War*, 335.

19 Funasaka Hiroshi, *Falling Blossoms*, trans. Funasaka Hiroshi and Jeffrey D. Rubin. (Singapore: Times Books International, 1986), 242.

20 Funasaka, *Falling Blossoms*, 22.

21 *Canadian Encyclopedia* 1 (1988): 78.

22 Tominaga Shozo, IJA, cited in Cook and Cook, *Japan at War*, 42.

23 Tominaga, Cook and Cook, *Japan at War*, 42.

24 Tominaga, Cook and Cook, *Japan at War*, 42.

25 Uno Shintaro, *Kempeitai* NCO, in Cook and Cook, *Japan at War*, 155.

26 Lewis Bush, *Clutch of Circumstance*, 197.

27 Adams, *No Time for Geishas*, 113.

28 Cook and Cook, *Japan at War*, 32.

29 Wellcome Institute for the History of Medicine, London, CMAC, RAMC Collection, RAMC 729, Miscellaneous Obituaries, Photographs, and other Memorabilia, 7.

30 Julien M. Goodman, *M.D.P.O.W.*, 29-30.

31 Ashton, *Bataan Diary*, 155.

32 IWM, Department of Documents, London, Item 86/89/1, Papers of A. Dandie, "The Story of 'J' Force," 188.

33 Dandie Papers, "The Story of 'J' Force," 42-43.
34 Muneo Shito (pseud.), "No Time For the Dying," in Soka Gakkai Youth Division, *Peace is Our Duty: Accounts of What War Can Do to Man*, trans. Richard L. Gage (Tokyo: Japan Times, 1982), 53.
35 Kiyoshi Obayashi, "Sires of Hatred," in Soka Gakkai, *Peace Is Our Duty*, 101.
36 Shohei Ooka, *Fires on the Plain*, trans. Ivan Morris (Baltimore: Penguin Books Inc., 1969), 3.
37 Bush, *Clutch of Circumstance*, 41.
38 Cook and Cook, *Japan at War*, 47.
39 Adams, *No Time for Geishas*, 38
40 IMTFE, Exhibit No. 1981A, Interrogation of Tojo Hideki, 26 March 1946.
41 Harding Interview, in Gustave Gingras and Carol Chapman, *Sequelae of Inhuman Conditions*, 7.
42 Sato Hideo, cited in Cook and Cook, *Japan at War*, 235.
43 IMTFE, Exhibits, Document 1960.
44 Uno Shintaro, an NCO in the *Kempeitai*, in Cook and Cook, *Japan at War*, 153.
45 Uno, in Cook and Cook, *Japan at War*, 153.
46 IMTFE, Exhibits, Document 1963, Instructions of War Minister Tojo Hideki to the Newly-Appointed Commanders of the Prisoner of War Camps, 7 July 1942.
47 On Haruku, see C. Roland, "Stripping Away the Veneer: POW Survival in the Far East as an Index of Cultural Atavism," *Journal of Military History* 53 (1989): 79-94.
48 Dewar Interview, in Gingras and Chapman, *Sequelae of Inhuman Conditions*, 7.
49 Abbott, *And All My War is Done*, 47.
50 William Allister, *Where Life and Death Hold Hands*, 80.
51 Allister, *Where Life and Death*, 90.
52 Inouye's complicated case has been synopsized cogently in Patrick Brode, *Casual Slaughters and Accidental Judgments: Canadian War Crimes Prosecutions, 1944-1948* (Toronto: Published for The Osgoode Society for Canadian Legal History by University of Toronto Press, 1997), 169-76.
53 Dr. Anthony Henry Coombes MBE, Interview, CGR, HCHM/OHA, HCM 5-94, 4 May 1994, Sussex, England, 44.
54 Ilza Veith, "Humane Warfare and Inhuman War: Japan and its Treatment of War Prisoners," *Bulletin of the History of Medicine* 19 (1946): 355-74.
55 Veith, "Humane Warfare," 357.
56 Veith, "Humane Warfare," 359
57 Haru Matsukata Reischauer, *Samurai and Silk: A Japanese and American Heritage*, 101.
58 Charles Burdick and Ursula Moessner, *The German Prisoners-of-War in Japan, 1914-1920* (New York: Lanham, 1984), 63.
59 Burdick and Moessner, *The German Prisoners-of-War*, 73ff.
60 Burdick and Moessner, *The German Prisoners-of-War*, 92.
61 Burdick and Moessner, *The German Prisoners-of-War*, 128.
62 Burdick and Moessner, *The German Prisoners-of-War*, 99.
63 Nogi Harumichi, in Cook and Cook, *Japan at War*, 113.
64 William Manchester, *Goodbye Darkness: A Memoir of the Pacific War*, cited in Mordecai Richler, ed., *Writers on World War II: An Anthology*, 228-230.
65 Joseph C. Grew, *Report from Tokyo*, 29. His book was based on Grew's 10-year period as Ambassador of the USA to Japan.
66 Dora Sanders Carney, *Foreign Devils Had Light Eyes: A Memoir of Shanghai, 1933-1939* (Toronto: Dorset Publishing, 1980), 175.
67 Ariyoshi Sawako, *The River Ki [Kinokawa]*, trans. Mildred Tahara (Tokyo: Kodansha International, 1981), 208-209.

68 Mrs. Hugh Fraser, *A Diplomatist's Wife in Japan: Letters from Home to Home* (London: Hutchinson, 1899), Vol. 2, 195-96.

69 Go Shizuko, *Requiem [Rekuiemu]*, trans. Geraldine Harcourt (Tokyo: Kodansha International, 1991), 17. Novel of a young woman, Oizumi Setsuko, dying of tuberculosis amid desolation in bombed-out Yokohama, 1945.

Chapter Ten

1 CWM, Ottawa, Item 58 A1 24.4, Diary of Lt. Henry White, entry for 4 September 1945, 46.

2 Richard Fuller, *Shokan: Hirohito's Samurai*, 44.

3 IWM, Department of Documents, London, Item 93/18/1, Papers of Mrs. D. Ingram [Sister D. Van Wart], Hong Kong, 9.

4 Charles P. Stacey, *Official History of the Canadian Army in the Second World War*, Vol. 1, *Six Years of War*, 488.

5 Stacey, *Six Years of War*, 489.

6 Stacey, *Six Years of War*, 489.

7 The *Awatea* was not part of this operation, having been sunk during the Allied landings in North Africa in November 1942.

8 C.R. Shelley, "HMCS *Prince Robert*: The Career of an Armed Merchant Cruiser," *Canadian Military History* 4 (1995): 57-58.

9 John E. Moss, "A Medical Survey of Allied Repatriates after Liberation from Japanese Prisons," 599.

10 Moss, "A Medical Survey of Allied Repatriates," 600.

11 CWM, White Diary, entry for 9 October 1945, 50.

12 Larry M. Dean, Frank N. Willis, and Robert Obourn, "Health Records of American prisoners of the Japanese during World War II," 841.

13 John B. Crawford, "A Preliminary Report on a Follow-up Study of Repatriates from Japanese Prisoner of War Camps," 165.

14 Crawford, "A Preliminary Report on a Follow-up Study," 166.

15 Crawford, "A Preliminary Report on a Follow-up Study," 160.

16 Kenneth Gaudin, Interview, in Gustave Gingras and Carol Chapman, *The Sequelae of Inhuman Conditions*, 6.

17 Red McCarron, in Anonymous, *The Royal Rifles of Canada in Hong Kong, 1941-1945* (Sherbrooke: Hong Kong Veterans' Association of Canada, Quebec-Maritimes Branch, 1980), 419.

18 Patrick Brode, *Casual Slaughters and Accidental Judgments: Canadian War Crimes Prosecutions, 1944-1948*, 199.

19 Bowie, "Captive Surgeon," 265.

20 CWM, White Diary, entry for 15 September 1945, 48.

21 Ellen M. Gee, "Veterans and Veterans Legislation in Canada: An Historical Overview," *Canadian Journal of Aging* 7 (1988): 204-17.

22 Chapter 7, "The Last Battle," in, Anonymous, *Royal Rifles of Canada*, 420-30.

23 Kenneth Cambon, *Guest of Hirohito*, 109.

24 See the documents submitted in 1987 in Gingras and Chapman, *The Sequelae of Inhuman Conditions*.

25 Selwyn Selwyn-Clarke, *Hong Kong Government: Annual Report of the Medical Department for 1946* (Hong Kong: Local Printing Press, Ltd.), 20.

Bibliography

Primary Sources

A: Archival Materials

Allied Translator and Interpreter Section, First Australian Army ATIS Advanced Echelon, ATIS Preliminary Interrogation Reports: (a) No. 259, 20-IR-259, interrogation of Ro, Kan Do, PW No. JA 162065, 10 June 1945, 6 pp.; (b) No. 86, 10-IR-86, 1943, Sawatari, Med.2nd/Lt., Official PW No. JA 145212, 10 pp; (c) 20-IR-227, 27 April 1945, interrogation of Tanaka Yoshio, PW No. JA 162042, 4 pp.; (d) 20-IR-236, 24 April 1945, interrogation of Nakamura Takesuke, PW No. JA 162047, 3 pp.; (e) No. 144, 10-IR-144, 1943, Murozoma Toru, Official PW No. JA 145209, 8 pp.; (f) No. 139, 10-IR-139, 1943, Koki Tsuneo, Official PW No. JA 145435, 9 pp.; (g) 10-IR-121, No. 121, March 1943, Raki Toshimi, Ldg Pte.; (h) No. 86, 10-IR-86, 1943, Sawatari Zengoro, Official PW No. JA 145212, 10 pp.; (i) No. 259, 10-RR-72, 29 April 1944, Japanese Violations of the Laws of War; (j) No. 54, 10-IR-54, interrogation of Imagaki Riichi, Official PW No. JA 145979, 1943; (k) No. 20-IR-227, 27 April 1945, Tanaka Yoshio, PW No. JA 162042; (l) No. 10-SR-37, Spot Report 37, translation of excerpts from diary of Acting Commander, No. 2 MG Company, 144 Infantry Regiment, 25 December 1942; (m) No. 20, 50-IR-20, interrogation of Tabata Kazuo, PW No. 41 Div P-9384 GP 289, 4 January 1945.

Australian Archives, Mitchell. A471/1, Item 81048. Record of Military Court (Japanese War Criminals). Trial of L/Cpl. Mena Hisano, IJA, for (1) mutilation of a body, New Guinea, ca. 20 July 1945, and (2) cannibalism, New Guinea, ca. 20 July 1945; tried at Rabaul, 28 May 1946.

_____. A1067/1, Item UN46/WC/8 Pt. 1. Record of Military Court (Japanese War Criminals). AWC No. 2344. Trial of Med. Lt. Tomiyasu Hisato for murder and cannibalism at Sowan, New Guinea between May and October 1944.

_____. A1067/1, Item UN46/WC/8, Pt. 1i. Record of Military Court (Japanese War Criminals) AWC No. 2309, Trial of 1/Lt. Tazaki Takehito for mutilation and cannibalism of the body of a dead Australian soldier at Soarin, about 19-20 July 1945; tried at Wewak, 30 November 1945.

_____. A471/1, File 80794. Trial of Med. Capt. Takahashi Takashi, Capt. Miyoshi Masahiro, Med. WO Aizawa Teuchiro, WO Yamamoto Kenji, Med. Sgt. Maj. Kinjo Tokuyei, Sgt. Fukushima Akita, and Med. Cpl. Nakamura Utaka, at Rabaul, 15-16 April 1946; Charge: Cannibalism at Tanours about 5 Apr 43 by eating the flesh of 2 Indian POWs.

Australian War Memorial (AWM), Canberra. Personal Records. PR 83, File 32. Report of Service from December 1941 to September 1945 of Capt. J.J. Woodward, IMS/IAMC.

_____. Personal Records. PR 84/99. Accounts by Capt. James W. Chisholm and Capt. A.K. Barrett on their Experiences at Naoetsu POW Camp 4B, Niigata, Japan.

_____. AWM 54, File 481/1/24. Items of Medical Interest from Captured Japanese Documents and Interrogations of Prisoners of War; Locations of Disease in Japanese-Occupied Territory.

_____. AWM 54, File 779/1/19. Papers of L.A.R. Evans Concerning His Time as a POW in Singapore and Japan; 9 Parts, Folder 2.

_____. AWM 54, Written Records, 1939-45 War, 481/8/10. Final Summary of the Medical Staff, August 10, 1943-August 28, 1945, Fukuoka Camp 17.

_____. AWM 54, File 779/1/21. Reports to 1 Australian Prisoner of War Contact and Inquiry Unit by Various; Report from Diary of Maj. H.G.G. Robertson, RAMC, Shamshuipo Camp.

_____. AWM 54, File 1010/9/94. Cannibalism—Murder of Indian Prisoners of War, New Guinea—1943-1944.

_____. AWM 54, File 1010/9/23. War Crimes: L/Cpl. Mena Hisatano and Sgt. Tazaki Takekiko, Charged with Mutilation of the Dead and Cannibalism near Soarin Ridge 20 July 1945.

_____. AWM 54, File 1010/9/4. Interrogation of War Criminals: Uchiyama Seiichi, Maj. Yamada Masato, Gen. Magata, Gen. Makata Isiochi, Col. Muta Toyoji, Capt. Wada Misae, and Pe. Nagano Hisaku, Re the Executions of American Airmen at Kieta and Numa Numa, and the Execution of a Padre at Keita; Cannibalism in Jaba River Area, Brief Mention of Killing and Eating a Native Child at Etu, 1946 [sic].

Birchall W/C Leonard. MS Biographical Notes. In Possession of the Author, undated but ca. 1970.

Caire, James A. Typed Letter, Signed to C.G. Roland re his experiences as a POW in Oeyama Camp, Japan. 25 September 1992.

Canadian War Museum (CWM), Ottawa. Acc. No. 1983-38/1. Diary of Donald Geraghty, Hong Kong POW.

_____. Acc. No. 1981-276/10, cat. no. 60-6-52. F.D.F. Martyn Papers.

_____. Item 58 A1 24.5. Diary of Delbert Louis William Welsh, 16 October 1941-5 October 1942.

_____. Item 58 A1 24.4. Diary of Lt. Harry L. White, Winnipeg Grenadiers, 30 December 1941-20 October 1945, 51 pp.

Channing, Muriel Jean (McCaw). Personal communication to C.G. Roland, 11 March 1996.

Gill, J., Assistant Curator, Regimental Museum, Royal Logistic Corps, Camberley, Surrey. Personal communication to C.G. Roland, 31 October 1994.

Goad, Dr. Lloyd. Personal communication to C.G. Roland, 3 July 1986.

Gomes, Arthur. Personal communication, Typed Letter, Signed, to C.G. Roland, May 1991.

Government Records Service, Public Records Office, Hong Kong. Hong Kong Manuscript Series No. 81, Papers of Dr. A.H.R. Coombes.

_____. Hong Kong Manuscript Series No. 113, Sworn Statements by Indian Soldiers Imprisoned in Hong Kong During the Japanese Occupation, D. & S. No. 1/1.

_____. Ref. No. AB/920, Acc. No. 4462 (B), Copy of Diary Kept by Dr. Isaac Newton, Hong Kong, 7 Dec 41 till 1 June 42.

_____. Hong Kong Manuscript Series No. 72, Papers of Mrs. Phyllis Ayrton, D. & S. No. 1/5. Letter, 22 August 1942, from Marion Dudley to "Friends of Mine."

Public Records Office, Hong Kong. Hong Kong Record Series No. 225, War Diary of Maj. E.G. Stewart, D & S No. 1/48(2), notes for 22 December 1941.

Guitard, Gabriel. Notebook, Niigata POW Camp 5B, October 1943 to February 1944. Copy in possession of the author. Guitard died 22 February 1944.

Hannah Chair Archives, McMaster University, Hamilton, ON. POW Papers, Maj. William Muir Stewart Memoirs, Typescript 22 pp., from handwritten original, 1945.

Hinder, David C.C. "Experiences and conditions in three small POW parties." MS prepared for Australian Government enquiry chaired by Mr. Justice Toose, 1973.

International Military Tribunal for the Far East (IMTFE). Exhibit No. 1591A. Statement of Sister Miss A.F. Gordon, Territorial Army Nursing Service, of Events that Occurred at St. Stephen's College Hospital during the Period 23rd to 26th December 1941, Sworn 11 December 1945.

_____. Exhibit No. 1515A. Affidavit of Maj. J.W.D. Bull, RAMC, re. Medical Experiences at Kranji No. 2 Camp, Singapore, 17 January 1945 [*sic*, 1946?].

_____. Exhibit No. 1446. Document Captured at Danmap, Aitape Area, North East New Guinea, 31 December 1944.

_____. Exhibit No. 1447. Extract from Interrogation of Japanese POW Yanagizawa Eiji, Captured at Marasupe, New Guinea, 25 December 1944.

_____. Exhibit No. 1982A. Extract from Testimony of Hideki Tojo, 27 March 1946.

_____. Exhibit No. 3140. List of POW Camps Visited, 1942-45.

_____. Exhibits No. 1967, 1969, and 1971A: 1967, Memorandum from Yeiichi Tatsumi to Hideki Tojo Re. POW Labor, 2 October 1942; 1969, Memorandum from Kaitaro Kondo to Kotaro Nakamura, same subject, 7 October 1942; 1971A, Excerpt from Foreign Affairs Monthly Report, September 1942, Re. POW Labour.

_____. Exhibit No. 3111, Investigation Squad of Army Medical College, Suggestions Regarding Improvement of Health Conditions of Prisoners of War Camp; Undated [On Internal Evidence, First Half of 1943], 5 pp.

_____. Defence Counsel Evidence. Vol. 37, No. 1594. Affidavit of Capt. S. Martin Banfill, Experiences at and Near the Salesian Mission, Hong Kong, 19 December 1941; dated 22 December 1945.

_____. Defence Counsel Evidence. Vol. 37, No. 1600A. Deposition of H 6047, L/Sgt. William Albert Hall, WG, 29 January 1946, 8 pp.

_____. Exhibit No. 3137. Deposition of Charles Ream Jackson re Medical and Other Conditions in Hamowa POW Camp, 11 August 1947, 6 pp.

_____. Exhibit No. 1981A. Interrogation of Tojo Hideki, 26 March 1946.

_____. Exhibits, Document 1963. Instructions of War Minister Tojo Hideki to the Newly Appointed Commanders of the Prisoner of War Camps, 7 July 1942.

_____. Exhibits, Document 1960. Instructions of War Minister Tojo Hideki to Commander, Zentsuji Division, 30 May 1942.

Imperial War Museum (IWM), Department of Documents, London. Item 84/42/1. Diary of Maj. Cecil Templer, RA, Battle of Hongkong December 1941, Prisoner of War Camps Hongkong Argyll Street and Shamshuipo, 1942 to 1945, 27 pp.

_____. Item PP/MCR/121, Diary of Adrian Richardson Billings, RN, 1941-1945, 104 pp.

_____. MS Diary of Maj. W.T. Carden re: his service as an NCO with Royal Army Pay Corps at Hong Kong.

_____. Item 87/34/1. Papers of Geoffrey C. Hamilton, "Prisoner of War in Hong Kong and Japan, 1941-1945."

_____. Item 73/671. Papers of Barbara C. Redwood.

_____. Item PP/MCR/121. Diary of Adrian Richardson Billings, RN, 1941-1945.

_____. Item PP/MCR/25. World War 2 Memoirs of Mrs M.W. Redwood. Microfilm of Typed Letter, Signed, MS entitled: "Incident at Jockey Club, Happy Valley, Hong Kong, Dec. '41."

_____. Item P324. Papers of Mrs. Day Joyce, Hong Kong.

_____. Item 93/18/1. Papers of Mrs. D. Ingram [Sister D. Van Wart], Hong Kong.

_____. Item 85/36/1. Diary of Lt.Col. R.J.L. Penfold, 5 January 1942 to 12 August 1945.

_____. Item 86/89/1. Papers of A. Dandie, "The Story of 'J' Force."

_____. Item 81/32/1. J. F. Chandler, Diary, 1943-45, re. POW life in Java and the Spice Islands.

_____. Item 86/67/1. Papers of Albert Kettleborough.

_____. Dr. Ross MacArthur, Diary, Singapore and Burma-Siam Railway, 1942-1945 (on loan).

_____. Item 456. Brigadier C.H. Stringer, Lists of Medical Personnel, Malaya.

_____. Item 82/32/1. C.G. Thompson, "Into the Sun." (Typescript, Warksworth, NZ).

_____. File PP/MCR/243. Diary of A.J. Alsey, 1942. Re-transcribed and annotated 1966.

_____. Item 85/42/1. Papers of CSM Ronald Alfred Edwards, HKVDC.

_____. Item 84/42/1. Diary of Maj. Cecil Templer, RA, Battle of Hongkong December 1941, Prisoner of War Camps Hongkong Argyll Street and Shamshuipo [sic], 1942 to 1945, 27 pp.

_____. Item 88/33/1. Papers of Don Peacock: MS "Banjo Mickey Mouse: An Erk's Diary of 1276 Incredible Days as Guest of the Emperor."

Kobayashi, N.C. Personal communication to C.G. Roland, 8 December 1993.

Leath, Norman J. "Report prepared for C.G. Roland, MD, History of Medicine, McMaster University, Hamilton, Ontario, by Mr. N.J. Leath, 17 Tees Court,

Ellesmere Port, South Wirral, Great Britain, on 1st February 1988." MS, 1988.

McMaster, Archie Lee. *Lo Joe*. MS, United States Military Academy Library, Special Collections, [1942-5].

Millbank, Royal Army Medical College Library, London. Muniment Room, Item 1291. Bowie Papers. Experiences in Hong Kong in World War II.

_____. Item 496. Medical Reports. Tamuang POW Camp, Thailand. Prepared by Lt.Col. W.G. Harvey, SMO.

Montgomery, William H. "I Hired Out to Fight." MS, n.d.; MS in possession of the author.

National Archives and Records Administration (NARA), Washington. Records of the Office of the Judge Advocate General (Army), War Crimes Section. RG 153, File 35-2100. Trial of Taradochi Miki and Nakayama Tarokichi for War Crimes Allegedly Committed at Oeyama POW Camp. Tried at Yokohama, 15 May 1947; Case No. 147.

_____. RG 153, File 35-2282. Trial of Funaki Eisaku, Hada Kyui, Harada Kichiji, Hori Sakuzo, Ishiyama Jinmatsu, Ito Shiroji, Ito Yoshichi, Iwanami Shamatsu, Karube Yuzo, Kawaguchi Shinnosuke, Kobayashi Koei, Kobayashi Ryoji, Kunikane Eihachi, Kurada Kuraichi, Matsuo Kyujiro, Mimura Tetsue, Morimoto Zenji, Minami Yoshisuke, Nakamura Rokushi, Nakayama Minoo Nasuno Yoshizo, Nishima Gontoro, Ogawa Zensaku, Onishi Soji, Ono Iwazo, Ono Takematsu, Ono Toshihiko, Sato Isao, Sato Kushiro, Sato Shinichiro, Seino Kiyoshi, Shimabara Nichiro, Dr. Shirai Ryoei, Suda Takesi, Sugazawa Kiyotaka, Takizawa Masaji, Watanabe Shohei, and Yamamoto Kitiji, on Numerous Counts of Forcing Prisoners to Work, Providing Inadequate Food, Clothing, Shelter, and Medicines, All Occurring at Niigata, Japan, Camp 5b and Associated Work Sites. Tried at Yokohama, 25 October 1948 to 6 September 1949; Case No. 351.

_____. RG 153, File 36-491. Trial of Sgt./Maj. Yasutake Hideo for Various Alleged War Crimes Committed at Fukuoka Camp No. 2.

_____. RG 153, File 35-997. Trial of Med.2/Lt. Fujii Hiroshi on 28 Charges. Tried at Yokohama 27 September to 31 December 1946; Case No. 111.

_____. RG 153, File 35-998. Statement of Robert Emerson Altman, 24 September 1946.

_____. RG 153, File 35-2213. Trial of Tanaka Shinishi, Civilian, for Alleged Offences Against Allied POWs at Umeda Bunsho Camp, April 1943 to May 1945. Tried at Yokohama, 1-12 August 1947; Case No. 211.

_____. RG 153, File 35-145. Trial of Yumita Kyogzo, Kondo Shoogo, and Ishige Michiharu for Alleged Offences Against Allied POWs at Kawasaki Camp 5D, Honshu, Japan. Tried at Yokohama, 11 April 1946; Case No. 28.

_____. RG 153, File 35-1697. Trial of Ninomiya Yutaka, Wakamatsu Manzo, and Ozawa Masaharu, for Alleged War Crimes Committed at Sendai POW Camp 2B, Yoshima, Honshu, Japan, 1944 and 1945. Tried at Yokohama 16 October to 13 November 1947; Case no. 225.

_____. RG 153, File 35-61. Trial of Okada Miyoroku, Commandant of Narumi POW Camp, 2B, Honshu, for War Crimes Allegedly Committed in 1945. Tried at Yokohama, 23-30 April 1946; Case No. 12.

_____. RG 153, File 35-1076. Trial of Nagahara Keiji, Capt., IJA, for Alleged War Crimes Committed while he was OC Tokyo Area POW Camp 21D, Takaoka City, Toyama, Honshu, Japan. Tried at Yokohama 30 September 1947 to 14 October 1947; Case No. 241.

_____. RG 153, File 58-82. File on Investigation of Alleged Japanese Atrocities against an American Airman, Including Murder and Cannibalism, August 1944.

_____. RG 153, File 42-16. Case of Mutilation, Leyte, 12 or 13 December 1944, 3 pp.

_____. RG 153, File 42-18. Case of Mutilation of Dead US Soldiers, Presumably to Obtain Meat for Food, 4-5 January 1945.

_____. RG 153, File 35-868. Trial of Kondo Kanechi, Accused of War Crimes against Several Canadian POWs at Tokyo Area 3D POW Camp, Yokohama, in 1943. Tried at Yokohama, 23-24 December 1946; Case No. 115.

_____.RG 153, File 51-26. Intelligence Report re Cannibalism in New Guinea, 8 February 1945.

_____. RG 153, File 51-49. Investigation of the Alleged Mutilations of the Bodies of 5 American Servicemen, Noemfoor Island, Dutch New Guinea, ca. 10 August 1945.

_____. RG 153, File 33-54. File of Affidavits relating to Niigata POW Camp No. 15D, Shintetsu. Deposition of LtCol. John Francis Breslin, MO at 15D 30 March 1944 to 5 September 1945; 3 February 1949, 4 pp.

_____. RG 153, File 35-408. Depositions with respect to Events in Oeyama POW Camp re Maltreatment of Pfc. J.C. Grant.

_____. RG 153, File 35-398. Trial of Takeuchi Hiroshi, Tanaka Kazuo, Sato Torao, Suzuki Keizo, Ozawa Kichihei, Maekawa Kazumasu, Miyazaki Hiroshi, and Emori Hidetoshi, for War Crimes Allegedly Committed against Various Allied POWs at Tokyo Area POW Camp No. 1, Kawasaki, 1944 to 1945. Tried at Yokohama, 28 March to 29 April 1946; Case No. 17.

_____. RG 153, File 35-621. Trial of Tanaka Hiroshi, Hitosugi Yukio, Kawai Shoji Tanaka Tokuichi, Nakagawa Tatsuo, Kawamura Kamaki, Hara Isamu, Yamagishi Masakazu, Sawano Yoshikazu, Yadoiwa Isao, Ieda Nakazo, Kondo Kinpachi, Mizuno Tatsuo, Kato Genzo, Kawamura Tomohisa, Kameda Jirokichi, Sakai Hideo, Kokubo Nobuo, Murase Akihisa, Hayashi Masao, Asakura Tadao, and Maeda Minoru, Charged with Numerous Offences against US, British, Canadian, and Australian POWs at Narumi POW Camp in 1944 and 1945. Tried at Yokohama, 2 September 1947 and thereafter; Case No. 182.

_____. RG 153, File 35-819. Trial of Lt. Sakai Tsuyoshi, 2nd Lt. Mori Kiyoichi, and Cpl. Kamayama Nubuo for War Crimes Allegedly Committed at Omine POW Camp, Japan. Tried at Yokohama, 5 March 1946; Case No. 13.

_____. RG 153, File 33-8. Photostats of Various Documents Relating to the Internal Operation of Kawasaki POW Camp, Japan, with Respect to the Orders of the IJA.

_____. RG 153, File 35-161. Trial of Civilian Attached IJA Narikawa Masanobu, on Charges of Brutality Meted out to Several Named American POWs at Kanagawa POW Camp, and to One British and Two

Canadian POWs at Oeyama POW Camp,dDuring 1945. Tried at Yokohama 24 February 1947; Case No. 68.

_____. RG 153, File 35-1097. Trial of Kojima Itchisaku for War Crimes Allegedly Committed at Niigata 5B POW Camp, Niigata, Honshu, Japan, between September 1943 and August 1945. Tried at Yokohama 9 June to 17 July 1947; Case No. 95.

_____. RG 153, File 35-103. Depositions re the Beating of Sam Moody at Narumi Camp #2, Nagoya, Japan, June or July 1945.

_____. RG 153, File 36-489. Trial of Lt. Yanaru Tetsutoshi, IJA, for War Crimes Allegedly Committed at Omine POW Camp, Also Called Fukuoka Dispatch Camp No. 8. Tried at Yokohama, 16 September 1946 to 23 January 1947; Case No. 84.

_____. RG 153, File 35-1730. Depositions re Alleged War Crimes at Sendai POW Camp 2B, Yoshima (near Tiara), Japan.

_____. RG 153, File 35-922. Trial of Lt. Kawabe Nagayasu, IJA, for War Crimes Allegedly Committed while he was OC, Sendai POW Camp No. 4, Ohasi, Honshu, Japan, August 1944 to April 1945. Tried at Yokohama, 22-28 May 1947; Case No. 132.

_____. File 35-483. Trial of Lt. Hazama Kosaku for War Crimes Allegedly Occurring while he was Commandant of Tanagawa Camp (January to August 1943) and of Oeyama Camp (August 1943 to August 1945). Tried at Yokohama, 3 February to 19 March 1947. Case No. 143.

_____. RG 153, File 48-36-1. Trial of Capt. Asano Shimpei, Surg/Lt. Ueno Chisato, Lt/Cmdr. Nakase Shohichi, Ens. Eriguchi Takeshi, WO Kobayashi Kazumi, and L/S Tanaka Sueta, all IJN. Tried at Guam, September-October 1947.

_____. RG 153, File 35-882. Trial of Yoshida Masato for War Crimes Allegedly Committed while Commandant of Niigata POW Camp 5B, 3 September 1943 to 5 February 1944. Tried at Yokohama, 12 May to 11 June 1948; Case No. 247.

_____. RG 153, File 33-76. Depositions on Niigata POW Camp. Depositions of Maj. Nelson N. Kaufmann, MC, USA, 23 April 1946, and Cpl. Elton Summers, USA, 7 October 1945.

_____. RG 153, File 35-1166. Depositions by Howard Sherman Swanson re Conditions at Kamioka POW Camp, 1944-1945.

_____. RG 153, File 35-1168. Four Depositions re Brutality of Japanese Captors in Kamioka POW Camp, Japan; Deposition of Sgt. Joseph Pase, 28 August 1946.

_____. RG 153, File 35-552. Trial of Lt. Nichizawa Masao, Lt. Chisuwa Takeichi, Pte. Kawamura Hiroshi, Civilian Kambe Hatsuaki, Sgt. Yamada Yoshitami,Civilian Shishido Shonusuke, and Civilian Ikeda Sukanobu, for Various War Crimes Allegedly Committed at Tokyo Area POW Branch Camp No. 2 and Mitsubishi Dockyard (Shipyard) Camp, Yokohama. Tried at Yokohama, 12 August to 1 November, 1946; Case No. 46.

_____. RG 338, Records of the US Eighth Army, Sugamo Prison Records, 1945-1952. 8132nd Army Unit, Sugamo Sup. Det., Box 231, File: Tokuda Hisakichi.

_____. RG 153, File 48-35-1. Trial of Surg/Capt. Iwanami Hiroshi, Surg/Lt. Kamikawa Hidehiro, Surg/Lt. Oishi Tetsuo, Ens. Asamura Shunpei, CPO Yoshizawa Kensaburo, CPO Homma Hachiro, CPO Watanabe Mitsuo,

CPO Tanabe Mamoru, CPO Mukai Yoshihisa, PO/1 Kawashima Tatsusaburo, PO/1 Sawada Tsuneo, PO/1 Tanaka Tokonusuke, PO/2 Namatame Kazuo, PO/1 Takaishi Susumu, PO/2 Akabori Toichiro, PO/2 Kuwabara Hiroyuki, PO/2 Tsutsui Kisaburo, and PO/2 Mitsuhashi Kichigoro, IJN.

_____. RG 153, File 35-921. Trial of Naganuma Seicki, Homma Nubuo, Iwabuchi Kiyomi, Sasaki Isamu, and Kintaichi Isami for Alleged War Crimes Committed at Sendai POW Camp #4, Ohasi, Honshu, Japan, between December 1943 and August 1945. Tried at Yokohama, 15 April 1947; Case No. 104.

_____. RG 153, File 35-2100. Trial of Taradochi Miki and Nakayama Tarokichi for War Crimes Allegedly Committed at Oeyama POW Camp. Tried at Yokohama, 15 May 1947; Case No. 147.

_____. RG 153, File 35-136. Depositions re. Atrocities Committed by Japanese Personnel Against POWs at Mitsushima POW Camp.

_____. RG 153, File 35-9. Depositions with Respect to Alleged Brutalities at Shinagawa POW Hospital, Zentsuji POW Camp, and Kawasaki Camp 1B.

_____. RG 153, File 35-508, Trial of Lt. Hirano Kenji, Medical Officer, for War Crimes Allegedly Committed in Eastern District Army Medical Department, Tokyo, March-April 1945. Tried at Yokohama, 7-19 April 1948; Case No. 295.

_____. RG 153, File 35-399. Trial of Furushima Chotaro for War Crimes Allegedly Committed at Funatsu Camp. Tried at Yokohama 28 December 1945 to 11 January 1946; Case No. 3.

_____. RG 153, File 35-205. Trial of Fujita Tatsuro, Hozumi Eiichi, Uchida Kanemasu, Maeda Kumaichi, and Yokoyama Kanzaburo for Killing Frank Spears, an American POW, by Bayoneting Him, at POW Camp 5B, Niigata, Japan, 19 July 1945. Tried at Yokohama, 23 May 1947; Case No. 176.

_____. RG 153, Far East Place Name Index, 1944-49. Box 5, Entry 139, File 35-9, Shinagawa Hospital.

_____. RG 153, File 35-153. Trial of Akamatsu Shigeo for War Crimes Allegedly Committed at Oeyama POW Camp, Honshu, Japan. Tried at Yokohama 30 March 1946; Case No. 19.

_____. RG 153, File 36-527. Trial of Aihara et al.

_____. RG 153, File 35-646. Conditions at Sendai POW Camp No. 3, Honshu, Japan.

_____. RG 153, File 35-956. Trial of Ishizawa Katsuo, Ota Koichi, Takasago Yasuchi, Koiwa Zenkichi, Sato Heikichi, Sasaki Kishio, and Tanifuji Nisa for Alleged War Crimes Committed while They Were on the Staff of Sendai Camp No. 3, and at Hosokura Mine of the Mitsubishi Mining Co. Tried at Yokohama, 7 January to 16 February 1948; Case No. 131.

_____. RG 153, File 35-1136. Statement of William Alfred Shayler re Beating Given to Joe Perdowski by CSM Tugby.

_____. RG 153, File 101-57-C. File on Trials of Harvey and Tugby in Winnipeg March 1946.

_____. RG 153, File 36-527. Trial of Capt. Aihara Kajuro; Col. Akita Hiroshi; Maj.Gen. Fukushima Kyusaku; Lt. Goiyama Shinju; Goshima Shiro, MD; Hirako Goichi, MD; Hirao Kenichi, MD; Maj.Gen. Hriuchi Kiyoma, MD; Lt.Gen. Inada Masazumi; Ishiyama Fukujiro, MD; Maj.Gen. Ito Shoshin

[Akinobu]; Lt.Col. Jin Iichiro; Komori Taku, MD; Kubo Toshiyuki, MD; Makino Reiichiro, MD; Mori Yoshio, MD; Morimoto Kenji, MD; Nogawa Nobuyoshi, MD; Ryu Miki, MD; Col. Sato Yoshinao; Senba [Semba] Yoshitaka, MD; Tashiro Jiro, MD; Tashiro Tomoki, MD; Torisu Taro, MD; Tsutsui [Tsutsue] Shizuko, RN; Lt. Gen. Yokoyama Isamu; and Others, on Numerous Charges, Especially Illegal Medical Experimentation, Vivisection, and Related Charges. Tried at Yokohama, 11 March to 27 August 1948; Case No. 290.

———. RG 153, File 33-15. Report on Visit of the Delegates of the Swiss Legation to Shinagawa POW Hospital (Higashi), 19 February 1945.

National Archives of Canada (NAC), Ottawa. Department of National Defence, RG 24, C 2 (f), vol. 8018, file TOK-1-4. Extracts from Diary of Maj. H.G.G. Robertson, RAMC, 1941-1943.

———. Department of National Defence, RG 24, C 2 (f), Vol. 8026, File 24-44. Oflag 79 (Formerly Oflag 8F).

———. Department of National Defence, RG 24, C 2 (f), Vol. 8018, File TOK-1-2-2. List of Minor Japanese War Criminals in Japan with Canadian Interest, 5 March, 1947.

———. Department of National Defence, RG 24, C 2 (f), Vol. 8019 File TOK-2-2. "Fukuoka Camp No. 5—Omine."

———. Department of National Defence, RG 24, Vol. 11251. Miscellaneous Reports on POW Camps in Germany, Italy, and the Far East.

———. Department of National Defence, RG 24, C 2 (f), Vol. 8018, File TOK-1-2-5; Part 1, Letter by E.H. Tinson, 4 April 1946, re Events at Shau Kie Wan on 19 December 1941, 2; Part 2. Despatches, R.O.G. Morton to Secretary, Dept. of National Defence (Army), 22 November 1946.

———. Department of National Defence, RG 24, C 2 (f), Vol. 8018, file TOK-1-2-11. Various Reports by Lt.Col. Oscar Orr Re. War Crimes Trials in the Far East, 1947.

———. Department of National Defence, Directorate of History, File 593(D17). Debriefing of Capt. John A.G. Reid, 31 October 1945.

———. Department of National Defence, RG 24, C 2 (f), Vol. 8027, File 28-12. Lecco Military Hospital, Italy.

———. Department of National Defence, RG 24, C 2 (f), Vol. 8020, File TOK-5-6. Chronological Chart of Ex-Prisoner of War Camps in Japan Proper. Undated but presumably late 1945.

———. Department of National Defence, RG 24, C 2 (f), Vol. 8020. File "Receipts from Affidavits from CRD."

———. Department of National Defence, RG 24, C 2 (f), Vol. 8023, File 19-44. Stalag 8B-Teschen, Germany

———. Department of National Defence, RG 24, Vol. 15290. War Diary, Winnipeg Grenadiers, 27 September 1939-23 September 1941.

———. Department of National Defence, RG 24, C 1, HQS 9050-12-15, reel C-5335. Cigarettes for POWs, 1943.

———. Department of National Defence, RG 24, Vol. 11251. Miscellaneous Reports on POW Camps in Germany, Italy, and the Far East.

———. MG30, E213, John Crawford Papers.

———. MG30, E181, Tom Forsyth, "Hong Kong Diary and Memories of Japan: Gleanings from the Diary of a Winnipeg Grenadier."

_____. Papers of Frank William Ebdon, MG 30, E 328. Letters, Ebdon to wife Bunny Ebdon, 18 November 1941 and 27 November 1941; Diary kept by CSM Ebdon, 26 December 1942 to 26 December 1943, at Sham Shui Po, Hong Kong, and Omine Camp, Japan.

_____. MG30, E437. Papers of Charles E. Price, "Notes on Contract Bridge." Compiled by W.F. Nugent, POW at Sham Shui Po POW Camp, 1943.

_____. Federal Records Centre, Ottawa. Locator No. G287-16. Trial of CSM Marcus Charles Tugby, Winnipeg Grenadiers, on 19 Counts Relating to Various Alleged War Crimes Committed against Allied POWs at Oeyama Camp, Japan, 1943-1945. Tried in Winnipeg, March 1946.

_____. Federal Records Centre, Ottawa. Locator No. G287-15. Trial of Cpl. (acting Sgt.) John Hugh Harvey, on Various Charges Arising from Events at Oeyama Camp, Japan, 1943-45, Including Manslaughter. Tried in Winnipeg, March 1946.

National Archives of Singapore, Singapore. Oral History Department. Oral History Interview No. 000103/10. Interview of Dato Haji Mohd Yusuf Bangs by Miss Yogini Yogarajah, 18 September 1981.

_____. Oral History Department. Oral Hisory Interview No. B119/003. Interview of Tsujimoto Sanosuke, formerly IJA, 25 October 1981.

_____. Oral History Department. Oral History Interview No. 000306/17. Interview of Mr Tan Wah Meng, 17 August 1983.

Naval Historical Center, Operational Archives, Washington, DC. J.S. Thiemeyer, Typescript Interrogation of Survivors Lt. Bookman (MC) USNR and Lt. Glusman (MC) USNR, Bureau of Medicine and Surgery. Records from Bilibid Prison and the Hospital Corps Archives, Box 4, Series IV: Hospital Corps Archives Publications.

_____. R.D. Millar, Narrative of Personal Experiences in the Far East. MS Prepared for Historical Records Section, Royal New Zealand Air Force, Wellington, New Zealand, 13 April 1946.

Public Record Office (PRO), London. War Office. War of 1939-1945: Reports of International Red Cross and Protecting Powers. File 188, Hong Kong.

_____. War of 1939-1945: Reports of International Red Cross and Protecting Powers. WO 224, File 192, Far East: Tokyo Group.

_____. War of 1939-1945: Reports of International Red Cross and Protecting Powers. WO 224, File 188, Hong Kong. Interrogation Report SKP/5/44, Lt. R.B. Goodwin, 20 October 1944, p. 16.

_____. Medical Historian's Papers. WO 222, File 22, Z.233, "POW Camps in Hong Kong and Japan," by Capt. A.J.N. Warrack, RAMC, 23 January 1946, 63 pp.

_____. Medical Historian's Papers. WO 222, File 117, Z.230, POW Camps in Thailand, by Major E.A. Smyth and Captain R.W. Lennon, RAMC.

_____. Medical Historian's Papers. WO 222, File 190, War Diary for No. 25 Prisoner of War Camp Commanded by Captain R.D. Wilkie, 2/SSVF, Fukuoka. 12 pp.

_____. War Crimes Papers. Judge Advocate General's Office. WO 235, File 892, Trial of Niimori Genichiro.

_____. War Crimes Papers. Judge Advocate General's Office. WO 235, File 1027, Trial of Lt. Sato Choichi, Hong Kong, 1 April to 5 May 1947.

_____. War Crimes Papers. Judge Advocate General's Office. WO 235, File 1012, Trial of Col. Tokunaga Isao, Capt. Saito Shunkishi, Lt. Tanaka Hitochi, Interpreter Tsutada Itsuo, and Sgt. Harada Jotaro, Hong Kong, 17 October 1946 to 14 February 1947.

_____. War Crimes Papers. Judge Advocate General's Office, WO 235, File 1015, Trial of Shoji Toshishige, Hong Kong, 10-17 March 1947.

_____. War Crimes Papers. Judge Advocate General's Office. WO 235, File 1030, Trial of Maj.Gen. Tanaka Ryosaburo for war crimes in December 1941, as OC 229th Regt. of 38th Div.; Tried at Hong Kong 8 April to 22 May 1947.

_____. WO 222, File 20A, War Diary of LtCol. C.O. Shackleton, RAMC, OC, Military Hospital, Bowen Road, Hong Kong, 1940-1 June 1943, pp. 32.

_____. War of 1939-1945: Reports of International Red Cross and Protecting Powers, WO 224, File 188, Hong Kong.

_____. War of 1939-1945: Reports of International Red Cross and Protecting Powers. WO 224, File 194, Far East: Java Camps. 304/1/Inf. CSDIC (India), Red Fort, Delhi: Information Section Report No. 85 dated 16 October 1944, 11 pp.

_____. War Crimes Papers. Judge Advocate General's Office. WO 235, File 1107, Trial of Lt.Gen. ITO Takeo, IJA, on Charges of Killing and Ill-treatment of Allied POWs, Wounded, and Sick Members of Allied Forces, by Members of Units under his Command in December 1941.

_____. WO 224, File 188. Hong Kong. Interrogation Report SKP/5/44, Lt. R.B. Goodwin, 20 October 1944.

Rhodes House Library, Oxford. MSS.Ind.Ocn.s.233. Dr. K.H. Uttley, MD, Hong Kong, "My Internment Diary: December 8th, 1941-August 1945."

_____. MSS.Ind.Ocn.s.76. Lance A. Searle, Diary, Wartime and Stanley Gaol, 1941-1943.

Ribiero, Luigi. [Reminiscences of a POW at Hong Kong]. MS, 1987.

Silliphant, William M. "Under the Japs in Bilibid." MS: Otis Historical Archives of the Armed Forces Medical Museum, 1946.

Steen, Harry E. "Recollections of Experiences as a POW in the Far East." MS, September 1982, in possession of the author.

University of Alberta Archives, Edmonton. Accession No. 77-1. Dr. Benjamin Wheeler Papers, Box 1, File 5, Memoir, "Some Experiences as a Prisoner-of-War of the Japanese," n.d.

Wellcome Institute for the History of Medicine, London. Contemporary Archives Medical Collection. Dr. Cicely Williams Collection. PP/CDW, Box 8, Folder 9; C.H.A., "The ABC of Vitamins."

_____. Current Medical Archives Collection. GC/131/18. Acc. no. 413, Papers of Surg/Cmdr. J.A. Page, RN.

_____. Current Medical Archives Collection. Medical Women's Federation Collection. SA/MWF, Box 21, C/195, Work of British Medical Women in POW Camps. Typed Letter, Signed, Report by Dr. Annie Sydenham, Nethersole Hospital, Hong Kong, 9 April 1950.

_____. Contemporary Medical Archives Centre. RAMC Collection. RAMC 729, Miscellaneous Obituaries, Photographs and Other Memorabilia.

B: Oral History Interviews

Adams, Robert Dewar. Interview by Charles G. Roland, Hannah Chair for the History of Medicine, Oral History Archive, McMaster University, Hamilton, Ontario, (HCHM/OHA). HCM 8-83, Winnipeg, MB, 27 May 1983.

Anderson, Dr. James William Anderson. Interview by Charles G. Roland, HCHM/OHA. HCM 43-85, Victoria, BC, 20 April 1985.

Ashton, William Stirling. Interview, in Gustave Gingras and Carol Chapman, *The Sequelae of Inhuman Conditions and Slave Labour Experienced by Members of the Canadian Components of the Hong Kong Forces, 1941-1945, while Prisoners of the Japanese Government.* Toronto: War Amputations of Canada, 1987.

Ateah, Joseph Ateah. Interview by Charles G. Roland, HCHM/OHA. HCM 16-83, Winnipeg, MB, 28 May 1983.

Atkinson, Harold Angus Martin. Interview by Charles G. Roland, HCHM/OHA. HCM 7-83, Winnipeg, MB, 27 May 1983.

Atkinson, Harold. Interview, in Gingras and Chapman, *The Sequelae of Inhuman Conditions.*

Ballingall, Arthur Thomas. Interview, in Gingras and Chapman, *The Sequelae of Inhuman Conditions.*

Banfill, Dr. S. Martin. Interview by Charles G. Roland, HCHM/OHA. HCM 27-83, Montreal, QC, 14 July 1983.

Banfill, Dr. S. Martin. Interview by Charles G. Roland, HCHM/OHA. HCM 4-90, Montreal, QC, 9 June 1990.

Bard, Dr. Solomon Matthew. Interview by Charles G. Roland, HCHM/OHA. HCM 7-87, Hong Kong, 7 September 1987.

Bard, Dr. Solomon Matthew. Interview by Charles G. Roland, HCHM/OHA. HCM 1-90, Burlington, ON, 7 May 1990.

Birchall, W/C Leonard Joseph. Interview by Charles G. Roland, HCHM/OHA. HCM 5-86, Kingston, ON, 22 February 1986.

Blaylock, Tom. Interview, Denton, TX, North Texas State University, Oral History Collection. No. 65, Dallas, TX, 22 March 1971.

Boyd, Robert. Interview by Charles G. Roland, HCHM/OHA. HCM 13-83, Winnipeg, MB, 28 May 1983.

Bras, Dr. Gerrit. Interview by Charles G. Roland, HCHM/OHA. HCM 24-86, Wageningen, Netherlands, 2 September 1986.

Brunet, Lucien Camille. Interview by Charles G. Roland, HCHM/OHA. HCM 40-85, Montreal, QC, 10 April 1985.

Bulmer, James Roy. Interview by Charles G. Roland, HCHM/OHA. HCM 2-82, Hamilton, ON, 15 January 1982.

Cake, Wallace Vivian. Interview by Charles G. Roland, HCHM/OHA. HCM 14-85, St. John's, NF, 12 February 1985.

Cambon, Kenneth G. Interview by Charles G. Roland, HCHM/OHA. OCM 23-83, Vancouver, BC, 10 June 1983.

Canivet, Leslie Malcolm. Interview by Charles G. Roland, HCHM/OHA. HCM 60-85, Grand Valley, ON, 29 June 1985.

Chatwell, John William. Interview, in Gingras and Chapman, *The Sequelae of Inhuman Conditions.*

Christie, Kathleen G. Interview by Charles G. Roland, HCHM/OHA. HCM 28-82, Toronto, ON, 8 December 1982.

Claricoates, Ronald Hugh. Interview by Charles G. Roland, HCHM/OHA. HCM 29-83, Kingston, ON, 24 September 1983.

Coombes, Dr. Anthony Henry, MBE. Interview by Charles G. Roland, HCHM/OHA. HCM 5-94, 4 May 1994, Sussex, England.

Cowling, Anthony Henry. Interview by Charles G. Roland, HCHM/OHA. HCM 48-85, Vancouver BC, 22 April 1985.

Crawford, Dr. John N.B. Interview by Charles G. Roland, HCHM/OHA. HCM 6-83, Ottawa, ON, 26 April 1983.

Cunningham, Dr. Winston Ross. Interview by Charles G. Roland, HCHM/OHA. HCM 18-83, London, ON, 28 June 1983.

Delbridge, Albert Henry. Interview, in Gingras and Chapman, *The Sequelae of Inhuman Conditions.*

Dewar, Thomas Joseph. Interview, in Gingras and Chapman, *The Sequelae of Inhuman Conditions.*

Doddridge, Philip. Interview by Charles G. Roland, HCHM/OHA. HCM 5-89, New Richmond, QC, 28 May 1989.

Duguay, Joseph John. Interview by Charles G. Roland, HCHM/OHA. HCM 6-89, St. Omer, QC, 28 May 1989.

Englehart, Harold Wilfred. Interview by Charles G. Roland, HCHM/OHA. HCM 37-85, Montreal, QC, 10 April 1985.

Evans, Frank. Interview by Dr. John Cule, HCHM/OHA. HCM 5-88, Llandysul, Wales, 27 September 1988.

Gale, Dr. Godfrey Livingstone. Interview by Charles G. Roland, HCHM/OHA. HCM 1-82, Weston, ON, 12 January 1982.

Garrison, John Breckenridge. Interview, North Texas State University, Denton, TX. Oral History Collection, No. 57.

Gaudin, Kenneth M. Interview, in Gingras and Chapman, *The Sequelae of Inhuman Conditions.*

Golden, David Aaron. Interview by Charles G. Roland, HCHM/OHA. HCM 1-84, Ottawa, ON, 12 January 1984.

Graham-Cumming, Dr. George. Interview by Charles G. Roland, HCHM/OHA. HCM 1-96, North Vancouver, BC, 3 February 1996.

Gregg, Robert. Interview, Denton, TX, North Texas State University, Oral History Collection. No. 69, Decatur TX, 24 March 1971.

Grey, Walter. Interview, in Gingras and Chapman, *The Sequelae of Inhuman Conditions.*

Harding, Frank Arnold. Interview, in Gingras and Chapman, *The Sequelae of Inhuman Conditions.*

Hardy, John Herbert. Interview by Charles G. Roland, HCHM/OHA. HCM 9-83, Winnipeg, MB, 27 May 1983.

Hourigan, Kenneth. Quoted by Studs Terkel in *The Good War.* Cited in Mordecai Richler, ed. *Writers on World War II: An Anthology.* Toronto: Penguin Books, 1993.

Jarcho, Dr. Saul. Interview by Charles G. Roland, HCHM/OHA. HCM 10-86, Rochester, NY, 2 May 1986.

Jenkins, Walter George. Interview by Charles G. Roland, HCHM/OHA. HCM 22-83, Victoria, BC, 9 June 1983.

Gregg, Robert. Interview. North Texas State University, Denton TX. Oral History Collection, No. 69.

Law, Reginald. Interview by Charles G. Roland, HCHM/OHA. HCM 7-89, Campbelltown, NB, 28 May 1989.

Leath, Norman J. Interview by Charles G. Roland, HCHM/OHA. HCM 11-89, Chester, England, 26 August 1989.

Lyons, Henry. Interview, in Gingras and Chapman, *The Sequelae of Inhuman Conditions.*

MacMillan, Angus A. Interview, in Gingras and Chapman, *The Sequelae of Inhuman Conditions.*

McRitchie, Angus. Interview by Charles G. Roland, HCHM/OHA. HCM 25-85, Winnipeg, MB, 9 March 1985.

Murray, Matthew William. Interview, in Gingras and Chapman, *The Sequelae of Inhuman Conditions.*

Overton, William James. Interview, in Gingras and Chapman, *The Sequelae of Inhuman Conditions.*

Palmer, George Thomas. Interview, in Gingras and Chapman, *The Sequelae of Inhuman Conditions.*

Peterson, George Nelson. Interview, in Gingras and Chapman, *The Sequelae of Inhuman Conditions.*

Pifher, Arthur Kenneth. Interview by Charles G. Roland, HCHM/OHA. HCM 1-89, Grimsby, ON, 10 February 1989.

Poirier, Pat. Interview by Charles G. Roland, HCHM/OHA. HCM 6-90, Montreal, QC, n.d.

Quirion, Joseph Roger Raymond. Interview by Charles G. Roland, HCHM/OHA. HCM 84-85, Montreal, QC, 22 November 1985.

Robinson, Roy. Interview by Charles G. Roland, HCHM/OHA. HCM 10-83, Winnipeg, MB, 27 May 1983.

Robinson, Roy. Interview, in Gingras and Chapman, *The Sequelae of Inhuman Conditions.*

Rodrigues, Sir Albert. Interview by Charles G. Roland, HCHM/OHA. HCM 8-87, Hong Kong, 8 September 1987.

Rousell, John. Interview by Charles G. Roland, HCHM/OHA. HCM 38-85, Montreal, QC, 10 April 1985, 21-23.

Sellers, Raymond Richard. Interview, in Gingras and Chapman, *The Sequelae of Inhuman Conditions.*

Simcoe, John. Interview, in Gingras and Chapman, *The Sequelae of Inhuman Conditions.*

Speller, Lionel Curtis. Interview by Charles G. Roland, HCHM/OHA. HCM 2-90, Victoria, BC, 27 May 1990.

Squires, Arthur Raymond. Interview by Charles G. Roland, HCHM/OHA. HCM 21-83, Victoria, BC, 9 June 1983.

Standish, Colin. Interview by Charles G. Roland, HCHM/OHA. HCM 9-89, Cookshire, QC, 30 May 1989.

Standish, Colin. Interview by Charles G. Roland, HCHM/OHA. HCM 3-90, Cookshire, QC, 8 June 1990.

Stewart, Dr. William Muir. Interview by Charles G. Roland, HCHM/OHA. HCM 62- 85, Burlington, ON, 6 July 1985.

Stroud, John Raymond. Interview by Charles G. Roland, HCHM/OHA. HCM 19-85, Toronto, ON, 26 February 1985.

C: Private Papers

Guitard, Gabriel. Notebook kept in pencil at Niigata POW Camp 5B, October 1943 to February 1944. (Book in possession of the author. Guitard died 22 February 1944.)

Leath, N.J. Data from lists maintained by Cpl. Leath as part of his duties as Chief Clerk at Bowen Road Hospital; copies sent by Leath to C.G. Roland, 1990.

Ricciuti, Flora. "Disease Statistics in Japanese Prisoners of War during World War Two." Manuscript presented on completion of a summer Hannah Studentship under the guidance of Dr. Charles G. Roland, September 1987.

Squires, Arthur Raymond. "War Diary, Hong Kong and Kowloon, 1941-1945." MS unnumbered pp., typescript 45 pp.

Steele, Randolph. "With the Royal Rifles of Canada in Hong Kong and Japan." MS Memoir in possession of the author, 18 pp.

Stewart, William. "Notes on Keeping Records. Camp 5B: Niigata," ALS, Brig. Wm. Stewart to Charles G. Roland, pp. 1-4, 1986.

D: Published

Pritchard, R. John and Sonia Magbanua Zaide, eds. *The Tokyo War Crimes Trial: Volume 6, Transcript of the Proceedings in Open Session, Pages 12,393-14,954* New York: Garland Publishing, 1981.

Personal Memoirs

Abbott, Stephen. *And All My War is Done.* Edinburgh: Pentland Press, 1991.

Adams, Geoffrey Pharoah. *No Time for Geishas.* London: Leo Cooper, 1973.

Allister, William. *Where Life and Death Hold Hands.* Toronto: Stoddart, 1989.

Arneil, Stan. *One Man's War.* Sydney: S.F. Arneil, 1981.

Ashton, Paul. *Bataan Diary.* Santa Barbara, CA: Paul Ashton, 1984.

Bertram, James. *Beneath the Shadows: A New Zealander in the Far East, 1939-46.* New York: John Day, 1947.

Bosanquet, David. *Escape through China: Survival after the Fall of Hong Kong.* London: Robert Hale, 1983.

Braddon, Russell. *The Naked Island.* London: Werner Laurie, 1952.

Bumgarner, John R. *Parade of the Dead: A US Army Physician's Memoir of Imprisonment by the Japanese, 1942-1945.* Jefferson, NC: McFarland, 1995.

Bush, Lewis. *Clutch of Circumstance.* Tokyo: Okuyama, 1956.

_____. *Land of the Dragonfly.* London: Robert Hale, 1959.

Caffrey, Kate. *Out in the Midday Sun: Singapore 1941-45.* London: New English Library, 1977.

Cambon, Kenneth. *Guest of Hirohito.* Vancouver: PW Press, 1990.

Carney, Dora Sanders. *Foreign Devils Had Light Eyes: A Memoir of Shanghai, 1933-1939.* Toronto: Dorset Publishing, 1980.

Chapman, F. Spencer. *The Jungle Is Neutral.* London, Chatto & Windus, 1949.

Charles, H. Robert. *Last Man Out.* Austin, Texas: Eakin Press, 1988.

Christie, Kay. "Behind Japanese Barbed Wire—a Canadian Nursing Sister in Hong Kong." *Royal Canadian Military Institute Year Book.* Toronto: RCMI, 1979.

Coates, Albert, and Newman Rosenthal. *The Albert Coates Story: The Will That Found the Way*. Melbourne: Hyland House, 1977.

Cook, Haruko Taya, and Theodore F. Cook. *Japan at War: An Oral History*. New York: New Press, 1992.

Cowling, Anthony. *My Life with the Samurai*. Kenthurst, NSW: Kangaroo Press, 1996.

Crawford, John N.B. "A Medical Officer in Hong Kong." *Manitoba Medical Review* 26 (1946): 63-68.

Curtin, A.P. "Imprisonment under the Japanese." *British Medical Journal* 2 (1946): 585-86.

Duncan, Ian L. "Life in a Japanese Prisoner-of-War Camp." *Medical Journal of Australia* 1 (1982): 302-306.

_____. "Makeshift Medicine: Combating Disease in Japanese Prison Camps." *Medical Journal of Australia* 1 (1983): 29-32.

Durrani, Mahmood Khan. *The Sixth Column: The Heroic Personal Story of Lt.-Col. Mahmood Khan Durrani, G.C.* London: Cassell, 1955.

Edge, Spence, and Jim Henderson. *No Honour, No Glory*. Auckland: Collins, 1983.

Edwards, Jack. *Banzai, You Bastards!* London: Souvenir Press, 1990.

Endo, Shusaku. *The Sea and Poison*. [Japanese title *Umi to Dokuyaku*] Trans. Michael Gallagher. Tokyo: Charles E. Tuttle, 1972.

_____. "The Last Supper." In *The Final Martyrs*, Trans. Van C. Gessel. London: Hodder and Stoughton, 1994.

Evans, Frank. *Roll Call at Oeyama: A P.O.W. Remembers*. Llandysul, Dyfed: J.D. Lewis & Sons, 1985.

Fisher, Les. *I Will Remember: Recollections and Reflections on Hong Kong 1941 to 1945 - Internment and Freedom*. Totton, Hampshire: A.L. Fisher, 1996.

Foster, Frank. *Comrades in Bondage*. London: Skeffington and Son, 1946.

Fraser, Mrs. Hugh. *A Diplomatist's Wife in Japan: Letters from Home to Home*. London: Hutchinson, 1899.

Funasaka, Hiroshi. *Falling Blossoms*. Trans. Funasaka Hiroshi and Jeffrey D. Rubin. Singapore: Times Books International, 1986.

Goodman, Julien M. *M.D.P.O.W.* New York: Exposition Press, 1972.

Goodwin, Ralph. *Passport to Eternity*. London: Arthur Barker, 1956.

_____. *Hongkong Escape*. London: Arthur Barker, 1953.

Gottlieb, M.L. "Impressions of POW Medical Officer in Japanese Concentration Camps." *US Navy Medical Bulletin* 46 (1946): 663-75.

Grew, Joseph C. *Report from Tokyo: A Message to the American People*. New York: Simon and Schuster, 1942.

Guest, Freddie. *Escape from the Bloodied Sun*. London: Hutchinson's Universal Book Club, 1957.

Hardie, Robert. *The Burma-Siam Railway: The Secret Diary of Dr. Robert Hardie, 1942-45*. London: Imperial War Museum, 1983.

Harrison, Kenneth. *The Brave Japanese*. Adelaide: Rigby, 1966.

Hubbard, Preston John. *Apocalypse Undone: My Survival of Japanes Imprisonment during World War II*. Nashville: Vanderbilt University Press, 1990.

Huxtable, Charles. *From the Somme to Singapore: A Medical Officer in Two World Wars*. Kenthurst, Australia: Kangaroo Press, 1987.

Jackson, Calvin G. *Diary of Col. Calvin G. Jackson, MD, Kept during World War II, 1941-1945.* Ada, OH: Ohio Northern University, 1992.

Jordan, Arnold. *Tenko on the River Kwai.* Launceston, Tasmania: Regal Publications, 1987.

Keith, Agnes Newton. *Three Came Home.* Introduction by Carl Mydans. New York: Time Inc., 1965.

Kell, Derwent. *A Doctor's Borneo.* Brisbane: Boolarong Publications, 1984.

Kelly, Terence. *FEPOW: The Story of a Voyage beyond Belief.* London: Robert Hale, 1985.

Lan, Alice Y., and Betty M. Hu. *We Flee from Hong Kong.* Grand Rapids, MI: Zondervan Publishing House, 1944.

Leiper, G.A. *A Yen for My Thoughts.* Hong Kong: South China Morning Post , 1982.

Levering, Robert W. *Horror Trek: A True Story of Bataan, the Death March and Three and One-half Years in Japanese Prison Camps.* Dayton: Horstman, 1948.

Levi, Primo. "October 1944." *Survival in Auschwitz.* Cited in Mordecai Richler, ed. *Writers on World War II: An Anthology.* Toronto: Penguin Books, 1993.

Li, Shu-Fan. *Hong Kong Surgeon.* New York: E.P. Dutton, 1964.

Lockhart, Terry. *A Colonial Boy.* Devonport, Tasmania: Terry Lockhart, 1989.

Lomax, Eric. *The Railway Man.* London: Vintage, 1996.

Maltby, C.M. "Operations in Hong Kong from 8th to 25th December, 1941." *London Gazette,* suppl., 27 January 1948, no. 38190, 699-725.

Manchester, William. *Goodbye Darkness: A Memoir of the Pacific War.* Boston: Little Brown, 1979. Cited in Mordecai Richler, ed. *Writers on World War II: An Anthology.* Toronto: Penguin Books, 1993.

Marsman, Jan H. *I Escaped from Hong Kong.* New York: Reynal, 1942.

Martin, Adrian. *Brothers from Bataan: POWs, 1942-1945.* Manhattan, KA: Sunflower University Press, 1992.

Moriya, Tadashi. *No Requiem.* Trans. Geoffrey S. Kishimoto. Tokyo: Hokuseido Press, 1968.

Norquist, Ernest O. *Our Paradise: A GI's War Diary.* Hancock, WI: Pearl-Win Publishing, 1989.

Nussbaum, Chaim. *Chaplain on the River Kwai: Story of a Prisoner of War* New York: Shapolsky, 1988.

Ogawa, Tetsuro. *Terraced Hell: A Japanese Memoir of Defeat and Death in Northern Luzon, Philippines.* Rutland, VT and Tokyo: Charles E. Tuttle, 1972.

O'Kane, Richard H. *Clear the Bridge!: The War Patrols of the USS Tang.* Chicago: Rand McNally, 1977.

Pape, Richard. *Boldness Be My Friend.* London, Panther Books, 1985.

Parkin, Ray. *Into the Smother.* London, Hogarth Press,1963.

Paul, Daniel, and John St. John. *Surgeon at Arms.* London: Heinemann, 1958.

Poole, Philippa. *Of Love and War: The Letters and Diaries of Captain Adrian Curlewis and His Family, 1939-1945.* London: Century, 1983.

Proulx, Benjamin A. *Underground From Hongkong.* New York, E.P. Dutton, 1943.

Ryan, Thomas F. *Jesuits under Fire in the Siege of Hong Kong, 1941.* London: Burns Oates & Washbourne, 1945.

Sakai, Saburo, Martin Caidin, and Fred Saito. *Samurai!* New York: E.P. Dutton, 1957.

Scott, R. Jackson. *90 Days of Rice*. Pioneer, CA: California Traveler, 1975.

Selwyn-Clarke, Sir Selwyn. *Footprints: The Memoirs of Sir Selwyn Selwyn-Clarke, KBE, CMG, MC, C.St.J., MD, BS, FRCP, MRCS, DPH, DTM and H, Bar-at-Law, Former Governor and Commander-in-Chief, Seychelles*. Hong Kong: Sino-American Publishing, 1954.

Smith, Stanley W. *Prisoner of the Emperor: An American POW in World War II*. Duane A. Smith, ed. Niwot, CO: University Press of Colorado, 1991.

Soka Gakkai Youth Division. *Peace Is Our Duty: Accounts of What War Can Do to Man*. Trans. Richard L. Gage. Tokyo, Japan Times, 1982.

Soka Gakkai Youth Division. *Cries for Peace: Experiences of Japanese Victims of World War II*. Tokyo: Japan Times, 1978.

Stamp, Loren E. *Journey through Hell: Memoir of a World War II American Navy Medic Captured in the Philippines and Imprisoned by the Japanese*. Jefferson, NC: McFarland, 1993.

Stening, S.E.L. "Experiences as a Prisoner of War in Japan." *Medical Journal of Australia* 1 (1946): 773-75.

Stewart, John. *To the River Kwai: Two Journeys—1943, 1979*. London: Bloomsbury, 1988.

Summons, Walter Irvine. *Twice Their Prisoner*. Melbourne: Oxford University Press, 1946.

Taylor, Vince. *Cabanatuan, Japanese Death Camp: A Survivor's Story*. Waco, TX: Texian Press, 1985.

Teel, Horace G. *Our Days Were Years: History of the "Lost Battalion," 2nd Battalion, 36th Division*. Quanah, TX: Nortex, 1978.

Tsuji, Masanobu. *Singapore. 1941-1942: The Japanese Version of the Malayan Campaign of World War II*. Trans. Margaret E. Lake. Oxford: Oxford University Press, 1988.

Ugaki, Matome. *Fading Victory: The Diary of Admiral Matome Ugaki, 1941-1945*. Trans. Chihaya Masataka. Pittsburgh: University of Pittsburgh Press, 1991.

Waldron, Ben D., and Emily Burneson. *Corregidor, "From Paradise to Hell": True Narrative of Ben Waldron, Prisoner-of-War*. Freeman, SD: Ben D. Waldron, 1989.

Wall, Don, ed., *Singapore and Beyond:The Story of the Men of the 2/20 Battalion, Told by the Survivors*. East Hills, Australia: 2/20 Battalion Association, 1985.

Weinstein, Alfred A. *Barbed-Wire Surgeon*. New York: Macmillan, 1948.

Whitecross, Roy H. *Slaves of the Son of Heaven*. Sydney: Dymock's Book Arcade, 1953.

Wright, John M. Jr. *Captured on Corregidor: Diary of an American P.O.W. in World War II*. Jefferson, NC: McFarland, 1988.

Wright-Nooth, George, with Mark Adkin. *Prisoner of the Turnip Heads: Horror, Hunger and Humour in Hong Kong, 1941-1945*. London: Leo Cooper, 1994.

Zia, I.D. *The Unforgettable Epoch (1937-1945)*. Hong Kong: Chi Sheng Publishing, 1971.

Secondary Sources

Allen, Louis. *The End of the War in Asia*. London: Hart-Davis, MacGibbon, 1976.

_____. *Burma: The Longest War, 1941-45*. New York: St. Martin's Press, 1984.

_____. "Japanese Literature of the Second World War." *Proceedings of the British Association for Japanese Studies* 2 (1977): 117-52.

Anonymous. *Report of the International Committee of the Red Cross on Its Activities during the Second World War (September 1, 1939 - June 30, 1947).* Vol. 1, General Activities. Geneva: International Red Cross, 1948.

_____. *A Record of the Actions of the Hongkong Volunteer Defence Corps in the Battle for Hong Kong, December, 1941.* Hong Kong: Ye Olde Printerie, [1954].

_____. *The Royal Rifles of Canada in Hong Kong, 1941-1945.* Sherbrooke: Hong Kong Veterans' Association of Canada, Quebec-Maritimes Branch, 1980.

Arthur, Anthony. *Bushmasters: America's Jungle Warriors of World War II.* New York: St. Martin's Press, 1987.

Beaumont, Joan. *Gull Force: Survival and Leadership in Captivity, 1941-1945.* North Sydney: Allen & Unwin, 1988.

Birch, Alan, and Martin Cole. *Captive Christmas: The Battle of Hong Kong, December 1941.* Hong Kong: Heinemann Asia, 1979.

Blair, Joan, and Clay Blair, Jr. *Return from the River Kwai.* New York: Simon & Schuster, 1979.

Blair, Lawrence, with Lorne Blair. *Ring of Fire.* Toronto: Bantam Books, 1988.

Bowers, John Z. *Medical Education in Japan: From Chinese Medicine to Western Medicine.* New York: Hoeber Medical Division, Harper & Row, 1965.

Brackman, Arnold C. *The Other Nuremberg: The Untold Story of the Tokyo War Crimes Trials.* New York: William Morrow, 1987.

Bridgewater, William, and Seymour Kurtz, eds. *The Columbia Encyclopedia,* 3rd ed.

Brode, Patrick. *Casual Slaughters and Accidental Judgments: Canadian War Crimes Prosecutions, 1944-1948.* Toronto: Published for the Osgoode Society for Canadian Legal History by University of Toronto Press, 1997.

Brown, Wenzell. *Hong Kong Aftermath.* New York: Smith & Durrell, 1943.

Brownmiller, Susan. *Against Our Will: Men, Women, and Rape.* New York: Simon and Schuster, 1975.

Bruce, Phillip. *Second to None: The Story of the Hong Kong Volunteers.* Hong Kong: Oxford University Press, 1991.

Burdick, Charles, and Ursula Moessner. *The German Prisoners-of-War in Japan, 1914-1920.* New York: Lanham, 1984.

Burrill, William, *Hemingway, The Toronto Years.* Toronto: Doubleday Canada, 1994.

Campbell, Kristine A. "Knots in the Fabric: Richard Pearson Strong and the Bilibid Prison Vaccine Trials, 1905-1906." *Bulletin of the History of Medicine* 68 (1994): 600-38.

Cary, Otis, ed. *From a Ruined Empire: Letters—Japan, China, Korea, 1945-46.* Tokyo: Kodansha International, 1984.

Chang, Iris. *The Rape of Nanking: The Forgotten Holocaust of World War II.* New York: Penguin Books, 1998.

Clark, Russell S. *An End to Tears.* Sydney: Peter Huston, 1946.

Condon-Rall, Mary Ellen. "Allied Cooperation in Malaria Prevention and Control: The World War II Southwest Pacific Experience." *Journal of the History of Medicine and Allied Sciences* 46 (1991): 493-513.

_____. "U.S. Army Medical Preparations and the Outbreak of War: The Philippines, 1941-6 May 1942." *Journal of Military History* 56 (1992): 35-56.

Cott, Jonathan. *Wandering Ghost: The Odyssey of Lafcadio Hearn.* New York: Kodansha, 1990.

Cuthbertson, Ken. *Nobody Said Not to Go: The Life, Loves, and Adventures of Emily Hahn*. Boston: Faber and Faber, 1998.

Dancocks, Daniel G. *In Enemy Hands: Canadian Prisoners of War, 1939-45* Edmonton: Hurtig, 1983.

Daws, Gavan. *Prisoners of the Japanese: POWs of World War II in the Pacific*. New York: William Morrow, 1994.

Deighton, Len. *Blood, Tears and Folly: In the Darkest Hour of the Second World War*. London: Cape, 1993.

Dexter, David. *The New Guinea Offensives*. Canberra: Australian War Memorial, 1961.

Dingman, Roger. *Ghost of War: The Sinking of the Awa Maru and Japanese-American Relations, 1945-1995*. Annapolis: Naval Institute Press, 1997.

Duff, Sir Lyman P. *Report on the Canadian Expeditionary Force to the Crown Colony of Hong Kong*. Ottawa: The King's Printer, 1942.

Dunning, A.J. *Extremes: Reflections on Human Behavior*. Trans. Johan Theron. New York: Harcourt Brace Jovanovich, 1992.

Endacott, George Beer. *Hong Kong Eclipse*. Hong Kong: Oxford University Press, 1978.

_____. *Fragrant Harbour: A Short History of Hong Kong*. Hong Kong: Oxford University Press, 1962.

_____. *A History of Hong Kong*. London: Oxford University Press, 1964.

Elphick, Peter and Michael Smith. *Odd Man Out: The Story of the Singapore Traitor*. London: Hodder and Stoughton, 1994.

Frank, Benis M., and Harry I. Shaw, Jr. *Victory and Occupation: History of the US Marine Corps in World War II*, Volume V. Washington: US Marine Corps, 1968.

Fuller, Richard. *Shokan: Hirohito's Samurai*. London: Arms and Armour, 1992.

Garrett, Richard. *P.O.W.* London: David & Charles, 1981.

Geddes, Gary. *Hong Kong Poems*. Oberon Press, 1987.

Gee, Ellen M. "Veterans and Veterans Legislation in Canada: An Historical Overview." *Canadian Journal of Aging* 7 (1988): 204-17.

Gibbs, John M. "Prisoner of War Camps in Japan and Japanese Controlled Areas as Taken from Reports of Interned American Prisoners. Osaka No. 3 Oeyama, Japan." *Liaison & Research American Prisoner of War Information Bureau* (31 July 1946), 1-3.

Gingras, Gustave, and Carol Chapman. *The Sequelae of Inhuman Conditions and Slave Labour Experienced by Members of the Canadian Components of the Hong Kong Forces, 1941-1945, while Prisoners of the Japanese Government*. Toronto: War Amputations of Canada, 1987.

Gold, Hal. *Unit 731 Testimony*. Tokyo: Yenbooks, 1996.

Goldsmid, Edmund, ed., *A Counter-Blaste to Tobacco*. (Written by King James I). Edinburgh: privately printed, 1884; originally published in London, 1604.

Greenhous, Brereton. *"C" Force to Hong Kong: A Canadian Catastrophe, 1941-1945*. Toronto: Dundurn Press, 1997.

Grew, Joseph C. *Report from Tokyo: A Message to the American People*. New York: Simon and Schuster, 1942.

Hane, Mikiso. *Peasants, Rebels, and Outcasts: The Underside of Modern Japan*. New York: Pantheon Books, 1982.

Hardy, Anne. "Beriberi, Vitamin B1 and World Food Policy, 1925-1970." *Medical History* 39 (1995): 61-77.

Harries, Meirion, and Susie Harries. *Soldiers of the Sun: The Rise and Fall of the Imperial Japanese Army, 1868-1945*. London: Heinemann, 1991.

Harris, Sheldon. *Factories of Death: Japanese Biological Warfare 1932-45 and the American Cover-up*. New York: Routledge, 1994.

Harrison, Gordon. *Mosquitoes, Malaria & Man: A History of the Hostilities Since 1880*. New York: E.P. Dutton, 1978.

Hibbert, Joyce. "Biscuit, Book, and Candle in Hong Kong." In *Fragments of War: Stories from Survivors of World War II*. Toronto: Dundurn Press, 1985.

Hicks, George. *The Comfort Women: Sex Slaves of the Japanese Imperial Forces*. London: Souvenir Press, 1995.

Hoyt, Edwin P. *Japan's War: The Great Pacific Conflict, 1853 to 1952*. New York: Da Capo, 1986.

Jeffrey, Betty. *White Coolies*. Sydney: Angus & Robertson, 1954.

Kahn, E.J. Jr. *The Stragglers*. New York: Random House, 1962.

LaForte, Robert S., and Ronald E. Marcello. *Building the Death Railway: The Ordeal of American POWs in Burma, 1942-1945*. Wilmington, Delaware: Scholarly Resources, 1993.

Long, Gavin. *The Final Campaigns*. Canberra: Australian War Memorial, 1963.

Longmate, Norman. *How We Lived Then: A History of Everyday Life during the Second World War*. London: Arrow Books, 1988.

Luff, John. *The Hidden Years*. Hong Kong: South China Morning Post, 1967.

MacDougall, Heather. *Activists and Advocates: Toronto's Health Department, 1883-1983*. Toronto: Dundurn Press, 1990.

Mackenzie, Compton. *Eastern Epic: Volume 1, September 1939-March 1943, Defence*. London: Chatto & Windus, 1951.

MacKenzie, S.P. "The Treatment of Prisoners of War in World War II" *Journal of Modern History* 66 (1994): 487-520.

Manaka, Yoshio, and Ian A. Urquhart. *The Layman's Guide to Acupuncture*. New York: Weatherhill, 1991.

McCarthy, Dudley. *South-West Pacific Area—First Year: Kokoda to Wau*. Canberra: Australian War Memorial, 1959.

McDonald, Donald. *Surgeons Twoe and a Barber: Being Some Account of the Life and Work of the Indian Medical Service (1600-1947)*. London: William Heinemann Medical Books, 1950.

Mestler, Gordon E. "A Galaxy of Old Japanese Medical Books with Miscellaneous Notes on Early Medicine in Japan: Part II. Acupuncture and Moxibustion, Bathing, Balneotherapy and Massage, Nursing, Pediatrics and Hygiene, Obstetrics and Gynecology." *Bulletin of the Medical Library Association* 42 (1954): 468-81.

Miller, John Jr. *The War in the Pacific: Guadalcanal: The First Offensive*. Washington: Department of the Army, 1949.

Miller, Robert W. "War Crimes Trials at Yokohama." *Brooklyn Law Review* 15 (1949): 191-209.

Milner, Samuel. *The War in the Pacific: Victory in Papua*. Washington: Department of the Army, 1957.

Muir, Augustus. *The First of Foot: The History of the Royal Scots (The Royal Regiment)*. Edinburgh: Royal Scots History Committee, 1961.

Neary, Peter. "Venereal Disease and Public Health Administration in Newfoundland in the 1930s and 1940s." *Canadian Bulletin of Medical History/Bulletin canadien d'histoire de la médicine* 15 (1998): 129-51.

Nelson, Hank. *P.O.W: Prisoners of War—Australians under Nippon.* Sydney: Australian Broadcasting Commission, 1985.

_____. "'A Bowl of Rice for Seven Camels': The Dynamics of Prisoner-of-War Camps." *Journal of the Australian War Memorial* 14 (1989): 33-42.

Newby, Eric. *A Short Walk in the Hindu Kush.* London: Picador, 1981.

Nolan, Liam. *Small Man of Nanataki: The True Story of a Japanese Who Risked His Life to Provide Comfort for His Enemies.* New York: E.P. Dutton, 1966.

Orwell, George. *Down and Out in Paris and London.* Harmondsworth, Middlesex: Penguin, 1970.

Paull, Raymond. *Retreat from Kokoda: The Australian Campaign in New Guinea, 1942.* Port Melbourne, Victoria: Mandarin Australia, 1989.

Perras, Galen Roger. "'Our Position in the Far East Would be Stronger Without This Unsatisfactory Commitment': Britain and the Reinforcement of Hong Kong, 1941." *Canadian Journal of History* 30 (1995): 231-59.

Piccigallo, Philip R. *The Japanese on Trial: Allied War Crimes Operations in the East, 1945-1951.* Austin: University of Texas Press, 1979.

_____. *In the Shadow of Nuremberg: Trials of Japanese in the East, 1945-1951.* Ph.D. Thesis, City University of New York, 1977.

Pritchard, R. John. "The Nature and Significance of British Post-war Trials of Japanese War Criminals, 1945-1948." *Proceedings of the British Association for Japanese Studies* 2 (1977): 189-219.

_____. "The Historical Experience of British War Crimes Courts in the Far East, 1946-1948." *International Relations* 6 (1978): 311-26.

_____. "Lessons from British Proceedings against Japanese War Criminals." *Human Rights Review* 3 (1978): 104-21.

_____. "An Overview of the Historical Importance of the Tokyo War Trial." In C. Hosoya, N. Ando, Y. Onuma, and R. Minear, eds., *The Tokyo War Crimes Trial: An International Symposium.* Tokyo: Kodansha International, 1986.

_____. "What the Historian Can Find in the Proceedings of the International Military Tribunal for the Far East." Suntory-Toyota International Centre for Economics and Related Disciplines, London School of Economics, Discussion Paper IS/89/197, pp. 8-25

Radford, R.A. "The Economic Organisation of a POW Camp." *Economica* 12 (1945): 189-201.

Reischauer, Haru Matsukata. *Samurai and Silk: A Japanese and American Heritage.* Cambridge: Belknap Press of Harvard University Press, 1986.

Roland, Charles G. "Stripping away the Veneer: POW Survival in the Far East as an Index of Cultural Atavism." *Journal of Military History* 53 (1989): 79-94.

_____. "Allied POWs, Japanese Captors, and the Geneva Convention." *War and Society* 9 (1991): 83-101.

_____. *Courage under Siege: Disease, Starvation, and Death in the Warsaw Ghetto.* New York: Oxford University Press, 1992.

_____. "Sunk under the Taxation of Nature": Malaria in Upper Canada. In C.G. Roland. *Health, Disease and Medicine: Essays in Canadian History.* Toronto: Hannah Institute for the History of Medicine, 1984.

_____. "Human Vivisection: The Intoxication of Limitless Power in Wartime." In Bob Moore and Kent Fedorowich, eds. *Prisoners of War and Their Captors in World War II*. Manchester: Manchester University Press, 1996.

_____. "Massacre and Rape at Hong Kong: Two Case Studies Involving Medical Personnel and Patients." *Journal of Contemporary History* 32 (1997): 43-61.

_____. "Medical Aspects of War in the West, 1812-1813." In K.G. Pryke and L.L. Kulisek, eds. *The Western District*. Windsor, Ontario: Essex County Historical Society, 1983.

_____., and Harry S. Shannon. "Patterns of Disease among World War II Prisoners of the Japanese: Hunger, Weight Loss, and Deficiency Diseases in Two Camps." *Journal of the History of Medicine and Allied Sciences* 46 (1991): 65-85.

Russell, Paul F. *Man's Mastery of Malaria*. London: Oxford University Press, 1955.

Saga, Junichi. *Memories of Silk and Straw: A Self-Portrait of Small-Town Japan*. Trans. Garry Evans. Tokyo: Kodansha International, 1990.

Sergeant, Harriet. *Shanghai*. London: John Murray, 1998.

Seifert, Ruth. "War and Rape: A Preliminary Analysis." In Alexandra Stiglmayer, ed. *Mass Rape: The War against Women in Bosnia-Herzegovina*. Trans. Marion Faber. Lincoln: University of Nebraska Press, 1993.

Shearer, G.P. "Stanley, Hong Kong: The First Three Years." *Royal Engineers Journal* 58 (1944): 161-74.

Shelley, C.R. "HMCS *Prince Roberts*: The Career of an Armed Merchant Cruiser." *Canadian Military History* 4 (1995): 47-60.

Stacey, Charles P. *Official History of the Canadian Army in the Second World War, Volume I: Six Years of War*. Ottawa: Edmond Cloutier, 1955.

Starling, Peter H. *In Oriente Fidelis: The Army Medical Services in the Battle of Hong Kong, December 1941*. Aldershot: RAMC Historical Museum [1986].

Steven, Walter T. *In This Sign*. Toronto: Ryerson Press, n.d.

Stewart, Jean Cantlie. *The Quality of Mercy: The Lives of Sir James and Lady Cantlie*. London: George Allen & Unwin, 1983.

Swinson, Arthur. *Four Samurai: A Quartet of Japanese Army Commanders in the Second World War*. London: Hutchinson, 1968.

Taylor, Vince. *Cabanatuan, Japanese Death Camp: A Survivor's Story*. Waco, TX, Texian Press, 1985.

United States Strategic Bombing Survey. *The War against Japanese Transportation, 1941-1945*. [Washington, DC]: Transportation Division, 1947.

_____. *The Japanese Wartime Standard of Living and Utilization of Manpower*. [Washington, DC]: Manpower, Food and Civilian Supplies Division, 1947.

Vance, Jonathan F. *Objects of Concern: Canadian Prisoners of War through the Twentieth Century*. Vancouver: UBC Press, 1994.

Van der Vat, Dan. *Stealth at Sea: The History of the Submarine*. Boston, New York: Houghton Mifflin, 1994.

Veith, Ilza. "Humane Warfare and Inhuman War: Japan and its Treatment of War Prisoners." *Bulletin of the History of Medicine* 19 (1946): 355-74.

Watt, Sir James, Eric J. Freeman, and William F. Bynum, eds. *Starving Sailors: The Influence of Nutrition upon Naval and Maritime History*. Greenwich: National Maritime Museum, 1981.

West, Rebecca. *The New Meaning of Treason*. London: Penguin Books, 1985.

Wigmore, Lionel. *The Japanese Thrust*. Canberra: Australian War Memorial, 1968.

Whitman, Walt. *Leaves of Grass*. Harold W. Blodgett and Sculley Bradley, eds. New York: New York University Press, 1965.

Campaign Histories

Anonymous. *The Royal Rifles of Canada in Hong Kong, 1941-1945*. Sherbrooke: Hong Kong Veterans' Association of Canada, Quebec-Maritimes Branch, 1980.

Ferguson, Ted. *Desperate Siege: The Battle of Hong Kong*. Toronto: Doubleday Canada, 1980.

Lindsay, Oliver. *The Lasting Honour: The Fall of Hong Kong 1941*. London: Hamish Hamilton, 1978.

Ride, Edwin. *BAAG: Hong Kong Resistance, 1942-1945*. Hong Kong: Oxford University Press, 1981.

Vincent, Carl. *No Reason Why: The Canadian Hong Kong Tragedy, an Examination*. Stittsville: Canada's Wings, 1981.

Wall, Don, ed. *Singapore and Beyond:The Story of the Men of the 2/20 Battalion, Told by the Survivors*. East Hills, Australia: 2/20 Battalion Association, 1985.

Medical Research or Clinical Medical Sources

Adamson, J.D., and D.C. Brereton. "Ultimate Disabilities in Hong Kong Repatriates." *Treatment Services Bulletin* ser.4, 3 (1948): 5-10.

Adamson, J.D., and C.M. Judge. "Residual Disabilities in Hong Kong Prisoners of War." *Canadian Services Medical Journal* 12 (1956): 837-51.

Adamson, J.D., P.K. Tisdale, D.C. Brereton, and L.W.B. Card, "Residual Disabilities in Hong Kong Repatriates," *Canadian Medical Association Journal* 56 (1947): 481-86.

Anonymous. "Quinine." http://www.bev.net/education/schools/ ahss cience/apbiol/quinine.html.

Aykroyd, W.R. "Beriberi and Other Food-deficiency Diseases in Newfoundland and Labrador." *Journal of Hygiene* 30 (1930): 357-86.

Bell, P.G., and J.C. O'Neill. "Optic Atrophy in Hong Kong Prisoners of War." *Canadian Medical Association Journal* 56 (1947): 475-81.

Belmonte, A. Colaco. "Ervaringen uit gevangenkampen op Java en in Japan." ["Experiences in the Prison Camps of Java and in Japan"] *Nederlands Tijdschrift van Geneeskunde* 89 (1945): 419-24; [reprinted same journal, 129 (1985): 1506-1509.] Translated by Dr. Jans Muller, 1989.

Bowie, Donald C. "Captive Surgeon in Hong Kong: The Story of the British Military Hospital, Hong Kong, 1942-1945." *Journal of the Hong Kong Branch of the Royal Asiatic Society* 15 (1975): 150-290.

Bras, Gerrit (trans. F.W. Klutzow). "Ziekten en hun behandeling in kampen langs de rivier de Kwai." *Nederlands Tijdschrift voor Geneeskunde* 129 (1985): 1529-32.

Brennan, D.J. "The Burning Feet Syndrome: Observations of Cases Among Prisoners of War in Manchuria." *Medical Journal of Australia* 2 (1946): 232-34.

Brooke, H.H.W. "Chest X-ray Survey of Repatriated Prisoners of War from Japanese Camps." *Canadian Medical Association Journal* 54 (1946): 141-44.

Carpenter, Kenneth J., ed. *Pellagra*. Stroudsburg, PA: Hutchinson Ross, 1981.

Clarke, C.A., and I.B. Sneddon. "Nutritional Neuropathy in Prisoners-of-War and Internees from Hong-Kong." *Lancet* 1 (1946): 734-737.

Crawford, John N.B. "A Preliminary Report on a Follow-up Study of Repatriates from Japanese Prisoner of War Camps." *Treatment Services Bulletin* 5 (1950): 158-68.

Crawford, John N.B., and John A.G. Reid. "Nutritional Disease Affecting Canadian Troops Held Prisoner of War by the Japanese." *Canadian Journal of Research* 25 (1947): 53-85.

Cruikshank, Eric K. "Painful Feet in Prisoners-of-War in the Far East." *Lancet* 2 (1946): 369-72.

Curtin, A.P. "Imprisonment under the Japanese." *British Medical Journal* 2 (1946): 585-86.

Dean, Larry M., Frank N. Willis, and Robert Obourn. "Health Records of American Prisoners of the Japanese during World War II." *Military Medicine* 145 (1980): 838-41.

Dekking, H.M. "Tropical Nutritional Amblyopia ('Camp Eyes')." *Ophthalmologica* 113 (1947): 65-92.

Denny-Brown, D. "Neurological Conditions Resulting from Prolonged and Severe Dietary Restrictions (Case Reports in Prisoners-of-War and General Review)." *Medicine* 26 (1947): 41-113.

Dixon, J.M.S. "Diphtheria in North America." *Journal of Hygiene* 93 (1934): 419-21.

Duncan, Ian L. "Life in a Japanese Prisoner-of-war Camp." *Medical Journal of Australia* 1 (1982): 302-306.

Duncan, Ian L. "Makeshift Medicine: Combating Disease in Japanese Prison Camps." *Medical Journal of Australia* 1 (1983): 29-32.

_____. "Ocular Signs in the Prisoner of War from the Far East." *British Medical Journal* 1 (1946): 626-27.

Everts, W.H. "Nutritional Disorders in Allied Repatriates and Japanese Prisoners of War." *Journal of Nervous and Mental Diseases* 106 (1947): 393-400.

Fisher, C. Miller. "Residual Neuropathological Changes in Canadians Held Prisoners of War by the Japanese (Strachan's Disease)." *Canadian Services Medical Journal* 11 (1955): 157-99.

Freemon, Frank R. *Causes of Neuropathy*. Copenhagen: Munksgaard, 1975.

Gill, Geoffrey V., and Dion R. Bell. "Persisting Tropical Diseases amongst Former Prisoners of War of the Japanese." *Practitioner* 224 (1980): 801-803.

_____. "Persisting Nutritional Neuropathy amongst Former War Prisoners." *Journal of Neurology, Neurosurgery, and Psychiatry* 45 (1982): 861-65.

Glusman, Murray. "The Syndrome of 'Burning Feet' (Nutritional Melalgia) as a Manifestation of Nutritional Deficiency." *American Journal of Medicine* 3 (1947): 211-23.

Gopalan, C. "The 'Burning-feet' Syndrome." *Indian Medical Gazette* 81 (1946): 22-26.

Gottlieb, M.L. "Impressions of a POW Medical Officer in Japanese Concentration Camps." *US Navy Medical Bulletin* 46 (1946): 663-75.

Grierson, J. "On the Burning in the Feet of Natives." *Transactions of the Medical & Physical Society of Calcutta* 2 (1826): 275-80.

Haimsohn, J.S. "Avitaminoses as Seen in Japanese Prisoners of War, with Review of Two Cases." *Memphis Medical Journal* 22 (1947): 196-200.

Hardy, John Herbert. Interview by Charles G. Roland, HCHM/OHA. HCM 9-83, Winnipeg, MB, 27 May 1983.

Harrison, George F. "Nutritional Deficiency, Painful Feet, High Blood Pressure in Hong Kong." *Lancet* 1 (1946): 961-64.

Hibbs, Ralph E. "Beriberi in Japanese Prison Camps." *Annals of Internal Medicine* 25 (1946): 270-82.

Hinder, David C.C. "Prisoners of War: Long-term Effects." *Medical Journal of Australia* 1 (1981): 565-66.

Hong, Chang-Zern. "Peripheral Neuropathy in Former Prisoners of War." *Quan* 41 (5) (1987): 7-9.

Katz, Charles J. "Neuropathologic Manifestations Found in a Japanese Prison Camp." *Journal of Nervous & Mental Diseases* 103 (1946): 456-65.

Leyton, G.B. "Effects of Slow Starvation." *Lancet* 2 (1946): 73-79.

Liebow, A.A., P.D. MacLean, J.H. Bumstead, and L.G. Welt. "Tropical Ulcers and Cutaneous Diphtheria." *Archives of Internal Medicine.* 78 (1946): 255-95

Maisey, C.W. "Some Observations on, and Methods of Dealing with, Medical Problems when a Prisoner of War of the Japanese, 1942-1945." *Journal of the Royal Army Medical Corps* 92 (1949): 244-64.

Malcolmson, J.G. *Observations on Some Forms of Rheumatism.* Madras: Vepery Mission Press, 1835.

May, Ella Louise. "Parasitologic Study of 400 Soldiers Interned by the Japanese." *American Journal of Tropical Medicine* 27 (1947): 129-30.

Morgan, Hugh J., Irving S. Wright, and Arie van Ravenswaay. "Health of Repatriated Prisoners of War from the Far East." *Journal of the American Medical Association* 130 (1946): 995-99.

Moss, John E. "A Medical Survey of Allied Repatriates after Liberation from Japanese Prisons." *US Naval Medical Bulletin* 47 (1947): 598-604.

Mukherjee, H.C. "Scope of a Medical Man while a Prisoner of War." *Antiseptic: A Monthly Medical Journal* 43 (1946): 635-39.

Murray, John, and Anne Murray. "Suppression of Infection by Famine and Its Activation by Refeeding—A Paradox?" *Perspectives in Biology and Medicine* 20 (1977): 471-83.

Nardini, J.E. "Vitamin Deficiency Diseases in Allied Prisoners of the Japanese." *US Naval Medical Bulletin* 47 (1947): 272-78.

_____. "Survival Factors in American Prisoners of War of the Japanese." *American Journal of Psychiatry* 109 (1952): 241-48.

Oomen, H.A.P.C. "Wanvoeding bij Europeanen in de oorlog in de Pacific, 1942-1945." ["Malnutrition among Europeans during the Pacific War, 1942-1945." Translated by Dr. F.W. Klutzow] *Ned. Tijdschr. Geneeskd.* 129 (1985): 1521-25.

Page, J.A. "Painful-feet Syndrome among Prisoners of War in the Far East." *British Medical Journal* 2 (1946): 260-62.

Pemberton, T. Max. "Observations on Diseases among British Prisoners of War in Japanese Hands in the Far East (1942-1945)." *New Zealand Medical Journal* 48 (1949): 145-50.

Pohlman, Max Edward, and Edward Francis Ritter, Jr. "Observations on Vitamin Deficiencies in an Eye, Ear, Nose, and Throat Clinic of a Japanese Prison Hospital." *American Journal of Ophthalmology* 35 (1952): 228-30.

Porter, Alexander. *The Diseases of the Madras Famine of 1877-78.* Madras: Government Press, 1889.

Rifkin, Harold. "Dengue Fever (Breakbone Fever). In Max Pinner and Benjamin F. Miller, eds. *When Doctors Are Patients.* New York: Norton, 1952.

Robinson, J.E.C. "Work and Problems of a Medical Officer Prisoner of War in the Far East." *Journal of the Royal Army Medical Corps* 91 (1948): 51-65.

Roman, Gustavo C., Peter S. Spencer, and Bruce S. Schoenberg. "Tropical Myeloneuropathies: The Hidden Endemias." *Neurology* 35 (1985): 1158-70.

Roman, Gustavo C. "Epidemic Neuropathies of Jamaica." *Transactions and Studies of the College of Physicians of Philadelphia* ser. 5, 7 (1985): 261-74.

Russell, Paul F. *Man's Mastery of Malaria.* London: Geoffrey Cumberlege, Oxford University Press, 1955.

Selwyn-Clarke, P. Selwyn. *Hong Kong Government: Annual Report of the Medical Department for 1946.* Hong Kong: Local Printing Press, 1947.

Sharples, L.R. "The Condition of 'Burning Feet' or 'Foot Burning" in Labourers on Sugar Plantations in the Corentyne District of British Guiana." *Journal of Tropical Medicine and Hygiene* 32 (1929): 358-60.

Simpson, John. "'Burning Feet' in British Prisoners-of-war in the Far East." *Lancet* 1 (1946): 959-61.

Smith, Dean A. "Nutritional Neuropathies in the Civilian Internment Camp, Hong Kong, January, 1942-August, 1945." *Brain* 69 (1946): 209-22.

_____, and Michael F.A. Woodruff. *Deficiency Diseases in Japanese Prison Camps.* London: His Majesty's Stationery Office, 1951.

Smith, Stanley W. *Prisoner of the Emperor: An American POW in World War II.* Duane A. Smith, ed. Niwot, CO: University Press of Colorado, 1991.

Smitskamp, Hendrik. *A Neuro-Vascular Syndrome Related to Vitamin Deficiency.* Amsterdam: Scheltema & Holkema's Boekhandel en Uitgeversmaatschappij N.V., 1947.

Stahlie, T.D. "'Kampogen,' een herinnering." *Ned. Tijdschr. Geneeskd.* 129 (1985): 1532-35.

Stannus, Hugh S. "Pellagra in Nyasaland." *Transactions of the Royal Society for Tropical Medicine and Hygiene* 5 (1911-12): 112-19.

Stening, S.E.L. "Experiences as a Prisoner of War in Japan." *Medical Journal of Australia* 1 (1946): 773-75.

Todd, K.W. "European into Coolie: Ps.O.W. Adapt Themselves to the Tropical Villagers' Diseases." *Journal of the Royal Army Medical Corps* 86 (1946): 179-85.

Veith, Ilza. "Humane Warfare and Inhuman War: Japan and its Treatment of War Prisoners." *Bulletin of the History of Medicine* 19 (1946): 355-74.

Vernon, Sidney. "Nutritional melalgia, a deficiency vascular disease." *JAMA* 143 (1950): 799-802.

Walker, Allan S. *Medical Services of the R.A.N. and R.A.A.F., with a Section on Women in the Army Medical Services.* Canberra: Australian War Memorial, 1961.

_____. *Middle East and Far East*. Canberra: Australian War Memorial, 1962.

Warrack, A.J.N. "Conditions Experienced as a Prisoner of War from a Medical Point of View." *Journal of the Royal Army Medical Corps* 87 (1946): 209-30.

White, J. Glyn. "Administrative and Clinical Problems in Australian and British Prisoner-of-war Camps in Singapore 1942 to 1945." *Medical Journal of Australia* 2 (1946): 401-403.

Whitfield, R.G.S. "Anomalous Manifestations of Malnutrition in Japanese Prison Camps." *British Medical Journal* 2 (1947): 164-68.

Wilcocks, Charles, and Philip E.C. Manson-Bahr. "Kuru." In Wilcocks and Manson-Bahr. *Manson's Tropical Diseases*. Baltimore, Williams & Wilkins, 1972.

Williams, Robert R. *Toward the Conquest of Beriberi*. Cambridge: Harvard University Press, 1961.

Tertiary Sources

Anonymous. *The Register of the George Cross*. Cheltenham: This England Books, 1985.

_____. *Canadian Prisoners of War and Missing Personnel in the Far East*. Ottawa: King's Printer, 1945.

_____. "Beriberi Heart Disease Regulation." *The Quan* [newsletter of the American Defenders of Bataan & Corregidor, Inc.] 49 (February 1995): 1.

Bercuson, Daniel J., and J.L. Granatstein. *Dictionary of Canadian Military History*. Toronto: Oxford University Press, 1992.

Dennis, Peter, Jeffrey Grey, Ewan Morris, Robin Prior, and John Connor, eds. *The Oxford Companion to Australian Military History*. Melbourne: Oxford University Press, 1995.

Haddock, David R.W. "Neurologic Illness in the Tropics." In Strickland, *Hunter's Tropical Medicine*. Toronto: W.B. Saunders, 1984.

King, W.L. Mackenzie "War Crimes: Canadian Representatives in Trials at Hong Kong." *Dominion of Canada: Official Report of Debates, House of Commons, Second Session—Twentieth Parliament. 10 George VI, 1946. Vol. 1, 1946*. Ottawa: King's Printer, 1947.

Low, Sir Francis, ed. *The Indian Year Book 1944-45: A Statistical and Historical Annual of the Indian Empire, with an Explanation of the Principal Topics of the Day*. Bombay: Bennett, Coleman [1945].

Fiction

Allister, William *A Handful of Rice*. London: Secker & Warburg, 1961.

Ariyoshi, Sawako. *The River Ki [Kinokawa]*. Trans. Mildred Tahara. Tokyo: Kodansha International, 1981.

Barker, Pat. *The Ghost Road*. London: Penguin Books, 1996.

Ford, James Allan. *Season of Escape*. London: Hodder & Stoughton, 1963.

Go, Shizuko. *Requiem [Rekuiemu]*. Trans. Geraldine Harcourt. Tokyo: Kodansha International, 1991.

Hahn, Agatha Dillard. *Commentary on Ooka Shohei's Prisoner of War Memoirs (Furyoki)*.

Ooka, Shohei. *Fires on the Plain*. Trans. Ivan Morris. Baltimore: Penguin Books, 1969.

Takeyama, Michio. *Harp of Burma*. Trans. Howard Hibbett. Rutland VT: Charles E. Tuttle Co., 1966.

Tanizaki, Jun'ichiro. *The Makioka Sisters*. New York: Vintage Books, 1995.

Yamasaki, Toyoko. *The Barren Zone*. Trans. James T. Araki. Tokyo: Kodansha International, 1985.

Index

Note: *Page numbers followed by "f" denote a figure. Page numbers followed by "t" denote a table. Page numbers in bold denote an illustration.*

Aberdeen FAP, 20-21
accidents, in Japan, 219
acute gastroenteritis, Argyle Street Camp, 83
Adams (Rfn.), 144
Adams, John H., 122
administration: Japanese, 49-55; POW camps, 227-28
agony ward, 238
agricultural production, decline of in Japan, 217
Ah Tim, survivor of execution, 34-35
air raids, Tokyo, 285
Allied bombers, attack on Hong Kong, 71
Allister, William, 62-63, 78, 97, 116-17, 245, 257, 263; dysentery, 174
Aloha Serenaders, 97
Alsey, Arthur A., 76-77, 79, 96, 137; *Lisbon Maru*, 210-11; and medical orderlies, 196
Ambon island, 78
amoebic dysentery, 171-72, 175; Kawasaki Camp 3D, 260; Niigata POW Camp, 238; Shinagawa POW Hospital, 296
amputees, food rations, 133
Anderson, James H., 34, 38, 159
Andrews-Levinge, Miss, 36

anesthesia, Hong Kong camps, 191
Anopheles mosquito, 177
Ansari, Mtreet Ahmed, vicious attack on, 88-89
anti-diphtheria serum, 160-61; supplies of, 161-64, 165
appendicitis, 191; Ma Tau Chung Camp, 88
Argyle Street Camp, 20, 47-48, 66-67, 79-85, 80f; caloric value of rations at, 133, 134t; officer's dog, 85; post-war, 326; Shackleton at, 50; surgery at, 191
ariboflavinosis, 147
Arisue, 122
Army Medical Store, 5; Salesian Mission, 31
Artemisia vulgaris (mugwort), 249, 302
Ascaris lumbricoides (tapeworm): during capitivity, 323
Ashton, Bill, 310; worms, 184
Ashton-Rose, Leopold W., 70, 80, 83, **87**, 87, 101, 145-46; dysentery, 173; malaria, 180; surgery, 191
Ateah, Joe, dengue, 184
Atkinson, Harry, 247; diphtheria epidemic, 166-67; weight loss, 224

atom bomb, effect of, 321
atrocities, 29-43; and demoralization
  in camps, 62-63; Japanese
  attitudes towards, 30
Auxiliary Nursing Service (ANS), 5,
  32; in Hong Kong, 17
avitaminosis: during captivity, 323;
  citation of, 137-38; and electric
  feet, 150-51; Niigata Camp 5B,
  250; Sagamigahara Hospital, 291;
  Sendai Camp 2B, 278
Awa Maru, 201, 264; sinking of, 198
HMT *Awatea*, 2, 9, **10**, 11

bacillary dysentery, 59, 171-74;
  Niigata Camp 5B, 247
bad eyes, Omine Camp, 266
Badger, George C., 204
banality, of torture, 314
Bando camp, 317-18
Banfill, Stanley Martin, 10, 31-36, **32**,
  80, 88, 204; diphtheria epidemic,
  166, 168
Baptista, 98
Barbour, Bill, 251
Bard, Solomon, 96, 118, 164
Bardal, Njall, 97
Barker (Sgt), 131
barley, and rice diet, 142
Barlow, "Red," 251
BBC news, 22, 123
BCG vaccine, 261
Beadnell, H.M.S.G., 227, 229-30, 232
beating of PWOs, Omori Camp, 281
Beaumont, Joan, 78
bedbugs: North Point POW Camp,
  58; Omori Camp, 288
Begg, Mrs. E.M., 36-37
Begg, Stewart Duncan, 37-38
belief system, Japanese, 215
beriberi, 87, 130; among Japanese
  people, 208; during captivity,
  323; causes and effects, 137-42;
  as disease of economics, 138;
  endemic disease, 137; in Japan,
  215-16; Kawasaki Camp 3D, 260;
  Narumi Camp, 274; Niigata
  Camp 5B, 248, 250; Oeyama
  POW Camp, 230; Omine Camp,

266; Omori Camp, 288;
  Sagamigahara Hospital, 291-92;
  Sendai Camp 2B, 278-79;
  Shinagawa POW Hospital, 296;
  (Randy) Steele, 300-301
"Beriberi" (poem), 138
Berry, 286
Bertram, James, 63-64, 214, 286; on
  Indian POWs, 86; nursing in
  POW camps, 194-95
Berzenski, George, 122
The Big Four, Oeyama POW Camp,
  228, 233
Billings, 77; typhoid fever, 186-87
Birchall, Leonard, 188, 264, 283
Black, G.D.R., 36-37
black market, anti-diphtheria
  serum, 165
Bleich, LaMoyne C., 227; medical
  records, 230-31
Blue Rose, 99
Boon, Cecil "Cissy", 76-77, 76f, 96,
  315; exoneration of, 325; sale of
  quinine to Japanese, 180
Bosanquet, David, 65; escape of, 119
Bose, Chandra, 86, 88
Boulton, Mrs., 26
Bowen Road Military Hospital, 5, **6**,
  34, 49, 50-55; casualties, 14;
  cigarette trading for food, 111;
  diphtheria, 158-60; dysentery,
  174; equipment, 54; food
  compared to North Point, 132;
  former POW site, 325; and
  invasion, 23; medical orderlies,
  196; post-war, 327; severely ill
  POWs, 157; surgery at, 191; ward
  in, **50**
Bowie, Donald C., 12, 42, 50-52, 111,
  146, 159; diphtheria epidemic,
  162; malaria, 178-79; on post-war
  trials, 325
Boxer, Charles, 75
Boyadere, 99
Boyce (Captain), 116
Boyd, Robert, 156
Bradbury, Charles, 41-42
Braddon (researcher), 139, 141
Braddon, Russell, 100

Brady (Sgt.), 202
Breslin, John Francis, 243-44
British Army Aid Group (BAAG), 34, 89, 166; drug source, 165; Intelligence work of, 118
British Burmese War (1823-26): burning feet syndrome, 148-49
British Military Hospital, Bowen Road, 5
British POWs, and escaping, 118
British Red Cross, 33
Britwell (Sgt.), 161
Brown, Kenneth, 243
Brown, Wenzell, 39; malaria, 180
Brownmiller, Susan, 40-41
brutality: definition of, 304; institutionalized, 318; Japanese, 303-309, 310; motivation, 304-305; Narumi Camp, 270; Niigata Camp 5B, 236; Omori Camp, 282; to patients, 313; Pavlovian conditioning, 309; against prisoners when captured, 30; Sagamigahara Hospital, 291
bugs and parasites, North Point POW Camp, 58-59
Burma-Siam Railway, 155, 172; injuries, 219-20; malaria, 182; POWs working on, 207-208; "Speedo" period, 93
burning feet syndrome, 147, 151
Bush, Lewis, 49-50, 115, 144, 169, 281, 287, 289, 312; dysentery, 174; Happy Valley Garden Project, 203; on Hong Kong draft, 213; on moxibustion, 299
bushido, 305, 371n. 5; cultural phenomenon of, 308
Buxton, Mrs. A., 36-37

Callahan (Commander), 243
calories: Argyle Street Camp, 84; and body weight, 297-98
caloric value: of rations, 133-43, 134t
Cambon, Kenneth, 59, 196, 236
Camp 3D, Kawasaki, 153
Camp 5B, Niigata, 214
camphor tree *(Cinnamomum camphora)*, 326

Camp "N," 85
Canada: and its Far Eastern POW nationals, 71-72; military involvement, 7-8; racial prejudice in, 315
Canada "C" Force, 4
Canadian Dental Corps (CDC), 9-10
Canadian Postal Corps, 10
Canadian POWs, deaths, 156
Canivet, Les, 42; surgery, 191
canteen, at Sham Shui Po Camp, 67-68
capitulation, 43-44
Carden, W.T., 69, 78-79, 203
card games, 101
cardiac cases, 142-43
Carter (POW), 52
Castro, Ferdinand Maria "Sonny," **98**, 98-99, **99**
casualties, 321-23
casuarina tree *(Casuarina stricta)*, 326
Central British School, 55, 327; casualties, 15-21
"C" Force personnel, 156
Changi Camp, 146, 312; diphtheria, 158; food supplies at, 131, 133
Chau (Chinese physician), 32
Chichibu (Prince), 289
Chinese, and escaping, 117
Chinese underground, 94
Chinese women, Kai Tak airport, 115
chloroform, 191
cholera: Argyle Street Camp, 83; Japanese soldiers, 310
Christie, Kathleen G., 10, 45, 54
Christmas: life in Hong Kong, 91; menu, 25 December 1942, 135; Niigata Camp 5B, 252
Churchill, Norman Eugene, 298-99
Churchill, Winston, 3
Churchman, 265
Church of England, 106
HMS *Cicala*, 4
cigarette paper, substitute for, 108
cigarettes, 102-14; brands, 103; as currency, 59, 72, 102-104, 105, 114; lighting strategies, 107-108; payment of fines, 110; and

punishments, 109; at Sham Shui Po Camp, 68; trading for food, 110-14

Cinnamomum camphora (camphor tree), 326

Clague, Douglas, escape of, 119

Cleave (doctor), 82, 296, 297

Clinton, Bill, 112

clothing: Furakawa Mining Company, 266; Kawasaki Camp 3D, 263; lack of proper, 220; Marutsu Dockyard, 241-42; Niigata Camp 5B, 239, 240; Omori Camp, 288-89; in winter, 270

Cmeyla, Patrick M., 278, 286

coal mines, 275-79

Coates, Albert, 93, 123; weight loss and food supplied, 134-35

collaborators, 75-76

communal baths, 245

communication, importance of, 314-15

concerts: in Hong Kong, 95-98, 104; North Point POW Camp, 104

Condy's gargle, for diphtheria, 158

conflict: cultural differences and, 311; POWs and camp administration, 256

Connaught Laboratories, 168

construction, POWs in, 207

consumers, distinctions between, 223

cookhouse staff, life of, 95

cooks, and trading food, 131

Coombes, Anthony Henry, 77, 100, 134, 159, 160-61, 316; diphtheria epidemic, 163; dysentery carrier, 211; pellagra, 152; and worms, 185

cost, of matches, 108

courts-martial, and cigarettes, 109-10

Cox, Albert, 293

Crawford, John N.B., 10, 12, 48, 53, 72, 118, 156, **169**, 323-24; on diphtheria, 160; diphtheria epidemic, 165, 168-69; malaria, 179-80; post-war Canadian medical files, 149-50; Saito's beating of, 70; typical POW, 152

Crerar, H.D.G., 7

cruelty: to animals, 308; to humans, 308; of Japanese, 62-63

cultural differences, and conflict, 311

cultures: clash of, 248; Japanese, 306

Cunningham, Winston R., 10, 191

currency, sugar as, 285

Dagenan, 81

Dairy Farm Storage Godown, 162-63

D'Arcy, Hyacinth, 196

Davis, J.R., 297-98

Deane, H.L., 228

deaths: and burial, 203-205, 252-53; from cigarette trading for food, 113; diphtheria, 322; from exposure, 234; from insufficient quantity of food, 216; Kawasaki Camp 3D, 264; Marutsu Dockyard, 242; at Niigata, 235f; Rinko coal party, 241; Sagamigahara Hospital, 292; Sendai Camp 2B, 279; in Sham Shui Po Camp, 72; Shinagawa POW Hospital, 296, 298; from starvation

deficiency diseases, North Point POW Camp, 60

Delbridge, Albert, 224

dengue, 184

Denny-Brown, D., 142

dentistry, 191; Niigata Camp 5B, 243; Omori Camp, 285

Dev, Jemadar Chetan, 88, 123

Dewar, T.J., 192

diagnostic categories, 237

diarrhea, 146; Niigata Camp 5B, 250; Niigata POW Camp, 238; Omine Camp, 267; Sendai Camp 2B, 278

Dickson, Miss (Hotel Nursing Sister), 19

diet, Argyle Street Camp, 83-84

dietary fat, shortage of, 134

dietary protein: deficiency of, 146; low levels of, 142

diphtheria, 157-71; among Canadians, 164-71; antitoxin, 158; Argyle Street Camp, 85; in

Canada, 168; during captivity, 323; carriers, 166-67; cause and affects, 157-58; deaths, 158; 322; epidemic 1942, 56, 157-71; Hong Kong, 156; Kawasaki Camp 3D, 260; Narumi Camp, 274

discipline: Omori Camp, 280, 282; POW camps, 228

diseases: among Japanese people, 208; among POWs in Japan, 219-20; during captivity, 323-24; caused by poor nutrition, 136-37; in Japan, 215-16; statistics, 249-51

Dixon (RNVR), 123

Dockweiler, E.V., 261

Doherty, Ian, 67

Dolyama, 71

Don Jose (American freighter), 11

Doull, Lloyd, 179

drafts, 207-24; organization of, 212-13

Drover, Freddy, 165, 168

drug addiction, 108

drugs: Argyle Street Camp, 84; North Point POW Camp, 61; POW camps, 54; Shinagawa POW Hospital, 295-96; shortage of, 223; smuggled by Helen Ho, 74; sources of, 165

Durran, John, 153

dysentery, 171-76; Argyle Street Camp, 81; during captivity, 323; in Japan, 215-16; Ma Tau Chung Camp, 88; Niigata Camp 5B, 247, 250; North Point POW Camp, 59; Omine Camp, 267; POWs in Japan, 259; rod test, 175-76; St. Teresa's Hospital, 56; Sham Shui Po Camp, 72

Ebdon, Frank William, 97, 212-13, 266, 268

edema, 141-42; former POWs, 324; Narumi Camp, 274; Niigata Camp 5B, 250; Sagamigahara Hospital, 291

Edomoto, 283

Edwards, R.A., 274; weight during captivity, 134

8 ball club, 247

Eijkman (researcher), 139

electrical system, at Sham Shui Po Camp, 67-68

electric feet, 60, 84, 143-51, 292; post-war follow-up, 149-51; pre-war observations, 148-49

Ellis, Percy J., 122

emetine, 175, 260; amoebic dysentery, 238; dysentery, 172

Endacott, George Beer, 86-87

enforced labour, 266

engineering, POWs in, 207

Englehart, Harold, 204, 258

entertainment: life in Hong Kong, 91, 95-101; Niigata Camp 5B, 251; Omori Camp, 283

epidemics: diphtheria (1942), 56, 70, 72, 160; dysentery, 81, 171-76; malaria, 176-84; typhoid fever, 186-87

equipment, hospital, 294-95

"Escape Me Not" paper, 120

escaping, 79, 117-24; Japanese response, 119; Japanese retaliation to, 119-20; life in Hong Kong, 91

Evans (physician), 70, 83, 87

execution, of escapees, 122-23

exhaustion, 258

Expeditionary Force, 8-12

eye problems, 112, 152-53, 266, 274, 278, 324

failure to communicate, 314-15

Falkner, Richard Guy, **98**

families, and POWs' life, 91

Far East, diphtheria in, 158

Far Eastern POWs, 71-72; compared to European, 106

Fearon, Lois, 32-33

Fehily (Irish doctor), 18

Fellows, Francis E., 247, 249; Prisoners' Representative, 236-37

Fernandez, 277

Fidoe, Elizabeth A., 36

field hockey, 101

Fires on the Plain (Ooka), 312

First Canadian draft, 211-13

Fischer, Mattheus, 200

fishery yield, decline of in Japan, 217
fleas: and lice, 67; Omori Camp, 288
Flowchart of movements of Canadian servicemen December 1941, 212f
fly-catching, 58
food: average daily per capita, 217, 223; and cigarette trading, 110-14; comparison of North Point with Bowen Road, 132; coping with too little, 127-54; and corruption, 77; culturally forbidden, 268; in Japan, 223-24; Kawasaki Camp 3D, 262-64; Niigata Camp 5B, 245; sale of, 296; supplies, 128-29; theft of, 131; trading as speculation, 246-47; unusual, 135-43
food consumption: Marutsu Dockyard, 242; and sickness and death rates, 183
food foraging, by Japanese, 218
food parcels, from Hong Kong relatives, 73
food rations, 260; caloric value of, 133-43, 134t; for cigarettes, 274; distribution of, 273; manipulation of, 274; North Point POW Camp, 60; Oeyama POW Camp, 230-31; Omine Camp, 268; Omori Camp, 286-87; proportionate to work level principle, 132-33; Sendai Camp 2B, 278-79
food supply, in Japan, 216-17
Foote, John, 109
forced labour, 322-23
Ford (Colonel), 120
Forfar Road, 49; IJA Prisoner-of-War Headquarters, 79
Forsyth, Tom, 92-93, 132, 144, 157, 242, 251; diphtheria epidemic, 163-64
Foster (Sergeant), 56
Fourth Canadian draft, 214-18
Francis, George, 251
French Mission Hospital, 55
Fujii Hiroshi, 235-38, 248, 281-82, 294; and surgery, 298; war crimes trial, 232, 234, 245-46, 286-87
Fujimake Shigeo, 238

Fujita Ruitaro, 1, 321
Fukuoka 2 POW Camp: electric feet at, 148; surgery, 220-21
Fukuoka 7 POW Camp, and food, 131
Fukuoka 17 POW Camp, 219-20; tuberculosis, 187
Furakawa coal-mining company, 266
Furukawa coal-mining company, 275-77

gambling: for food, 113; for tobacco, 218
gangrene, response of medical orderly to, 311
gardening: Argyle Street Camp, 82; by officers, 93; Omori Camp, 284
Garrison, 220
gastrointestinal disease, in Japan, 232; former POWs, 324
Gaudin, Ken, 259-60
Geneva Convention on Prisoners of War, 35, 51, 54, 123, 207, 270, 276, 317; on escaping, 120
George VI, King, 8
Geraghty, Donald, 106, 144
gift parcels, from Hong Kong relatives, 73
Gill, Geoffrey, parasites, 184-85
Gin-Drinkers Line, malaria, 178
Glusman, Murray, 150, 151
Goad, Lloyd H., 285-86, 295
Gomes, Arthur, 39, 97, 115
Goodnough, 264
Goodwin, R.B., 61-62, 66, 79, 84
Gopalan, 150
Gordon, A.F., 36
Gottlieb, 296
Gozano (doctor), 18, 80
Grasett, A. Edward, 7, 7-8
Gray, Gordon Cameron, 10, 20
Gray, Hector, 73
Greater East Asia Co-Prosperity Sphere, 304
Green, Eric John, 74
Grey, Walter, 152-53
Gripsholm (Swedish ship), 106
USS *Grouper*, 210

Guadalcana, sick and wounded in, 182-83
Guam, ex-POWs from Japan, 323
Guangzhou (Canton), 3
Guitard, Gabriel, 2, 247-48
Gull Force, survivors of, 78
Gun Club Hill Barracks, 87
Gunn, W.D., 55
Guy, Lewis, 170

Hague Conventions, 35, 202, 317
Hahn, Emily "Mickie," 75
Haiashi, 272-73
Hainan island, 78
Hakusan Maru, 198, 201
Hall, William A., 122
Hanawa Camp, 218; death at, 252-53
A Handful of Rice (Allister), 78
happy feet, 60, 292; Narumi Camp, 274
Happy Valley Garden Project, 202-203
Happy Valley Racetrack, casualties, 14
Happy Valley Racetrack Emergency Hospital: and invasion, 23-26; rape at, 25-26, 30; sanitation, 24-25
Hara, 82
harassment, at work sites, 94-95
Harcourt, Sir Cecil Halliday Jepson, 1, 321
Harding, Frank, 153, 312-13
Hargreaves (doctor), 18, 80
Harrison, Argyll C., 31, 109
Harrison, G.F., 163
Harvey, John Hugh, 100, 228-29; courts-martial, 229
Hawaii, 323
Hawes, Mac, 242
Hazama Kosaku, 227-28, 229; abuse of POWs, 232; war crimes trial, 227
Hearn, Lafcadio, 215
hemorrhoids, 172
Henson, Carl, 193
Here Comes Charlie, 99
Hibbs, Ralph: beriberi, 147; on electric feet, 143
Higochi, 282

Hindu women, burning feet syndrome, 149
Hironaka, 279
Hiscox, Sydney, North Point POW Camp, 46-47
histological laboratories, 222-23
Ho, Alice, 28
Ho, Helen, food and clothing for POWs, 74
Ho Kai, 28
homosexuality, 100, 116-17, 262, 285
Honda (commandant), 35, 50
Hong Kong: before 8 Dec 1941, 1-12; attack on, 14-15; census 1941, 85-90; Colony of, 2-4; hospital admissions, 156; invasion 18-19 December, 21-23; malaria, 179, 182; rape in, 40-41; survival of Canadians at, 78
Hong Kong and New Territories, map, 14f
Hong Kong and Shanghai Bank, thiamine hydrochloride in, 129
Hong Kong and Singapore Royal Artillery, 4, 13, 86; POWs, 87
Hong Kong Chinese Symphony Orchestra, 96
Hong Kong Eye Hospital, 326
Hong Kong Field Ambulance, 5, 12, 14
Hong Kong Hotel, 26; casualties, 14
Hong Kong Hotel, Victoria, 5
Hong Kong Mule Corps, 13, 86
Hong Kong Naval Volunteer Reserve, 4, 13
Hong Kong Portuguese, and escaping, 117
Hong Kong POWs: drafts to Japan, 207-209; electric feet, 149; transporting to Japan, 209-18
Hong Kong Red Cross, food stores to camps, 197
Hong Kong University, 194
Hong Kong veterans, medical files of, 323-24
Hong Kong Volunteer Defence Corps (HKVDC), 4, 5, 12, 13, 326; nurses of, 39-43; Portuguese members, 98-100; rape of nurses, 37

Honshu Island, 234
Hook, Henry W., 53
Hopkins, 140
Hoshi Maru, 201
hospitals: admissions, Hong Kong,
    156; conditions in, 69; on Hong
    Kong Island, 23-43; Ma Tau
    Chung Camp, 82; volunteer
    officers, 83
Ho Tung, Sir Thomas, 64
housing, shortage of, 223
Hua, T.J., 73
Hubbard, 273
hunger: among Japanese people,
    275; impact of long-continued,
    136
Huxtable, Charles, 220

Ichiki, 82
I Gill, 304
immunization, 190; against
    diphtheria, 168
Imperial Japanese Army (IJA), 3,
    17-18; and POWs, 303-309;
    prisoners taken, 46
Imperial Japanese Army Prisoner of
    War Headquarters, 326-27
Imperial Japanese Navy (IJA), 3-4
Indian Hospital, Whitfield Barracks,
    5; casualties, 15
Indian Hospital Corps, 86
Indian Medical Department, 87
Indian Medical Service, 86
Indian National Army (INA), 82, 86
Indian nationals, incarceration of, 48
Indian officers: intimidation by
    Japanese, 88; segregation by
    Japanese, 82
Indian POWs: condition of, 86; and
    escaping, 117; Ma Tau Chung
    Camp, 86
Indian troops, contact with British,
    88; death toll, 86
inequality, between officers and
    other ranks, 79
Infantry Regiment (238th), 189-90
infectious diseases, decreased
    immunity to, 350n. 8
informers, 75

injuries, 190; Argyle Street Camp,
    80-81; Furukawa coal-mining
    company, 277; in Japan, 232;
    Niigata Camp 5B, 250;
    self-inflicted, 219-20
Ino (Sgt.), 258
inoculations, and isolation, 214
Inoue (doctor), 254
Inouye Kanao "The Kamloops Kid":
    brutality of, 315-16; death
    sentences of, 315-16; judicial
    execution of, 316
insensitivity, institutionalized, 311
International Committee for the
    Red Cross (ICRC), 72, 196-202,
    296; and Japanese authorities,
    200; Japanese hindrance of, 106;
    Narumi Camp, 275; tuberculosis
    data, 188
internees, treatment of, 45
iron foundry, Shintetsu Camp, 243-44
Isogai Rensuke, Governor of Hong
    Kong, 49
Ito (Captain), 213

Jackson, Calvin A., 55, 158, 218;
    dysentery, 176; and his pet
    chicken, 136
Jamaica, TAB inoculations, 168
Japanese: attitudes of, 245, 306; and
    bribes, 229; complexities of
    working with, 199-202; medical
    involvement, 238; and theft of
    food, 133; treatment of their
    servicemen, 309-18
Japanese Army medical college,
    health problems of POWs, 257,
    259
Japanese Army Regulation, 276
Japanese casualties: indifference
    towards, 310; killed by medical
    staff, 310
Japanese people, 318-20; attitudes
    of, 290; contacts with, 244-49
Japanese Prisoner of War Bureau,
    275
Japanese prisoners, as dishonourably
    dead, 306
Japanese Red Cross, 317

Japanese servicemen, malaria, 182-83
Japan Red Cross, 289
Japan Transport Co. Inc., 233
Jockey Club emergency hospital, 24
Joyce, Mrs. Day, 18, 20
Jubilee Buildings, **64**, 64-65; Canadians in, 164-65
justice, war crimes trials, 324-25

Kagy, E.S., 235-36, 261
Kai Tak, aerodrome at, 3
Kai Tak airport, construction of, 93-94
Kaneko, 265-66
Kano, 282
Kasayama Yoshikichi, 304
Kato (Lt.), 237, 247, 280-81
Kaufmann, 281-82
Kawasaki Camp 3D, 153, 181, 211, 213, 224, 253-64
Keil, George, 67
Keith, Agnes Newton, 194, 303
Kelly (driver), 31-32
Kempeitai, 298-99; brutality of, 313-14
Kengelbacher, C.A., 199; on Sham Shui Po Camp, 72
Kerr, Reg, 165
King, William Lyon Mackenzie, 8
Kinjo Shigeaki, 307
Kinkaseki Camp (Taiwan), 124
Kirk (doctor), 21
Kobe House, homosexuality at, 116
Kondo Kanechi, 255
Kondo Shoogo, 301
Koreans, in Japan, 304
Kowloon, mainland hospitals in, 15-21
Kowloon Hospital, 15-18, 15f
Kowloon Hotel, 18
Kowloon Military Hospital, casualties, 15
Kramer, Milton L., 301-302
Kravinchuk, Samuel, 96; Sham Shui Po Camp, 47
Kubo, 142
Kumagaya Tobuichi, 312
Kwong Wah Hospital, 73; casualties, 15

labourers, Japanese need for, 207
labour shortage, Japan, 71
La Czigane, 99
Laite, Uriah, 23
Land, Roy, 42
Lane Crawford department store, 129
Larsen, William, 221
La Salle College, 21; casualties, 15-21
La Salle College Temporary Hospital, 20, 74; latrines: sea, 59; Shinagawa POW Hospital, 295
Laurie (Capt.), death of, 242
Lavarie, Cecil F., 193
lawn bowling, 101
Lawson, John K., 9, 13
Leath, Norman, 34, 146
Lee, Maynard, 240
Letitia (hospital ship), 323
Levi, Primo, 192
lice: in camps, 67; North Point POW Camp, 58; Omori Camp, 288
Lisbon Maru, 96; torpedoed by US, 210-11
Loa Kikan, 119
loss of sight, 152-53
lugow (barley porridge), 245

McCarron, Joseph M. "Red," 324
McCaw, Muriel, 27, 56
McEwen, 301
Mackenzie (Hong Kong resident), 162-63
Mackenzie, Compton, 89
McKnight, Mel, 259
McLeod, Bobby, 243
McMasters, T.Y., 158
McRitchie, Angus, 284
Magistracy, casualties, 15-21
magnesium sulphate, 61; dysentery, 173
Mainland Brigade, 13
Maizuru Naval College, malnutrition among students, 223
The Makioka Sisters (Jun'ichiro), 140
malaria, 176-84; Bowen Road Military Hospital, 6; during captivity, 323; Oeyama POW Camp, 231; St. Teresa's Hospital, 56; symptoms, 176-77

Malcolmson, J.G., 148-49
malnutrition: and electric feet, 144, 148; Kawasaki Camp 3D, 262-64; and diseases, 223; Niigata Camp 5B, 250; Sham Shui Po Camp, 72, 84
Maltby, C.M., 4
Maltby, Christopher M., 7, 82, 119, 123
Manchester, William, 318
Manners (Major), 171
Manryu Maru, 213, 281
Marr, Thomas, 293
Martyn, Francis D.F., 46
Marutsu Dockyard, 240; work at, 241-43
Ma Tau Chung Camp, 47, 85-90; dysentery, 174; Indian officers moved to, 81; post-war, 326; surgery at, 191
Matheson, 259
Matilda Hospital, The Peak: casualties, 14
Matsuda, "Cardiff Joe," 213, 281
Matsusaki San, 282
Matsuzawa Psychopathic Hospital of Tokyo, drug shortage, 222
Mattseau, 204-205
medical assessments, on former POWs, 323
medical cost, of imprisonment, 323-24
medical experimentation, 202-203; Tokuda Hisakichi, 189
medical involvement, by Japanese, 238
medical planning, 4-7
medical records, Niigata Camp 5B, 249-51
medical services, Omori Camp, 285
medical supplies: Kawasaki Camp 3D, 261-62; Niigata Camp 15D, 243-44; shortage of, 222
medicines, 261; Argyle Street Camp, 84; Nihon Kokan, 258; shortage of, 223
mental health, post-war toll, 324
menu, Sham Shui Po Camp, 128

Middlesex Regiment: 1st Battalion, 4; "A Prisoner's Prayer at Bowen Road," 54-55
military duty, as prison sentence, 312
military hospitals, map (Hong Kong Island and Kowloon), 16f
Millar, R.D., and maggots, 136
mining: employment in, 207, 209; Oeyama POW Camp, 227
Miranda, Carmen, 98
miso beer, Omori Camp, 287
Mitsubishi Kasei, beriberi at, 208
Mitsubishi Mining Company, 223
Mitsubishi warehouses, 284
Mitsushima POW Camp, 142
Miyazu, 226
Monthly Returns (1942), 156t
morale, at Sham Shui Po Camp, 66-67
Morgan, 259
Morioka Maru, 299
SS *Morning Star*, 213
mortality statistics: Allied POWs in Asia, 318; Allied POWs in Europe, 318; of German and Austrian POWs, 318
HMS *Moth*, 4
Mount Austin Barracks, 46
moxibustion, 298-302; Japanese folk remedy, 248-49
mugwort (*Artemisia vulgaris*), 249, 302
Mulcahy, 259
murder, banality of, 309
Murray, James, 96
My Lai, 309

Nakom Patan POW Hospital, 123-24
Narumi Camp, 214, 269-75; camp population, 270; factory work, 271-72
Nazarin, Razee, 170
Nethersole Hospital, 28, 29
Neufeld, Benny, 127
Newfoundland and Labrador, beriberi in, 138-39
Newman, Samuel A., 301
Newnham, L.A., 123

news-sheet, Sham Shui Po Camp, 214
Newton, Isaac, 17-20, 30, 66-67, 79-81, 316; on Saito, 171
niacin, 147
nicotinic acid, 145, 147
Nihon-Kokan Shipbuilding Yard, 254, 257
Niigata Camp 15D/15B, 236
Niigata Camp 5B, 2, 233-53; aerial view, **239**; camp conditions, 238-40; collapse of roof at, 234-35, 252; hospital, 238; post-war, 327; punishments and cigarettes, 109; theft of food at, 133
Niigata Ironworks Inc., 233-34
Niigata Land and Sea Transport Company, 233
Ninomiya Yutaka, war crimes trial, 276
Nishihara Wakana, 307
Nishino, 281
Niwa Naomi, 319-20
Nixon (Peninsula Hotel manager), 19
Nohara Teishin, 310
Norquist, 288
Northcote, Sir Geoffrey, 7
North Point POW Camp, 30, 34, 46-48, 56-63; Banfill at, 35; daily food log, 130; demoralization of, 61-62; diphtheria, 158; electric feet, 144; escape from, 122; food compared to Bowen Road, 132; hospital admissions, 156; hospital at, 60-61; living quarters, 59; Martyn at, 46; plan of, 57f, 60f; post-war, 325-26; severely ill POWs, 157
Nosu (doctor), 221, 232
Novak, 276-77
Novocaine hydrochloride, 191
Nugent, W.F., 101
Numano, 301
nursing, in POW camps, 194-96
nutrition, at Stanley Internment Camp, 146

Oakley, Raymond J., 31, 32-33
Oeyama (Osaka Camp No. 3), 225-33

Oeyama Nickel Company, 148
Oeyama POW Camp, 100, 214; Canadians in, 226f; maggoty rice, 217; Martyn at, 46; medical conditions at, 230-33; NCOs in control of, 228; plan of, 226f; Red Cross parcels, 224; weight loss at, 135
Officer, J., 55
officers: electric feet, 144; and enlisted men, 77-78; inequality with other ranks, 84; money for food, 133; at Oeyama POW Camp, 229-30; survival data, 78
officer's POW camp, Argyle Street Camp, 81
Ofuna (interrogation camp), 283
Oguri, 282
Okada Miyoroku, war crimes trial, 270
Okada Umekichi, 1, 321
Omine Camp, 213, 264-69; living quarters, 268-69
Omori Camp, 279-90; camp population, 280-81; homosexuality at, 116; living quarters, 280-81; medicinal gargles, 219; plan of, 280f
Omuta Camp, sale of food, 110-11
Omuta Camp 17, 220
Once in a Lifetime, 100
O'Neill, Huck, 100
Ooka Shohei, 307, 312
optic atrophy: former POWs, 324
optic neuritis, 112; Narumi Camp, 274
orderlies, 194-96; volunteer, 196
Orloff (Russian doctor), 32
Orwell, George: impact of hunger, 136; on starvation, 127-28
Overseas League (Canada) Tobacco and Hamper Fund, efforts and failures of, 106
Overton, William, 279
Ozawa, 278-79

padi (red rice), 141
Page, J.A., 55, 200, 221, 254, 294; draft, 212

pantothenic acid, 150
parades, 51
parasites, 184-85
Paravicini, S., 200
Parker, Maurice A., 96, **98**
Pattingale, James Reuben, 255
Payne, John O., 122
Peak Mansions, 46
Pearce, John, escape of, 119
Pearl Harbor, 9
Peasegood, H., 38
pellagra, 87, 151-52; endemic disease, 137; in Japan, 215-16; Oeyama POW Camp, 230
Penfold, 86
Peninsula Hotel Temporary Hospital, 18-20
pensions, as ex-POWs, 151, 325
Percival (general), 44
perforated ulcer, operation for, 83
Perras, Galen, 9
Perrault, Isadore, 277
Philippines: beriberi, 147; diphtheria, 158; trading with Japanese, 107
physical work, 219; although unfit, 214
Pinnock, William, 292
Plasmodium parasites, 177
pneumonia, 261-62; during captivity, 323; medical procedures to combat, 248; Omori Camp, 286; Shinagawa POW Hospital, 296
Poirier, Pat, 256-57
Pollak, 261
Porteous, George, 100, 101
postal communication, 257; and POWs' life, 91-92
postlude, 325-27
potassium permanganate, 158
POW administration, Japanese, 49-55
POW camps: economic activity in, 103-107; Japanese Home Islands, 225-302; life in Hong Kong, 91-125; microcosm of human social order, 102-104; warranty not to escape, 52
POW medical officers: ethical and moral concerns of, 123-24; and restrictions on diagnosis, 137-38

POWs: abuse of, 232; behaviour of, 324-25; after capitulation of Hong Kong, 155-56; aid for, 201; diseases suffered during captivity, 181-82; guinea pigs at Sagamigahara Hospital, 292; Indian, 47-48; Japanese treatment of, 276-77; Red Cross supplies, 198t; theft among, 75; working alongside Japanese women, 244-45; working for the Japanese, 314; before World War Two, 317-18
Pratt, surgery without anesthetic, 221
HMCS *Prince Robert*, 9, **322**, 323
Prisoners' Representative, Fellows, Francis E., 236-37
psychiatric disease, Niigata Camp 5B, 249
psychiatry, 192-94
psychology, 192-94
public health measures, 213
pulmonary disease, in Japan, 232
punishments, 109-10; in the IJA, 311-12; Japanese, 110; for stealing food, 247
Punjab Regiment (2nd/14th), 13, 86, 88; POWs, 87
Punjab Regiment (14th), 2nd Battalion, 4

USS *Queenfish*, 202, 264
Queen Mary Hospital, 29, 34; casualties, 14; and invasion, 23
quinine, malaria, 176

R.J. Reynolds Tobacco Company, 112
R.N. Dockyard, 186
Rabbit Commission, 274
rackateers, at Oeyama POW Camp, 230
radio broadcasting, 92
5/7 Rajput Regiment, 13, 31, 86, 88
Ralston, James Layton, 7-8
RAMC [Rob All My Comrades], 195
rape: following invasion, 40-41; Happy Valley Racetrack Emergency Hospital, 25-26; ubiquity of during wartime, 40-41

Red Cross, 33; Omori Camp, 283-84
Red Cross parcels, 72; difficulties getting, 197-99; expenditures on, 106-107; food supplements, 224; illegal use of, 72-73; Japanese retention of, 289; Kawasaki Camp 3D, 264; Narumi Camp, 274; Oeyama POW Camp, 229; received, 246; traded for cigarettes, 218
Redwood, Barbara, 23-24, 26, 211
refinery, Oeyama POW Camp, 227
refugee camps, in Hong Kong, 85
229th Regiment, 31; murder of surrendered personnel, 35
Reid, John A.G., 10, 38-39, 253-64, 294; on diphtheria, 160; draft, 212; at Guam, 323; illness in camps, 181; typical POW, 152
Report on Rations, December 1943, 134t
respiratory disease: in Japan, 215-16; Niigata Camp 5B, 250
retribution, 324-25
Ribiero, Luigi, 193-94; surgery, 191
rice, 128; cooking methods, 288; inadequate supplies, 218; polished, 218; quality of, 216; unpolished (brown), 218
"The Rice-O" program, 104
Ride, Sir Lindsay, 12, 48; escape from Sham Shui Po, 118
Riggs, 298
Riley, Norman, 271-72, 274
Rinko Coal Company, 233
Rinko coal yard, 240-41
Roberts, 265
Robertson, H.G.G., 65, 158, 254, 265, 267-68; dysentary, 172-73
Robertson, R.C., 194
HMS *Robin*, 4
Robinson, J.E.C., 212, 278
Robinson, Roy, 104
Rodgers, 270
Rodrigues, Sir Albert, 97; surgery, 191
Rogers (MQMS), 228
Rogers (WO2), Oeyama POW Camp, 233

Roland, Paul S., surgery, 221
Ross, Lance, 165, 245-46, 266-67, 300
Royal (Captain), 100
Royal Air Force, 4
Royal Army Medical Corps (RAMC), 5, 31; murder at Shau Kei Wan, 30
Royal Army Service Corps, 86
Royal Artillery, 4
Royal Canadian Army Medical Corps (RCAMC), 10
Royal Canadian Corps of Signals, 10
Royal Naval Hospital, casualties, 14
Royal Rifles of Canada (Quebec), 8, 31; venereal disease, 12
Royal Scots, 11; 2nd Battalion, 4; 8-25 December 1945 (18-day war), 13; malaria, 6-7
Rubia, 301
rumours, and morale, 67
Russo-Japanese War (1904-5), 317

sabotage: Japanese war effort, 258; Mitsubishi factory, 272
Sagamigahara Hospital, 290-93
Saikanu, "George," 49
St. Albert's Convent, 5, 49; casualties, 14; and invasion, 26-28
St. John's Ambulance Brigade, 12, 32
St. John's Ambulance personnel, decapitation of, 30
St. Stephen's College, 5, **36**; casualties, 14; malaria, 181; massacre at, 36-39; murder and rape at, 30
St. Teresa's Hospital, 55-56; casualties, 15; diphtheria, 158-59
St. Vincentius Hospital, dysentery, 174
Saito Shunkichi, 53-54, **70**, 70-71, 83, 202-203, 214; beating of PWOs, 169-70; war crimes trial, 71, 170-71
Sakai Takashi, 49
Saldivar, 298
Salesian Mission, 5, 31, **31**; area drawing, 33f
Samuel, Philip, dysentery, 174
Sanderson, Ralph, 104

sanitary conditions, North Point POW Camp, 57

sanitation, Happy Valley Racetrack Emergency Hospital, 24-25

Sato Hideo, on slapping, 313

Sawamori, 82

scarlet fever, 187

Schrage, David M., 2, 10

Schultz, Elack, 273

Scott, 220

Second Canadian draft, 213-14

Second World War, end of, 302

Seifert, Ruth, 41

Selby, J.A., 26

Sellers, Raymond, 193

Selwyn-Clarke, Mrs. "Red Hilda," and volunteers to deliver food parcels, 74-75

Selwyn-Clarke, Selwyn, 20, 73, 75, 81, 84, 129-30, 162, 326; and ICRC, 197; on the mental hospital, 194; on Saito, 171

Sendai Camp, tuberculosis, 187-88

Sendai Camp 2, 215

Sendai Camp 2B, 275-79; beating of PWOs, 276-77; camp population, 275-76; hospital, 278; living quarters, 275-76

Senryo Camp, 67

serum, anti-diphtheritic, 159

Setsuko, 319-20

7th Rajput Regiment, 4

sex, 115-17; life in Hong Kong, 91

Shackleton, C.O., 23, 48, 50, 52, 83-84

Sham Shui Po Camp, 10, 47-48, 49, 63-75, 166; aerial view, 63f; Canadian hospital at, 68-69; concerts at, 97; corruption, 77; daily schedule, 65; dentistry at, 191; diphtheria epidemic, 158, 160-61, 163-64, 166; draft to Japan, 209-10; dysentery, 174; electric feet, 144-45; escape from, 117, 120-21; extra rations, 129; interior of barracks, 69f; Isolation Hospital, Christmas menu, 135; layout of, 66f; operating table sketch, 189f; post-war, 326; Red Cross food supplies, 134; surgery at, 191; theft at, 65-66

Sham Shui Po Park, 326

Sharples, L.R., burning feet syndrome, 149

Shau Kei Wan, 18, 31-36

Shaw (medical NCO), 235-36

Sheffer, S., 100

Sheldon, Mrs., 20

Shinagawa Camp: food trading at, 131; POW hospital, 260; tuberculosis records, 188-89

Shinagawa POW Hospital, 293-98; "bad" period, 297-98

Shintetsu Camp, 243-44

Shintetsu Clinic, 236

Shintetsu iron foundry, 240

Shirai (doctor), 244

shortages, of doctors, 223

Show Draft, 211

Shumshuipo, robbery at, 195

sickness, Kawasaki Camp 3D, 262-64

sick prisoners, in mine or factory, 237

sight, loss of, 152-53

sign at Stewart, BC, **316**

Simmons, R., 100

Singapore, fear of Japanese, 44

skin, and diphtheria, 157-58

skin diseases, 186; in Japan, 215-16, 232; Niigata Camp 5B, 250; Omine Camp, 266; Sendai Camp 2B, 278

Smart, Jack, 203

Smith, Dean, 15, 18, 146-47

Smith, Mrs. W.J.L., 36-37

Smith, Stanley W., 299-300

smoking, *See also* cigarettes; as addiction, 114; problem, 102

smuggling: of drugs, 54, 295; Mitsubishi warehouses, 284-85

The Snake and Staff, 52-53

social process, in camps, 114

Soroka, Mitchell, 110, 255

Sources of Funds to Purchase Supplies for POWs, 198t

Spears, Frank, 249

Speller, Lionel, 255, 257

Spence, James C.M., 10, 191

Spencely, Walter, 190

spinal meningitis, Sham Shui Po Camp, 53-54
sports, 100-101; life in Hong Kong, 91
Squires, Ray, 105, 134, 165; dysentery, 173; skin diseases, 186; surgery, 191
Standish, Colin, 166, 263, 270-71, 273; weight loss, 134
Stanley Civilian Internment Camp, 56
Stanley Gaol, 86, 89
Stanley Internment Camp: cigarettes as currency, 104; nutritional state at, 146
Stanley Peninsula Internment Camp, 20; atrocities at, 38-39; malaria, 181; nursing sisters at, 45; Uttley at, 28
Stanley Prison, 120; death of Gray at, 73
Stanley Prison Hospital, casualties, 14
Star Ferry, 3
starvation: from cigarette trading for food, 112, 113; and disease, 183; Sham Shui Po Camp, 72
stealing. *See* theft
Steele, Randolfe (Randy), 39, 193, 244, 250-51, 300; agony ward, 238
Stening, S.E.L., 148, 227-28
Stericker, John, 22
stevedores, POWs as, 207
Stewart, William, 235-36, 243, 247, 300-301; medical records, 249-51
stockpiles: of Red Cross materials, 221-22; of supplies, 171
Strachan, burning feet syndrome, 148
Strahan, Arthur, 53-54, 83, 87
Suffiad, Mary, 32
Sugamo Prison, 237
suicide, 192-94
sulfa drugs, dysentery, 172-73
sulfanilamide, 61
sulfapyridine, 61; dysentery, 174
Sundaram, 87
surgery, 191-92, 220-24; Niigata Camp 5B, 250-51; at Sham Shui Po, 53; without anesthetic, 220-22, 259-60
surgical patients, treatment of, 82-83

surgical supplies, in Japan, 219
surrender, as a dishonour, 307
survival data: "Gull Force," 78; Royal Australian Navy, 78
Sutcliffe, J.L.R., 179
Suwa POW Camp, 264
Suzuki, 234, 246
Swinson, Arthur, 305
Swisher, 298
Swiss Red Cross volunteers, risk, 200
Sword, Staff, 242
Sydenham, Annie, 28-29

Taisho POW camp, 299
Takaki Kenkan, 140
Tanaka Butai, 31; war crimes trial, 35-36
Tanaka Hiroshi, 271-73; war crimes trial, 270
Tanaka Hisakichi, 49
Tanaka Hitochi, 82
Tanaka Ryosaburo, 31, 35
Tanizaki Jun'ichiro, 140
tapeworm, during captivity, 323
Tatsuo Maru, 265
Tatsuta Maru, 211
Tatu Maru, 211
Tatuta Maru, 254
Teague, Claude, 112
tenko, 51
tennis, 101
HMS *Tern*, 4
tests and immunizations, 190
theft: among POWs, 75; of food, 109, 247, 284-85; Hamowa POW Camp, 109; from Japanese, 275; at Oeyama POW Camp, 114; by officers, 66; POW camps, 228
thiamine, 141, 147
thiamine hydrochloride, in Hong Kong and Shanghai Bank, 129
Third Canadian draft, 214
Thomas, 298
Thomas, Arthur, 2
Thomas, Osler Lister, 31-32; survivor of execution, 34
Thompson, 230
HMS *Thracian*, 4

throat, and diphtheria, 157-58
Tinkler, 278
Tinson, Mrs., 31-33
tobacco, *See also* cigarettes; as addiction, 108-109, 112; substitutes, 109; traded for rice, 218; vs drugs and alcohol, 108-10
toilets, North Point POW Camp, 61
Tojo Hideki, 233, 312-13; on POWs working, 314; war crimes trial, 303, 306
Tokuda Hisakichi, **188**, 189, 293; "bad" Shinagawa, 297-98; and surgery, 295, 298; war crimes trial, 298
Tokugawa Yoshichika, 289
Tokugawa Yoshitomo, 289
Tokunaga, 200
Tokunaga Isao, 120, **121**
Tominaga Shozo, 30; trial of courage, 308-309
Tomlinson (doctor), 20-21
Toronto *Star*, Fly-Catching Contest of 1912, 58
torture, 298-99; of Indian officers, 89; Kawasaki Camp 3D, 255; moxibustion as, 298
Toyama Maru, 214, 270
tracheotomies, diphtheria, 159
trading, 101-102; food for cigarettes, 274; hazards of, 110-14; with one's captors, 107-108
treatment: dysentery, 56, 172-73; of POWs by Japanese prior to WW2, 317
trestle gang, 240
tropical diseases, ignorance of, 138
tropical nutritional amblyopia "camp eyes," 112
Tsang Fook Chor (Chinese physician), 32-33
Tsuneo Muramatsu, 222
tuberculosis, 187-90; Kawasaki Camp 3D, 260-61; Shinagawa POW Hospital, 296
Tucker, 96
Tugby, Marcus Charles (Mark), 100, 228, 230; courts-martial, 229; trial of, 325

Tung Wah Eastern Hospital, 5, 29; casualties, 14
typhoid fever, 186-87

Uehara, 307
Ugaki Matome, 182
United States, institutionalized brutality in, 318
University Hospital, casualties, 14
Uno Shintaro, 313-14
urination, frequency of from rice diet, 130
US advance airfield (Wai Chow), 123
US Marine Corps, 318
US Strategic Bombing Survey, 209
Uttley, K.H., 16-19, 79-80; and ICRC, 197; at St. Albert's Convent, 28
Uwamori, 254, 258-59, 260

van Boxtel, 172
Vance, Jonathan, 71
Van Wart, D., 26, 56, 159
Veale, 259
Veith, Ilza, 317
venereal disease (VD), 12, 185-86; Royal Scots, 6-7
Vernon, Sidney, 150-51
vision, loss of, 152-53
vitamin A deficiency, 130
vitamin B1, 141, 146-47
vitamin B complex, 147
vitamin B deficiency, 84, 112, 146; from polished rice, 130
vitamin deficiencies, 137, 142, 216; in Japan, 231; Sagamigahara Hospital, 292; Sham Shui Po Camp, 84
vitamin deficiency syndrome, 130
VJ Day, prisoners in Oeyama Camp, 227
Volunteer Aid Detachment Nurses (VADs), 23
volunteer orderlies, 196

Wada (camp commandant), 49-50
wages: of POWs, 208; Rinko Coal Company, 233

Wakasennin (American POW), 220
Wallace, death of, 237-38
Wallis, C., 13
Wallis, "Willie," 191-92
Wan Chai girls, 74
war crimes trials, 324-25; illegal use
    of Red Cross parcels, 72-73;
    Tanaka Butai, 35-36; Tanaka
    Hitochi, 82
War Memorial Casualty Clearing
    Station, 28-29
War Memorial Hospital, The Peak,
    casualties, 14
Warrack, A.J.N., 83-84, 170, 295, 297;
    on bacillary dysentery, 172
Warsaw Ghetto, decreased
    immunity, 350n. 8
Watanabe Kiyoshi "Uncle Jon," 67,
    162, 162; drug carrier, 74
Watanabe Mutsuhiro (The Bird),
    280-82, 284-85
The Water Jump, 209
Waters, May, 45, 323
Watson & Co., 170
weak eyes, Sendai Camp 2B, 278
weight loss: average, 216; during
    capitivity, 323; Kawasaki Camp
    3D, 260-61, 263; Narumi Camp,
    274; Oeyama POW Camp,
    230-31, 231f
Weight Loss among POWs at
    Oeyama Camp, 135t
Weinstein, Alfred, 142, 280, 289, 294
Weir, Tom, 96
Welsh, D.L.W., 164
West (Sgt), 110
West, Ernest M., 255
Wheeler, Benjamin, 44; dysentery, 175
White, Harry, 58, 65, 69, 75, 85, 94,
    96, 101, 144-45, 158-59, 200, 204,
    325; malaria, 179-80
White, Lynton, 120; escape of, 119
White, S.E.H., **121**
Whitfield, 294
Whitney, P.N., 36

Williams, Amy, 24
Williamson (Winnipeg Grenadiers),
    30
Wilson, F., 158
Winnie the Pooh, 100
Winnipeg Grenadiers, 2, 8, 10, 12,
    92; capture at Jardine's Lookour,
    41; "D" Company, 23; training
    deficiencies, 9
women: and food parcels, 74;
    liaisons with, 73-74; in the
    workforce, 244-45
Woodruff, Michael, 146
Woods (Sgt), typhoid fever, 186
Woodward, J.J., 15, 70-71, 82, 83, 87,
    123, 195; malaria, 180; Omori
    Camp, 281-82
work, 224; life in Hong Kong, 91,
    93-95; of medical personnel,
    93-94; Narumi Camp, 272;
    Shinagawa POW Hospital, 296;
    and sick men, 181
Work Performed by POWs, by
    Industry, 209t
World War One, Japanese treatment
    of POWs, 317-18
worms, 184-85; in camps, 59

Yamaji, 246
Yamata, 271-72
Yanaru Tetsutoshi, 265
Yaroogsky (doctor), 18
yeast substances, 287-88; against
    vitamin deficiencies, 137
Yeo (Chinese physician), 16
Yomisu Omae, 40-41
Yoshida Masato, 244; war crimes
    trial, 237
Young, Sir Mark, 7, 10
Yu (Chinese physician), 16
Zentsuji Camp, American POWs as
    stevedores, 207
Zia (physician in Hong Kong), 40
Zindel, Rudolf, 197, 199, 200
Zytaruk, 261